THERAPEUTIC TARGETS FOR INFLAMMATION AND CANCER

Novel Therapies for Digestive Diseases

THERAPEUTIC TARGETS FOR INFLAMMATION AND CANCER

Novel Therapies for Digestive Diseases

Editor

Chi Hin Cho

School of Biomedical Sciences, Faculty of Medicine
The Chinese University of Hong Kong, Hong Kong, China
Laboratory of Molecular Pharmacology, School of Pharmacy
Southwest Medical University, Luzhou, Sichuan, China

World Scientific

NEW JERSEY • LONDON • SINGAPORE • BEIJING • SHANGHAI • HONG KONG • TAIPEI • CHENNAI • TOKYO

Published by

World Scientific Publishing Co. Pte. Ltd.

5 Toh Tuck Link, Singapore 596224

USA office: 27 Warren Street, Suite 401-402, Hackensack, NJ 07601

UK office: 57 Shelton Street, Covent Garden, London WC2H 9HE

Library of Congress Cataloging-in-Publication Data
Names: Cho, C.-H. (Chi-Hin), editor.
Title: Therapeutic targets for inflammation and cancer : novel therapies for digestive diseases / edited by Chi Hin Cho.
Description: New Jersey : World Scientific, 2016. | Includes bibliographical references and index.
Identifiers: LCCN 2016030116 | ISBN 9789813148567 (hardcover : alk. paper)
Subjects: | MESH: Digestive System Neoplasms--therapy | Gastroenteritis--therapy | Digestive System Neoplasms--genetics | Carcinogenesis--genetics
Classification: LCC RC280.D5 | NLM WI 149 | DDC 616.99/43--dc23
LC record available at https://lccn.loc.gov/2016030116

British Library Cataloguing-in-Publication Data
A catalogue record for this book is available from the British Library.

Desk Editors: Suraj Kumar/Joy Quek

Typeset by Stallion Press
Email: enquiries@stallionpress.com

Printed in Singapore

Foreword

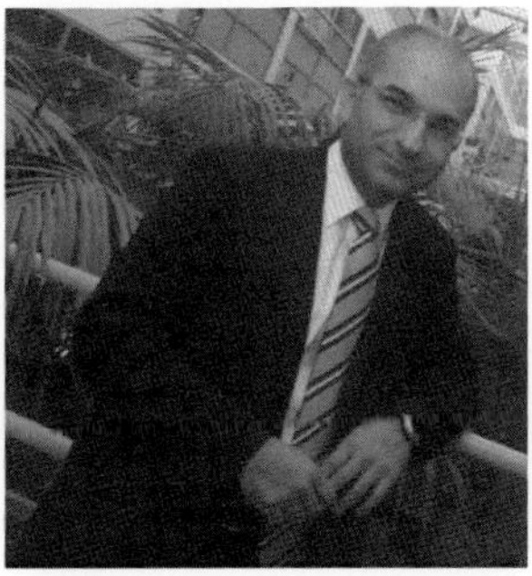

It gives me great pleasure to write this short foreword for this outstanding book. Chronic inflammation is the "root of all evil" and in the context of cancer plays the most prominent role in initiating, promoting and spreading the disease. Gastrointestinal and liver cancers exert the largest global health burden of any malignant disease and as such require a concerted international effort to unravel the pathophysiology and identify novel strategies for prevention, treatment and ultimately cure. This book is an excellent compendium of state-of-the-art knowledge on the role of chronic inflammation in gastrointestinal cancer and the novel strategies for treating it. The strength lies in the outstanding faculty of authors who hail from the best research laboratories in Asia-Pacific, Europe and North America. The content is comprehensive, authoritative and translational. The first section gives an excellent account of therapeutic approaches in treating inflammatory GI disorders and this is followed by similar approaches for gastrointestinal tract cancer. The last section deals with the exciting new field of autophagy and microRNAs as therapeutic targets in digestive cancer.

This is an essential book for all researchers interested in inflammation and cancer. It is also a particularly useful book for clinicians from different disciplines including oncology gastroenterology and clinical pharmacology. The editor and authors are highly commended on producing this invaluable book.

Professor Emad M El-Omar
Professor of Medicine
Editor in Chief, *Gut*
St George and Sutherland Clinical School
University of New South Wales
Sydney, NSW
Australia
e.el-omar@unsw.edu.au

About the Editor

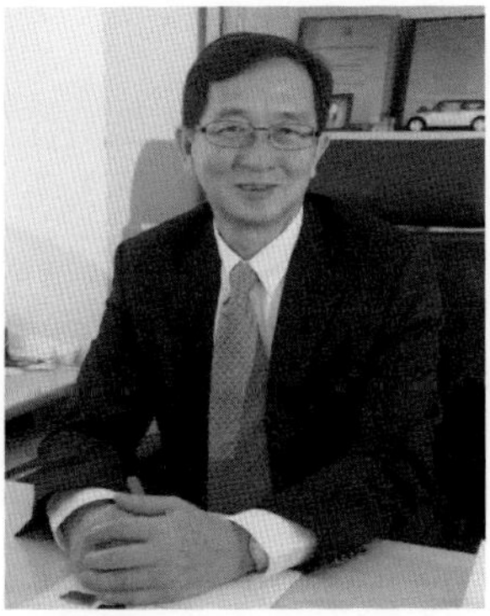

Professor Chi Hin Cho received his undergraduate and master training in Taiwan and USA. He graduated with a PhD in Pharmacology from the University of Hong Kong (HKU) in 1978. He went through his postdoctoral training in Canada and started his first faculty position in the National Yang Ming Medical College and Taipei Veterans General Hospital in 1981 as associate professor and investigator, respectively, in Taiwan. He returned back to HKU as a lecturer in the Department of Pharmacology in 1984 and became Chair Professor of Pharmacology in 2000. Later in his career, Prof. Cho joined the Chinese University of Hong Kong (CUHK) in 2007 as a Chairman and Professor of Pharmacology in the Department of Pharmacology. Thereafter, he has been the Research Professor and Associate Director in the School of Biomedical Sciences, Faculty of Medicine in CUHK. He became the Emeritus Professor of Pharmacology in the same university in 2016. Professionally, he was the President (2006–2010) and Chair of Presidential Council (2012–2015) of the Gastrointestinal Pharmacology Section of the International Union of Basic and Clinical Pharmacology and also council members in a number of professional bodies in ulcer research and gastrointestinal pharmacology. Prof. Cho has been the

Visiting and Honorary Professor in a number of renowned universities in China, Hong Kong, and USA. He is now the Distinguished Professor of Pharmacology in the Southwest Medical University in China. His current research interests focus on drug development for inflammation and cancers in the gastrointestinal tract. Prof. Cho has served as the editorial board member, associate editor, and also editor in more than 55 journals in the fields of gastroenterology and pharmacology.

Prof. Chi Hin Cho, BPharm, PhD
School of Biomedical Sciences, Faculty of Medicine,
the Chinese University of Hong Kong, Hong Kong & Laboratory
of Molecular Pharmacology, School of Pharmacy, Southwest Medical
University, Luzhou, Sichuan, China
chcho@cuhk.edu.hk

List of Contributors

Aladdin Alswaifi, MBBS
Concord Hospital
Level 1 West, Hospital Rd
Sydney, New South Wales, Australia

Tetsuo Arakawa, MD, PhD
President
Osaka City University
Osaka City, Osaka, 558-8585, Japan

Kathy K. Auyeung, PhD
Centre for Cancer and Inflammation Research
School of Chinese Medicine
Hong Kong Baptist University, Hong Kong, China

Hideo Baba, MD, PhD
Department of Gastroenterological Surgery
Graduate School of Medical Science
Kumamoto University, Kumamoto 860-8556, Japan

Jean-Philippe Babeu, PhD
Department of Anatomy and Cell Biology
Faculty of Medicine and Health Sciences
Université de Sherbrooke, Quebec, Canada

François Boudreau, PhD
Department of Anatomy and Cell biology, Faculty of Medicine and Health Sciences, Université de Sherbrooke, Quebec, Canada
Email: francois.boudreau@usherbrooke.ca

Tomasz Brzozowski, PhD
Department of Physiology, Jagiellonian University Medical College
Cracow, Poland
Email: mpbrzozo@cyf-kr.edu.pl

Yi Chen, MD, PhD
Department of Gastrointestinal Surgery, West China Hospital, Sichuan University, Chengdu 610041, China
Email: 2264199@qq.com

Tzyy-Wen Chiou, PhD
Department of Life Science
Graduate Institute of Biotechnology
National Dong Hwa University, Hualien, Taiwan

Chi Hin Cho, BPharm, PhD
School of Biomedical Sciences, Faculty of Medicine, the Chinese University of Hong Kong, Hong Kong & Laboratory of Molecular Pharmacology, School of Pharmacy, Southwest Medical University, Luzhou, Sichuan, China
Email: chcho@cuhk.edu.hk

Hong-Meng Chuang, MS
The Buddhist Tzu Chi Bioinnovation Center
Department of Life Sciences
National Chung Hsing University, Taichung, Taiwan

Ágnes Fehér, MD
Department of Pharmacology and Pharmacotherapy
Faculty of Medicine, Semmelweis University
Nagyvárad tér 4
1089 Budapest, Hungary

Andrew Fesler, B.S.
Department of Pathology, Stony Brook Medicine
Stony Brook University
Stony Brook, New York, USA

Yasuhiro Fujiwara, MD, PhD
Department of Gastroenterology and Samurai GI Research Centre
Osaka City University Graduate School of Medicine
Osaka City, Osaka, 545-8585, Japan

Vânia Gonçalves, PhD
Department of Human Genetics
National Health Institute 'Dr. Ricardo Jorge'
Lisbon, Portugal

BioISI (Biosystems & Integrative Sciences Institute)
Faculty of Sciences, University of Lisbon, Portugal

Klara Gyires, MD, PhD, DSc
Department of Pharmacology and Pharmacotherapy
Faculty of Medicine, Semmelweis University
Nagyvárad tér 4
1089 Budapest, Hungary
Email: gyires.klara@med.semmelweis-univ.hu

Horng-Jyh Harn, MD, PhD
The Buddhist Tzu Chi Bioinnovation Center
Department of Pathology
Buddhist Tzu Chi General Hospital
Tzu Chi University, Hualien, Taiwan
Email: arthewduke@gmail.com

Li-Ing Ho, MD
Division of Respiratory Therapy
Department of Chest Medicine
Taipei Veterans General Hospital, Taipei, Taiwan

Mao-Hsuan Huang, MS
Department of Life Sciences
National Chung Hsing University, Taichung, Taiwan

The Buddhist Tzu Chi Bioinnovation Center Hualien, Taiwan

Takatsugu Ishimoto, MD, PhD
Department of Gastroenterological Surgery, Graduate School of Medical Science, Kumamoto University, 1-1-1 Honjo, Kumamoto 860-8556, Japan
Email: taka1516@kumamoto-u.ac.jp

Peter Jordan, PhD
Department of Human Genetics
National Health Institute 'Dr. Ricardo Jorge'
Lisbon, Portugal

BioISI (Biosystems & Integrative Sciences Institute)
Faculty of Sciences, University of Lisbon
Lisbon, Portugal
Email: peter.jordan@insa.min-saude.pt

Jingfang Ju, PhD
Professor of Pathology
Department of Pathology
State University of New York at Stony Brook (Stony Brook University)
Stony Brook, New York, 11794-8693
Email: jingfang.ju@stonybrookmedicine.edu

Philipp Kaldis, PhD
Institute of Molecular and Cell Biology (IMCB)
A*STAR (Agency for Science, Technology and Research)
61 Biopolis Drive, Proteos #3-09
Singapore 138673, Republic of Singapore

Department of Biochemistry
National University of Singapore (NUS)
Singapore 117597, Republic of Singapore
Email: kaldis@imcb.a-star.edu.sg

Joshua K. S. Ko, PhD
Center for Cancer and Inflammation Research, School of Chinese Medicine
Hong Kong Baptist University, 7 Baptist University Road, Kowloon Tong
Hong Kong, China
Email: jksko@hkbu.edu.hk

Ava Kwong, MD, PhD
Department of Surgery, Faculty of Medicine
The University of Hong Kong
Hong Kong, China

Department of Surgery
Hong Kong Sanatorium and Hospital
Hong Kong, China

Rupert W. Leong, MBBS, MD
Concord Hospital, Level 1 West, Hospital Road, Sydney
New South Wales, Australia
Email: rupertleong@hotmail.com

Ming Xing Li, PhD
Laboratory of Molecular Pharmacology
School of Pharmacy, Southwest Medical University
Luzhou, Sichuan, China

Shinn-Zong Lin, MD, PhD
Department of Neurosurgery
Buddhist Tzu Chi General Hospital
Tzu Chi University, Hualien, Taiwan

The Buddhist Tzu Chi Bioinnovation Center Hualien, Taiwan

Zhihua Liu, PhD
State Key Lab of Molecular Oncology, National Cancer Center/Cancer
Hospital, Chinese Academy of Medical Sciences, Chaoyang District,
Beijing 100021, P.R. China
Email: liuzh@cicams.ac.cn

Gang Ma, PhD
Department of Gastrointestinal Cancer Biology
Tianjin Medical University Cancer Institute and Hospital
National Clinical Research Center for Cancer
Key Laboratory of Cancer Prevention and Therapy
Tianjin 300060, China

Li Ma, MD, PhD
Department of Science Education
Hofstra Northwell School of Medicine
500 Hofstra University
Hempstead, NY 11549, USA
Email: Li.Ma@hofstra.edu

Jolanta Majka, MD, PhD
Department of Physiology
Jagiellonian University Medical College
31-531 Cracow, Poland

Stefano Mancini, MD
Department of Diagnostic and Clinical Medicine, and Public Health
University of Modena and Reggio Emilia
I-41125, Modena, Italy

Francesco Mariani, PhD
Department of Diagnostic and Clinical Medicine, and Public Health
University of Modena and Reggio Emilia
I-41125, Modena, Italy

Paulo Matos, PhD
Department of Chemistry and Biochemistry
Faculty of Sciences, University of Lisbon, Portugal

BioISI (Biosystems & Integrative Sciences Institute)
Faculty of Sciences, University of Lisbon, Portugal

Department of Human Genetics
National Health Institute 'Dr. Ricardo Jorge'
Lisbon, Portugal

Hidenori Matsui, PhD
Kitasato Institute for Life Sciences
Kitasato University, Tokyo, Japan

Nikola Mitrev, B.Med.Sc., MBBS
Concord Hospital
Level 1 West, Hospital Rd
Sydney, New South Wales, Australia

Sebastian Mueller, MD, PhD
Centre of Alcohol Research (CAR)
University of Heidelberg, Heidelberg, Germany

Department of Medicine (Gastroenterology & Hepatology)
Salem Medical Centre, Heidelberg, Germany

Masahiko Nakamura, MD
School of Pharmacy, Kitasato University
Tokyo, Japan
Email: mngast@mac.com

Anders Øverby, PhD
School of Pharmacy
Kitasato University, Tokyo, Japan

The Center of Education in Kongsvinger
Kongsvinger, Norway

Nathan Palmer, BSc
Institute of Molecular and Cell Biology (IMCB)
A*STAR (Agency for Science, Technology and Research)
61 Biopolis Drive, Proteos #3-09
Singapore 138673, Republic of Singapore

Department of Biochemistry
National University of Singapore (NUS)
Singapore 117597, Republic of Singapore

Luca Roncucci, MD, PhD
Department of Diagnostic and Clinical Medicine, and Public Health
University of Modena and Reggio Emilia, Policlinico, Via Del Pozzo, 71
I-41125 Modena, Italy
Email: roncucci.luca@unimore.it

Helmut Karl Seitz, MD, AGAF
Centre of Alcohol Research (CAR), University of Heidelberg
Heidelberg, Germany & Department of Medicine (Gastroenterology & Hepatology), Salem Medical Centre, Heidelberg, Germany
Email: helmut_karl.seitz@urz.uni-heidelberg.de

Paola Sena, PhD
Department of Biomedical, Metabolic and Neural Sciences
Section of Human Morphology
University of Modena and Reggio Emilia
I-41125, Modena, Italy

Gautam Sethi, PhD
Department of Pharmacology, National University of Singapore
Singapore 117597, Republic of Singapore
Email: gautam_sethi@nuhs.edu.sg

Muthu K. Shanmugam, PhD
Department of Pharmacology
National University of Singapore (NUS)
Singapore 117597, Republic of Singapore

Masatsugu Shiba, MD, PhD
Department of Gastroenterology and Samurai GI Research Centre
Osaka City University Graduate School of Medicine
Osaka City, 545-8585, Osaka, Japan

Vivian Y. Shin, PhD
Department of Surgery, Faculty of Medicine, The University of Hong Kong
Hong Kong, China
Email: vyshin@hku.hk

Hong-Lin Su, PhD
Department of Life Sciences
National Chung Hsing University, Taichung, Taiwan

Aleksandra Szlachcic, MD, PhD
Department of Physiology
Jagiellonian University Medical College
31-531 Cracow, Poland

Shogo Takeda, MD, PhD
Department of Gastroenterology and Samurai GI Research Centre
Osaka City University Graduate School of Medicine
Osaka City, Osaka, 545-8585, Japan

Tetsuya Tanigawa, MD, PhD
Department of Gastroenterology and Samurai GI Research Centre, Osaka City University Graduate School of Medicine, 1-4-3 Asahimachi, Abeno-ku
Osaka City, Osaka 545-8585, Japan
Email: ttanigawa@med.osaka-cu.ac.jp

Hiroshi Tatsuwaki, MD, PhD
Department of Gastroenterology and Samurai GI Research Centre
Osaka City University Graduate School of Medicine
Osaka City, 545-8585, Osaka, Japan

Kazunari Tominaga, MD, PhD
Second Department of Internal Medicine
Osaka Medical College
Takatsuki City, Osaka 569-8686, Japan

Sheng-Feng Tsai, MS
Department of Life Sciences
National Chung Hsing University, Taichung, Taiwan

Jinhui Wang, PhD
College of Pharmacy, Xinjiang Medical University
Urumqi 830011, China

Peiqi Wang, PhD
Department of Gastrointestinal Surgery, West China Hospital
Sichuan University, Chengdu 610041, China

State Key Laboratory of Oral Diseases
West China Hospital of Stomatology
Sichuan University, Chengdu 610041, China

Toshio Watanabe, MD, PhD
Department of Gastroenterology and Samurai GI Research Centre
Osaka City University Graduate School of Medicine
Osaka City, Osaka, 545-8585, Japan

Ssu-Yin Yen, PhD
Department of Life Science
Graduate Institute of Biotechnology
National Dong Hwa University, Hualien, Taiwan

The Buddhist Tzu Chi Bioinnovation Center Hualien, Taiwan

Yuanyuan Yin, PhD
Department of Gastrointestinal Surgery, West China Hospital
Sichuan University, Chengdu 610041, China

State Key Laboratory of Oral Diseases
West China Hospital of Stomatology
Sichuan University, Chengdu 610041, China

Yaxin Zheng, PhD
State Key Laboratory of Biotherapy and Collaborative Innovation
Center of Biotherapy
West China Hospital
Sichuan University, Chengdu 610041, China

Contents

Section I

General Introduction to Inflammation and Cancer in the Digestive Tract

Ming Xing Li and Chi Hin Cho

Inflammation and cancer are the major disorders in mankind. They are the most common diseases known in clinical practice and are the major causes of morbidity as well as mortality in humans. Unfortunately their underlying pathogenesis is still not well defined and the most difficult part is that they are likely to recur during remission. Pathologically both inflammation and cancer are causally linked. In fact, it has been established that almost all organs that suffer from chronic inflammation would eventually have an increased risk of cancer. This is particularly true for the malignancies in the digestive system, including those in the liver and gastrointestinal tract.[1]

Studying the pathogenic processes in inflammation and cancer and their causal relationship has been overwhelmed in the literatures in the past decade. Over thirty five thousand studies both from experimental and clinical investigations from PubMed have been reported. With these enormous efforts, we now understand better than ten years ago about the pathogenesis and literally identify the potential biomarkers for the diagnosis and therapeutic targets for both diseases.

In the advance of both basic sciences and biotechnology research, there has been huge development in the discoveries of drugs and therapeutic modalities against the different pathogenic targets in the prevention and treatment of inflammation and cancer. In this book, researchers and clinicians from 12 different regions and countries share their extensive professional and research experiences in studying the different important pathogenic modulators and also drugs used either clinically or still under experimental investigations for both diseases in the digestive tract.

This book aims to capture these discoveries and experiences to shed new light on future therapeutic options for both inflammation and cancer in the digestive system. In this regard, it begins with the description of the brain/gut interaction and also the phenomenon of microbiota–gut–brain axis in the pathogenesis of cognitive disorders and inflammation in the gastrointestinal tract. Also, nesfatin-1 an appetite peptide is introduced to demonstrate its therapeutic efficacy to prevent acute hemorrhagic lesions and accelerate ulcer healing in the stomach. The current prophylactic treatment in patients with inflammatory bowel disease is also discussed. The established therapies and the therapeutic strategies in the treatment of alcoholic liver disease are compared for the better options of therapy. Experimentally, the importance of hepatocyte nuclear factor-4-α in gastrointestinal inflammation is also emphasized in the first part of the book.

Cancers in the upper gastrointestinal tract, including those in the esophagus and stomach to the lower intestine are the major focuses in this book. The epigenetics and microenvironment, the nuclear factor-κ and the hypoxia-inducible factor-1α and also the involvement of prostaglandins and their metabolism and receptors in the carcinogenesis and treatment for gastrointestinal cancers are extensively reviewed in the hope that new therapeutic targets can be identified. The later development of herb/drug interactions and their pros and cons in the treatment of gastrointestinal cancer and also the progression of therapeutic agents from bench to bedside in esophageal cancer, are also fully discussed in the second part of the book.

There is no doubt that there has been a great advancement in studying the contributory roles of both microRNAs and autophagy in the pathogenic processes of inflammation and cancer, especially in the past ten years. The actions of microRNAs and autophagy are the two sides of a sword, either promoting or inhibitory to these diseases. This dichotomy phenomenon is especially appreciated in different types of cancer and also their clinical stages of the diseases. It is envisaged that studying their causal relationship will be the important research direction in the years to come. As such, modulation of the expression of different microRNAs and autophagy processes including autophagosome and lysosome interaction in cancer cells will be the potential therapeutic targets and strategies in the treatment of inflammation and cancer in the digestive tract.

Reference

1. CW Wu, J Yu (2012) General introduction. In: CH Cho & J Yu (eds.). *From Inflammation to Cancer: Advances in Diagnosis and Therapy for Gastrointestinal and Hepatological Diseases*, pp. 3–14. World Scientific, Singapore.

Section II
Inflammation and Therapeutics in the Digestive Tract

Chapter 1

Brain–Gut Relationship on Mucosal Inflammation in the Gastrointestinal Tract

Klara Gyires and Ágnes Fehér

Abstract

Central nervous system (CNS) communicates with the gastrointestinal (GI) tract through the so-called brain–gut axis and has impact on GI physiology and pathophysiology. Brain–gut axis is a bidirectional communication network, and through this axis the information from the gut to the brain may modify brain function and behavior. Several convincing data suggest that mental diseases as well as stress may play a central role in the development of gastric and activation of intestinal mucosal lesions and inflammation (e.g. inflammatory bowel diseases (IBDs)). On the other hand, human and animal studies suggest that inflammatory processes in the GI system, particularly in the gut may trigger central changes. These may lead to altered brain function and comorbidity of psychological/psychiatric disorders. It has been recognized that changes in microbiome composition can be manifested in alterations of cognitive and emotional functions. This has significantly contributed to the establishment of a new concept from the well-accepted gut–brain axis to the microbiota–gut–brain axis. The present chapter aims to give an overview on the mechanisms potentially involved in the brain–gut and gut–brain axis as well as the microbiota–gut–brain pathway in mammals.

Introduction

The role of central nervous system (CNS) in gastrointestinal (GI) mucosal integrity as well as in the development of gastric erosions has long been known. The relation between peptic ulceration and intracranial disease was suggested already in the middle of 19th century by Schiff and by Rokitansky. Both found a peculiar kind of gelatinous gastromalacia associated with intracranial lesions in newborn infants and also a relationship between third ventricular tumors and discrete gastric ulcers was observed.[1] In the 20th century, in 1932 Cushing published that patients with head injury, cerebral stroke or tumor had a high incidence of gastritis.[2] Selye recognized more than 70 years ago the occurrence of stress-related ulcers in humans, based on clinical reports on the huge increase in the number of perforated gastric and duodenal ulcers during bombings of London in World War II.[3] Furthermore, certain mental diseases may modify the risk for developing peptic ulcer. For example, a significant association was observed between schizophrenia and lower risk for duodenal (but not for gastrojejunal) ulcers in a case-control study.[4] Recent studies showed that people with mental illnesses (anxiety disorder, panic disorder, panic attacks, and social phobia) exhibited high risk for developing subsequent peptic ulcer disease.[5] Similarly, patients with bipolar disorders have a substantially higher risk for ulcer disease.[6] The above cited data are only some examples from the numerous experimental and human investigations which provide convincing evidence on the role of brain–gut axis in GI mucosal integrity and lesions.

The aim of the present work is to give a short overview on the basis of literatures how brain–gut axis influences the gastric and intestinal inflammation, mucosal injury or ulceration. On the other hand, this chapter also aims to analyze the gut–brain axis that is how the gastric or intestinal inflammatory, injurious processes may affect the CNS function and initiate pathological reactions.

Overview of brain–gut relationship

The CNS communicates with the GI tract through the so-called brain–gut axis. This axis is a bidirectional communication system, which involves the brain and spinal cord (CNS), the autonomic nervous system (vagal and spinal afferent neurons which convey information from the GI tract to the

CNS and efferent signals from CNS to the GI system), the enteric nervous system and the hypothalamic pituitary adrenal (HPA) axis.

Afferent neurons have a basic role in the regulation of GI functions. Beside intrinsic sensory neurons which have their cell body within the GI tract and originate in the myenteric or submucosal plexus, there are two groups of extrinsic sensory neurons: the vagal and spinal afferents. 75–90% of the axons in vagus nerve are afferent fibers (see Refs. 7 and 8) which originate in the jugular and nodose ganglia and project to medullary brain stem. Vagal afferents seem topically deliver information from the GI tract to the brain, and this sensory input is supposed to be relevant in the autonomic regulation and may influence the emotion, attitude, and behavior.[9,10]

The chemical and mechanical (contraction and distention) signals in the gut are conveyed to the nucleus tractus solitarii (NTS) via the vagal ascending fibers. Strong evidence supports the idea that glutamate is a transmitter in afferent vagal fibers conveying information from the gut to the brain.[11] After integration of the incoming information, neuronal communication between the NTS and the dorsal motor nucleus of vagus (DMV) results in modulation of DMV activity, and the vagal efferent output regulates GI functions such as secretion, absorption, motility,[7] and as a consequence of the previous actions, may affect also mucosal homeostasis.

Furthermore, besides the dorsal vagal complex (DVC), hypothalamus seems to have a particularly important role in central regulation of GI functions. Neuronal connection between hypothalamus and the central autonomic system have been described. The different viscero and somatosensory signals reach the hypothalamus through catecholaminergic and non-catecholaminergic neuronal pathways relayed in the spinal cord and the medulla oblongata. Vice versa, hypothalamus also influences autonomic activities through humoral and neurohumoral pathways. The descending efferent projections of the hypothalamus terminate on parasympathetic nuclei of the brainstem such as the DMV. The descending axons are mainly peptidergic (corticotropin-releasing factor (CRF), vasopressin, oxytocin, somatostatin, enkephalin, proopiomelanocortin (POMC)) and carry feedback signals to viscerosensory and brainstem catecholaminergic neurons and regulatory inputs to parasympathetic (DMV) and sympathetic (thoracolumbar intermediolateral cell column) preganglionic neurons. The ascending fibers are both peptidergic (enkephalin, NPY, neurotensin, dynorphins) and catecholaminergic.[12]

Activation of HPA axis may also influence several functions of the GI tract. In response to different psychological, physical stressors, CRF is released from neurons of the parvocellular part of the paraventricular nucleus (PVN) and through CRF1 receptors it induces the release of adrenocorticotropin (ACTH) from the anterior lobe of the pituitary. ACTH stimulates the release of glucocorticoids in the adrenal cortex, such as cortisol in humans and corticosterone in rodents. Glucocorticoids induce profound alterations in several functions of the organism. In addition, CRF stimulates the release of POMC products (e.g. β-endorphin). Consequently, the stress stimulus through glucocorticoids, CRF, ACTH, β-endorphin, as well as through additional neurohormones (such as substance P, vasoactive intestinal polypeptide, neuropeptide Y and cholecystokinin (CCK)) induces profound alterations in several functions of the organism, including the GI tract.[13]

Brain–Stomach Axis

The brain–gut axis is a bidirectional communication system between the CNS and the gut (Table 1). However, early observation suggested the relationship between CNS disorders and gastric ulcers formation.[1–3] On the other hand, also gastric mucosal insult signals the CNS. Therefore the brain–gut and brain–stomach axis and vice versa will be discussed separately in different parts of the chapter. This will be discussed separately in different parts of the chapter regarding the brain–stomach and brain–gut axis and vice versa in animals and humans.

Mental diseases, stress and gastric mucosal injury

The role of mental diseases, however, seems to be contradictory in the light of different literatures. For example, a significant association was observed between schizophrenia and diminished risk for duodenal ulcers but not for gastrojejunal ulcers,[4] while other mental illness, e.g. anxiety and panic disorders exhibited high risks for developing subsequent peptic ulcer disease.[5] In addition, bipolar disorders are likely to represent a substantially higher risk for ulcer disease.[6]

As mentioned above, Selye recognized the occurrence of stress ulcers in humans, based on clinical reports on the huge increase in the number of perforated gastric and duodenal ulcers during bombings of London in World War II,

Table 1. Human and experimental evidence for brain–stomach and stomach–brain axis.

Type of CNS–GI axis	Type of stimulus that alters brain–gut axis	Responses
Brain–stomach	*Humans*:	
	→ Acute stress	→ Perforated gastric and duodenal ulcers[3]
	→ Schizophrenia	→ Diminished risk for duodenal but not for gastrojejunal ulcers[4]
	→ Anxiety and panic disorders	→ High risks for developing subsequent peptic ulcer disease[5]
	→ Bipolar disorders	→ Higher risk for ulcer disease[6]
	→ Stress	→ Higher risk for gastric ulcer disease[16]
	Experimental animals:	
	→ Central injection of neuropeptides to the rat (i.c.v., i.c., DMV)	→ Inhibition of the gastric mucosal lesions induced by different ulcerogenic challenge[8,17–19]
	→ Leptin injected into the PVN (rat)	→ Gastric mucosal damage[26]
	→ Angiotensin II injected into the PVN (rat)	→ Inhibition of gastric ischemia/reperfusion-induced injury[25]
	→ Agmatine injected into lateral hypothalamus (rat)	→ Inhibition of the ethanol-induced gastric mucosal lesions[20]
Stomach–brain	*Experimental animals*:	
	→ Minimally injurious concentration of HCl (0.15–0.5 M) (rat)	→ Expression of c-Fos mRNA and c-Fos protein in the NTS[27]
	→ NaCl (0.15 M) or HCl (0.15 and 0.25 M) (mouse)	→ Expression of c-Fos protein in NTS[28]
	→ Mild gastritis by DSS or iodoacetamide (mouse)	→ Significantly enhanced the c-Fos response to HCl in NTS[28]
	→ i.p. injection of IL-1β and TNF-α (rat)	→ Significantly higher c-Fos mRNA expression in the NTS than to acid challenge[29]
	→ RWIS (rat)	→ c-Fos expression in the DMV during the stress, followed by NA, NTS and AP[30]

Abbreviations: DMV: dorsal motor nucleus of vagus; DSS: dextran sulfate sodium; i.c.: intracisternally; i.c.v.: intracerebroventricularly; i.p.: intraperitoneally; NTS: nucleus tractus solitarii; PVN: paraventricular nucleus; TNF-α: tumor necrosis factor-α; RWIS: restraint water-immersion stress.

more than 70 years ago.[3] However, the mechanism of stress-related gastric mucosal injury is not fully understood and clarified even now. Gastric acid is essential for the development of gastric mucosal injury and antisecretory drugs are basically important in the pharmacologic manipulation of intraluminal pH as a therapeutic possibility. However, both in humans and animals, gastric acid secretion can be decreased during stress and it was suggested that reduction of gastric acid secretion is a defense mechanism during stress mediated by a central neuronal mediator including nitric oxide (NO) specifically in the DMV.[14] Furthermore, though glucocorticoids have generally been accepted as ulcerogenic hormones, Filaretova *et al.* suggested that glucocorticoids released during activation of the HPA axis act as gastroprotective hormones.[15]

The stress-related mucosal lesions may be mainly due to the decrease of gastric mucosal adaptive mechanisms and reduction of gastric mucosal circulation as a consequence of redistribution of blood flow from the visceral region to the vital organs.[16] The reduced mucosal perfusion can result in a splanchnic ischemia, and reperfusion injury, which may induce directly mucosal damage of gastric mucosa. In addition, gastric hypomotility, a further factor contributes to mucosal injury in stress.[16]

Experimental evidence for the role of CNS in gastric mucosal homeostasis

Gastric mucosal injury provoked by different stressors (e.g. cold restraint stress or forced swimming stress in rats) is one of the most widely used models in ulcer research.[8,16]

Moreover, in the last 25 years increasing numbers of experimental evidence have indicated that also gastric mucosal protection can be initiated centrally. Several neuropeptides have been shown to exert gastric mucosal protection against ethanol-induced mucosal injury given intracisternally (i.c.), into DMV or intracerebroventricularly (i.c.v.), such as thyrotropin-releasing hormone (TRH), opioid peptides, nociceptin, nocistatin (i.c.v.), substance P and angiotensin II (i.c.v.) (see Refs. 17–19). Recently, the gastroprotective effect of agmatine, an endogenous aminoguanidine, ligand of imidazoline and α_2 adrenergic receptors given i.c.v. was published.[20] In addition, some neuropeptides, besides possessing a key role in regulation of food intake, are likely to play a role in gastric mucosal defense as well, for example amylin (i.c.v.), adrenomedullin (i.c.), peptide YY (PYY) (i.c.v.), orexin-A (i.c.), leptin (i.c.v., ethanol- and ischemia-reperfusion-induced lesions), nesfatin-1 (i.c.v.) and TLQP-21 (i.c.v.), a vascular endothelial growth factor (VEGF)-derived peptide (i.c.v.).[17–19]

However, it should be emphasized that the dose-response curves of several neuropeptides, such as RX 77368 (a stable TRH analog), adrenomedullin, nociceptin and nocistatin, substance P and angiotensin II proved to be partly sigmoid, partly bell-shaped. Common characteristic of the bell-shaped dose-response relationships is that the reduction of the effect may be expected typically to be 10- and 100-fold the effective dose range (though the range can also be much wider).[19,21]

Moreover, neuropeptides were shown to inhibit gastric mucosal damage induced by stress or non-steroidal anti-inflammatory drugs as well.[8,19]

Conveying the centrally initiated effect to the periphery

How can the central action of different neuropeptides be conveyed to the periphery and to induce gastric mucosal protection? Convincing evidence suggests the basic role of DVC and vagal nerve in centrally initiated gastric mucosal protection. Namely, vagal nerve was shown to play a fundamental role in maintaining gastric mucosal integrity and gastric mucosal defense. TRH injected at low doses into the cisterna magna or the DMN was the first peptide reported to protect the gastric mucosa against ethanol injury through stimulation of vagal cholinergic pathways (see Ref. 17). Vagal dependent mechanism of mucosal protection has been described for most of the neuropeptides mentioned above.[17,19]

The peripheral mechanism of vagal-mediated gastroprotective effect has been well documented by biochemical and pharmacological studies, suggesting that the activation of vagal cholinergic pathways stimulates the release of gastric mucosal prostaglandins (PGs) and NO, as well as the effector function of capsaicin-sensitive afferent fibers containing calcitonin gene-related peptide (CGRP).[17] However, it should be kept in mind that vagal nerve has a dual role. It can mediate both mucosal damaging and protective effects. For example through the activation of parasympathetic outflow to the stomach TRH in higher dose range than the gastroprotective one stimulated gastric acid and pepsin secretion, gastric emptying and induced ulceration acting centrally in DVC.[22]

Several data suggest that besides vagal nerve the adrenergic system may also play a role in conveying the centrally initiated effect to the periphery.[19,23] For example, the gastroprotective effect of centrally injected ghrelin could be significantly decreased by blocking both cholinergic and adrenergic systems.[24] Furthermore, the centrally induced gastroprotective effect of opioid peptides is likely to be mediated also by both systems, since both bilateral cervical vagotomy and chemical sympathectomy by 6-hydroxydopamine (i.c.v.) antagonized the protective effect. The later action correlated with the reduction of the noradrenaline content in the NTS.[23] In contrast, angiotensin II injected into the paraventricular nucleus (PVN) dose-dependently inhibited gastric ischemia/reperfusion-induced injury, and the protective effect was not affected by subdiaphragmatic vagotomy or atropine, but was abolished by propranolol or disconnection of the nerves innervating the adrenal glands indicating that the central effects of angiotensin II are mediated in the periphery by a sympathetic — adrenal gland/β-adrenoceptor — pathway.[25]

Neuronal connection between hypothalamus and the central autonomic system has been well documented and consequently hypothalamic areas are also involved in the regulation of GI function and gastric mucosal integrity. For example, leptin injected into the PVN resulted in significant gastric damage indicating that leptin acting at a functionally specific population of PVN neurons may be involved in the control of GI function. It may also act as a humoral factor involved in gastric ulceration.[26] It should be emphasized that this effect of leptin is site specific, namely injected into non-PVN sites failed to induced mucosal lesions, even leptin exerted protective effect against ethanol- and ischemia-reperfusion-induced lesions injected i.c.v.[19] On the other hand, angiotensin II injected into the PVN dose-dependently inhibited gastric ischemia/reperfusion-induced injury (see above).[25] Similarly, the endogenous imidazoline and α_2-adrenoceptor agonist agmatine injected into lateral hypothalamus exerted gastroprotective action against ethanol-induced mucosal damage in a similar dose range that proved to be effective following i.c.v. administration.[20] The above studies indicate the role of hypothalamus and its connection with the centers of autonomic system in gastric mucosal injury/defense. However, activation of different hypothalamic areas induces different mucosal actions, both mucosal defense and lesion can be developed.

Stomach–Brain Axis

Vagal afferents have a basic role in delivering information from the GI tract to the brain. This sensory input is supposed to be relevant in the autonomic regulation as well as influencing the emotion, attitude and behavior.[7,9,10] Besides the vagal afferents, the spinal afferents also have fundamental importance in the transmission conducted from the GI tract to CNS. The cell body of spinal afferents is located in the dorsal root ganglia. Transmission of mechanical (e.g. distension) and chemical (e.g. increased H^+ ion concentration) stimuli was shown to be mediated by two distinct afferent pathways, the spinal and vagal ones, respectively.[27]

Afferent signaling of gastric acid challenge is not only directly related to the formation of mucosal injury, but also correlated with the back-diffused H^+. H^+ back-diffusion may be due to supraphysiological concentrations of intragastric hydrochloric acid (HCl) or to the insufficient function of gastric mucosal barrier, whose permeability may be increased by inflammation, stress, irritating food or liquid, infection, and non-steroidal anti-inflammatory drug use.[10] Signaling of gastric mucosal irritation to the CNS has been visualized by c-Fos mRNA expression in different brain areas. The functional c-Fos expression is supposed to reflect a valid image of brain activity. For example, exposure of the rat gastric mucosa to HCl in minimally injurious concentration (0.15–0.5 M HCl) resulted in a rapid expression of c-Fos mRNA and c-Fos protein in the NTS, but not in the spinal cord.[27] The c-Fos response to gastric acid challenge in NTS is suppressed by bilateral subdiaphragmatic vagotomy, suggesting that the chemostimulus of afferent nerves in gastric mucosa is conveyed to the NTS and area postrema (AP) of the brainstem predominantly by vagal afferents.[27]

Moreover, oral administration of NaCl (0.15 M) or HCl (0.15 and 0.25 M) induced c-Fos expression in NTS 2 hours later, as a result of activation of afferent neurons. Induction of mild gastritis by dextran sulfate sodium (DSS) or iodoacetamide (IAA) in the mouse significantly enhanced the c-Fos response to HCl. The gastritis-induced increase in the gastric acid-evoked c-Fos expression in the NTS was related to disruption of the gastric mucosal barrier, mucosal inflammation, mucosal acid influx and consequently, to enhanced activation of the afferent stomach–NTS axis. The results suggest that exposure of gastric mucosa to excess HCl signals NTS neurons express c-Fos. This afferent input is significantly enhanced when the stomach is inflamed.[28] Similarly, pretreatment of rats systemically (intraperitoneally) with pro-inflammatory cytokines, interleukin-1β (IL-1β) and tumor necrosis factor-α (TNF-α) resulted in a significantly higher c-Fos mRNA expression in the NTS than the gastric HCl challenge *per se*. This sensitizing effect seems to arise from a peripheral action on vagal afferents.[29]

Furthermore, the effect of restraint water-immersion stress (RWIS) on neuronal activities of the DVC and the nucleus ambiguous (NA) in rats has been examined. The most intense c-Fos expression was observed in the DMV during the stress, followed by NA, NTS and AP. These results indicate that the neuronal hyperactivity of DMV, NA, NTS and AP (especially DMV and NA), are the primary centers that control gastric functions. This may play an important role in the restraint-stress-induced gastric disorders on stomach motility, secretion and mucosal lesions.[30]

Brain–Gut Axis

Increasing evidence suggests that the brain may be involved in the pathogenesis of inflammatory bowel disease (IBD). The crosstalk between the nervous and immune systems could play a crucial role in the regulation of the immune response and consequently, the inflammatory processes. CNS interacts dynamically with the immune system to modulate inflammation through humoral and neural pathways. The interaction between the brain and gut is bidirectional. The CNS can affect gut function, and alteration in gut function in turn can influence the normal CNS activity and function (Table 2).

IBD is a chronic and relapsing inflammatory condition of the GI tract. The two main forms of IBD are Crohn's disease (CD) and ulcerative colitis (UC). The cause of IBD is not exactly known. The recent consensus is that IBDs are initiated and perpetuated by an impaired immune response against the gut microbiota in genetically susceptible individuals and the disease is caused by a combination of different factors, including genetics, immune dysregulation, barrier dysfunction, change in microbial flora and environmental influences.

UC and CD were initially considered as classic examples of psychosomatic diseases and association between IBD and psychiatric disorders was suggested. The results and conclusions of different previous studies that aimed to analyze potential association between adverse life events or psychiatric disorders and

Table 2. Human and experimental evidence for brain–gut and gut–brain axis.

Type of CNS–GI axis	Type of stimulus	Response
Brain–gut	*Humans*:	
	→ Traumatic events in childhood	→ Development of psychiatric diseases and functional bowel disorders later in life[32]
	→ Mental depression and negative psychological stress	→ Contribution to an increased risk of relapse in IBD[33,34]
	→ Depression, panic and generalized anxiety	→ More common in IBD patients than in the control population[33,34]
	→ Major depression	→ Can contribute to failure of the successful treatment with infliximab[35]
	→ Stress and negative psychosocial factors	→ Negative impact on the course of IBD[44,45]
	Experimental animals:	
	→ Induction of depression by chronic i.c.v. injection of reserpine or olfactory bulbectomy (mouse)	→ Reactivated quiescent colitis induced by DSS or dinitrobenzene-sulphonic acid[37,38]
	→ Exposure to restraint stress for four days (rat)	→ Increased mucosal inflammatory reaction induced by TNBS[46]
	→ Restraint stress (rat)	→ Partial reactivation of mucosal inflammation[47]
Gut–brain	*Humans*:	
	→ IBD	→ Impaired mental health[53]
	→ Disturbances of the gut microbial community	→ Potential contribution to the development of neuropsychiatric diseases[66]
	Experimental animals:	
	→ DSS colitis (mouse)	→ Changes in stress-associated behavior and neuropeptide gene expression in limbic system[54]

Abbreviations: DSS: dextran sulfate sodium; i.c.v.: intracerebroventricularly; IBD: inflammatory bowel disease; TNBS: 2,4,6-trinitrobenzenesulfonic acid.

disease activity in IBD are mixed (see Ref. 31). In the last 10–15 years, however, considerable evidence has accumulated that occurrence of mental disorders are more frequent in IBD patients than in the control population. For example, traumatic events in childhood (such as general trauma, physical punishment, emotional abuse, and sexual events) have been associated with the development of psychiatric diseases and functional bowel disorders later in life.[32] Moreover, mental depression and negative psychological stress were found to contribute to an increased risk of relapse in IBD.[33,34]

Depression and IBD

It has been well established that mental depression may coexist with IBD, and IBD is often exacerbated in the presence of psychiatric disturbances. Several psychiatric diseases, such as major depression, panic and generalized anxiety are more common in IBD patients than in the control population.[33,34] In addition, major depression can also be responsible for the failure of the successful treatment with infliximab.[35] These findings also confirm the concept that the diagnosis and management of major depression should be part of the clinical approach to treat patients with IBD.

Previous analysis showed that the associations between IBD and depression were the strongest when the mental conditions were diagnosed shortly before UC, although the association between depression and UC was also significant when depression preceded UC by five or more years. It was speculated that development of depression or anxiety one year or less before diagnosis of UC might be considered as a consequence of early symptoms of the yet undiagnosed GI condition. On the other hand, the data may also indicate, that the psychiatric disorders could be aetiological factors in the development of UC.[36] Experimental data also suggest correlation between the two diseases: induction of depression by chronic i.c.v. injection of reserpine or by olfactory bulbectomy reactivated quiescent colitis induced by DSS (lymphocyte-independent model of chronic colitis) or dinitrobenzenesulfonic acid (lymphocyte-dependent model) in mice.[37,38]

Why can depression negatively influence the course of IBD?

Research focused on the mechanism how nervous system may influence the immune system revealed that the vagal innervation of the GI tract plays a major role in controlling intestinal immune activation since the release of acetylcholine reduces the immune cell activation by interacting with α-7 nicotinic acetylcholine receptors (α7nAChR).[39] It has been demonstrated that depression results in autonomic imbalance, with impaired parasympathomimetic functions.[40] Experimental findings also confirm that impaired cholinergic function may play a causal role in gut inflammation; disease activity index, macroscopic and histologic scores, myeloperoxidase activity, level of serum amyloid-P, and colonic tissue levels of IL-1β, interleukin-6 (IL-6), and TNF-α were increased significantly in vagotomized mice in DSS and hapten-induced colitis when compared with sham-operated mice that received DSS or the hapten.[41] These results suggest that vagal nerve is likely to exert a tonic inhibition on acute inflammation. In accordance with this finding, vagotomy as well as experimental depression, resulted in reactivation of inflammation in mice with chronic colitis.[38] The vagus-induced inhibition of inflammatory process may be correlated with a selective suppression of pro-inflammatory cytokine secretion from the macrophages via the activation of α7nAChR, which are located on the macrophages and immune cells (see Ref. 42).

Human data are in harmony with the experimental findings. In patients with major depression, increased the inflammatory parameters, such as C-reactive protein (CRP) and TNF-α, as well as the leukocytes counts also increased. Antidepressant treatment with selective serotonin reuptake inhibitors resulted in a decreased level of TNF-α, CRP, and leukocyte counts comparable with those of the control patients and it was suggested that TNF-α could be considered as a potential state marker in major depression.[43]

Stress and IBD

In humans, psychosocial factors and stress are also likely to influence the course of IBD. Reviews, studied the international evidence-based guidelines on the management of IBD concluded that there is a strong evidence on comorbidity of IBD and psychosocial factors such as mental disorders or stress. Stress and psychosocial factors may have a negative impact on the course of the disease, although they are not likely to play a major role in the aetiology of IBD.[44] Similar conclusion was drawn by Bonaz and Bernstein[45] on the effect of stress or other negative psychological factors in the course of IBD. Identification of biomarkers of brain–gut interactions, for example serum/salivary cortisol (as a marker of the HPA axis), variability of heart rate (as an indicator of balance between the sympathetic and vagal activities), could clarify the contribution of psychosocial influence and stress to the reactivation of IBD.[45]

Experimental psychological stress is likely to contribute to the reactivation of GI inflammation in animal models of colitis. Rats produced an increased mucosal inflammatory reaction induced by 2,4,6-trinitrobenzenesulfonic (TNBS) acid when they were exposed to restraint stress for four days prior to induction of colitis.[46] Similarly, restrain stress resulted in partial reactivation of mucosal inflammation (increased colonic myeloperoxidase production, but not signs of mucosal inflammation) in rats which had recovered from TNBS colitis 6 weeks previously.[47] Furthermore, it has been shown that in mice recovered from TNBS colitis, colitis could be provoked by giving lower dose range of TNBS if they were exposed to restraint stress.[48]

Why does stress negatively influence the course of IBD?

Several mechanisms have been raised regarding the stress-related deleterious mucosal action. Stress-induced alterations in IBD may be mediated by activation of HPA axis as well as by alterations in bacterial–mucosal interactions, and mucosal mast cells function.[31] For example, chronic sustained stress in humans causes a prolonged increase in cortisol over several days which may exert immunosuppressive action.[49] On the other hand, acute stress stimulus results in a prompt increase of catecholamines and cortisol, but only for few hours. The serum levels of inflammatory cytokines, which are important in the pathogenesis of IBD (TNF-α, IL-6, and interferon-γ) were higher, and also cytokine production by whole blood proved to be elevated. Thus acute stress is associated with immune enhancement (see Ref. 31).

Moreover, acute and chronic stress leads to disruption of intestinal mucosal tight junctions, which enhances mucosal permeability, facilitates microbial translocation into the intestinal wall. The increased number of microbes in the colonic tissue provokes an immune response with excessive cytokine release and the consequent inflammation. Thus, stress results in a negative impact on IBD.[50]

Change of composition of microflora is recognized as one of the main mechanisms in the pathogenesis of IBD. Dopamine and noradrenaline increased enterohemorrhagic *E. coli* O157:H7 adherence compared to untreated control tissues in murine cecum under *ex vivo* condition. Results suggest that conditions associated with elevated catecholamine release, such as stress exposure, may influence host susceptibility to *E. coli* O157:H7 infection. Furthermore, exposure to a social stressor was reported to affect microbial populations, including the *lactobacilli* in the mouse. Because the *lactobacilli* can have beneficial effect in human intestinal homeostasis, stress-induced reduction of their population could initiate pathological alterations. Thus, stress disrupts the community structure of the gut microbiota.[51,52]

Mast cells may also play a basic role in stress-induced activation of intestinal inflammation. Namely, CRF and substance P released from enteric neurons in response to stress stimuli may induce the release of mast cell mediators, which promote bacterial mucosal adherence and microbial translocation into the intestinal wall resulting in sensitization of T cells and the production of IFN-γ and TNF-α. These cytokines may initiate inflammation and cause a secondary increase in permeability (see review of Ref. 31).

Gut–Brain Axis

Over the past decade, increasing number of experimental data suggested a complex and bidirectional interaction between the GI tract and the CNS, the so-called gut–brain axis. Convincing evidence has accumulated from both human and animal studies indicating that inflammatory processes in the gut may trigger central changes that lead to altered brain function. Comorbidity of psychological/psychiatric disorders and IBD influence the course of each other when they coexist. IBD impairs the quality of life of the patients not only because of the intestinal (such as abdominal pain associated with diarrhea, rectal bleeding, and malnutrition) and extraintestinal (among others fever, weight loss, arthritis, arthralgia, mucocutaneous, ophthalmologic lesions) symptoms, but also because of the impaired mental health (see Ref. 53). Recent experimental findings suggested that dextran sulfate sodium-induced colitis in the mice influences the stress-associated behavior and neuropeptide gene expression in the limbic system of mice.[54]

Moreover, inflammation in any peripheral organ may induce a common pattern of CNS response, the so-called "sickness syndrome", which includes fever, sleepiness, anorexia, hyperalgesia, fatigue, mood alterations, cognitive dysfunction and corticosteroid release.[55]

Mechanism of intestinal inflammation-induced brain alterations

Cytokines and prostaglandins

Several mechanisms have been raised to play a role in the gut–CNS communication during the course of intestinal inflammation.[56] Different cytokines, e.g. IL-1β, IL-6, and TNF-α, have a profound role in the pathogenic mechanisms of IBD and these cytokines also appear in the circulation. For example, secretion of IL-1β and TNF-α from polymorphonuclear leukocytes (PMN) of patients with CD and UC stimulated by lipopolysaccharide was higher than that from normal control cells, though these changes were not specific for IBD but rather reflected intestinal inflammation in general.[57] These cytokines are too bulky to cross the blood–brain barrier (BBB) in large amounts, however, inflammatory cytokines can be actively transported into the CNS[58] in minor amounts. The physiological/pathophysiological importance of this active transport has not been clarified yet. In addition, at the BBB through their receptors on perivascular and endothelial cells cytokines can increase the expression of cyclooxygenase-2 (COX-2) and biosynthesis of PGE_2.[59] Prostaglandins are supposed to be a key mediator responsible for brain responses to systemic inflammation by their ability to cross the BBB.[55] In addition, proinflammatory messengers activate cell adhesion molecules on the cerebral endothelium resulting in rolling, adhesion, and migration of leukocytes into the parenchyma. Peripheral TNF-α is likely to play a critical role in initiating this interaction between leukocytes and endothelial cells.[60]

These signaling mechanisms from the periphery promote additional synthesis of cytokines inside the brain, such as IL-1, IL-6, and TNF-α, most probably by activating the microglial cells (see reviews of Refs. 61 and 62). These cytokines play a role in the pathogenic mechanisms of several diseases associated with inflammation, like behavior-disorders, cognitive changes, and affective disorders,[61,62] since cytokines may alter neurotransmission in the brain. In this regard, it has been suggested that cytokines, as signaling molecules of the immune system, may be involved also in the provocation or exacerbation of mood disorders such as mental depression. This assumption is supported by several observations; for example severe depression is accompanied by increased cytokine production/levels, or immunotherapy with IL-2 or interferon-α promotes development of depressive symptoms that are reduced by antidepressive agents. Furthermore, as mentioned above, cytokines may elicit neuroendocrine and neurotransmitter changes centrally that are the characteristics also for depressive disorders.[63]

An additional mechanism of how peripheral inflammation may signal to CNS was suggested by the findings that cytokines can sensitize and/or stimulate vagal and spinal afferent neurons and thus contribute to a rapid propagation of immune signals.[53] On the other hand, the cytokine-stimulated vagal afferents could activate the vago-vagal anti-inflammatory reflex through the cholinergic vagal efferents, and the released acetylcholine via the α7nAChR on macrophages and other immune cells to inhibit inflammation within the gut.[39,41,42]

Gut–microbiota

Gut microbiome is an integral part of the gut–brain axis. It is becoming increasingly recognized that the presence of a healthy and diverse gut microbiota is important for the normal cognitive and emotional processing. It was known that altered emotional state, depression and chronic stress can change the composition of gut microbiome. However, it is becoming evident that the interaction is bidirectional, and gut microbiome can alter neuropsychological functions (see Ref. 64).

IBD is caused by a combination of genetic factors, immune dysregulations, barrier dysfunction, and change in microbial flora. Under normal condition, the intestinal barrier prevents the invasion of microbes and toxins. Mucosal permeability is regulated by several factors such as microbiota composition, diet, infection, drugs, toxins, decreased internal perfusion, stress, depression, etc. The recognition that differential microbiome composition can be manifested in alterations of behavior and cognition, has significantly contributed to the establishment of a concept, to extend the well-accepted gut–brain axis to the microbiota–gut–brain axis.[53,65] In supporting this new concept, a recent detailed experimental analysis indicates that the gut microbiota regulates the development and function of the brain, and that disturbances of the microbial community may contribute to the development of neuropsychiatric diseases.[66] Information of the microbiota–gut–brain communication axis can be forwarded from the gut to the brain by the vagal and spinal afferents, immune mediators, gut hormone- and gut microbiota-derived molecules (see Refs. 53 and 67).

Microbial factors, such as polysaccharide A derived from *Bacteroides fragilis* or components of *Lactobacillus rhamnosus* (JB-1), can stimulate the vagal afferent neurons demonstrated by voltage recordings from intestinal primary afferent neurons.[68] In addition, a recent paper reviewed the role of microbial endocrinology in the microbiome–gut–brain axis. The microbiome is able to produce a variety of neuroactive substances, such as catecholamines, histamine, and other compounds, that binding to their receptors can influence the host neurophysiology and neurotransmission in the GI tract. On the other hand, following absorption these substances can enter into the systemic circulation where they can induce receptor-mediated actions. Toxins produced by intestinal pathogenic microorganisms and the focal inflammation induced by immune responses developed against these pathogens, can increase gut permeability (see Ref. 69). The non-specific factors such as lipopolysaccharide (LPS), can influence the CNS directly by activating toll-like receptor 4 (TLR4) on microglial cells causing the release of inflammatory cytokines by them within the CNS, or indirectly by inducing release of inflammatory cytokines from the GI tract.[70]

Summary and Conclusion

The CNS communicates with the GI tract through the so-called brain–gut axis and has a significant impact on GI physiology and pathophysiology. Brain–gut axis is a bidirectional communication network, and through this gut–brain axis, information from the gut may modify the brain function and behavior. This bidirectional communication system includes the CNS (both brain and spinal cord), the autonomic nervous system, the enteric nervous system and the HPA axis. The autonomic system involves vagal and spinal afferent neurons which play an important role to convey the information from the GI tract to the CNS, and the efferent neurons from CNS to the GI system. The HPA axis has a fundamental role to coordinate the adaptive responses of the organism to different stress stimuli.[71]

The brain–gut axis has been implicated in the pathogenesis of several GI disorders. Increasing evidence suggests that mental diseases (e.g. schizophrenia, anxiety, depression) play a role in the development of both gastric and intestinal mucosal lesions and inflammation (e.g. IBD). Activation of HPA axis by different stressors may also influence several functions of GI tract. It could contribute to the development of gastric mucosal erosion, ulceration and activation of IBD through the releases of CRF, ACTH, glucocorticoids and other hormones and mediators.

In recent years, convincing evidence has accumulated from both human and animal studies suggesting that inflammatory processes in the gut may trigger central changes and alter brain function. Comorbidity of psychological/psychiatric disorders and IBD influence the course of the each other when they coexist. Moreover, it is becoming increasingly recognized that the presence of a healthy and diverse gut microbiota is important for the normal cognitive and emotional processing.[64] Therefore, it is conceivable that the well-accepted gut–brain axis concept is now extended to the new phenomenon of microbiota–gut–brain axis.[53,65]

There are multiple mechanisms involved in the pathogenetic role of CNS in gastric mucosal injury and intestinal inflammatory diseases. Vice versa, also diverse effects have been suggested that CNS alterations may be elicited by GI inflammatory processes. For example, impaired cholinergic function, that is a characteristic for mental depression, may play a causal role in gut inflammation, since activation of vagal nerve results in selective suppression of pro-inflammatory cytokine secretion from the macrophages via the α7nAChR receptor.[39,41] Stress-induced alterations in IBD may be mediated by activation of HPA axis as well as by disruption of mucosal tight junctions, which results in enhancement of mucosal permeability, facilitation of microbial translocation into the intestinal wall, and development of immune response and inflammation.[50]

Moreover, different cytokines (e.g. IL-1β, IL-6, and TNF-α) having a role in the pathogenic mechanism of IBD, directly or indirectly through the formation of PGE_2 promote additional synthesis of cytokines (e.g. IL-1, IL-6, and TNF-α) in the brain. These cytokines modify the neurotransmission in the brain resulting in behavior disorders, cognitive changes, and affective disorders (see Refs. 61 and 62). In addition, the microbiota–gut–brain communication axis can forward the information from the gut to the brain by vagal and spinal afferents, immune mediators, gut hormones and gut microbiota-derived molecules.[53,67]

While well-tolerated, effective pharmacological therapies are available for the treatment of gastric mucosal injury, ulceration, IBD is still a major health problem, which can severely impair the quality of life and negatively affect mental health. On the other hand, the gut inflammation can be exacerbated by psychiatric disorders, adverse life events, negative stress stimulus, which, in turn, can aggravate disease course, prognosis and attenuate the response to the therapy.

Further studies are needed to obtain more information about microbial products, gut hormones, immune mediators and neuropeptides involved in neuro-immune interactions in intestinal inflammation. Mast cell mediators, cannabinoids, opioids, NPY, PYY, CRF, and other neuropeptides, TRP channels and their receptors are among the many factors which are the potential targets for the therapeutic intervention of IBD.[53]

References

1. DM Long, AS Leonard, SN Chou, LA French (1962) Hypothalamus and gastric ulceration I. Gastric effects of hypothalamic lesions. *Arch Neurol* **7**: 167–175.
2. H Cushing (1932) Peptic ulcers and the interbrain. *Surg Gynecol Obstet* **55**: 1–34.
3. H Selye (1943) Perforated peptic ulcer during air-raid. *Lancet* **20**: 252.
4. V Ozdemir, MM Jamal, K Osapay, MR Jadus, Z Sandor, M Hashemzadeh, S Szabo (2007) Cosegregation of gastrointestinal ulcers and schizophrenia in a large national inpatient discharge database: Revisiting the "brain–gut axis" hypothesis in ulcer pathogenesis. *J Investig Med* **55**: 315–320.
5. RD Goodwin, NJ Talley, M Hotopf, RA Cowles, S Galea, F Jacobi (2013) A link between physician-diagnosed ulcer and anxiety disorders among adults. *Ann Epidemiol* **23**: 189–192.
6. YC Hsu, CC Hsu, KH Chang, CY Lee, LW Chong, YC Wang, CH Kao (2015) Increased subsequent risk of peptic ulcer diseases in patients with bipolar disorders. *Medicine* (*Baltimore*) **94**: 1203.
7. HR Berthoud, WL Neuhuber (2000) Functional and chemical anatomy of the afferent vagal system. *Auton Neurosci* **85**: 1–17.
8. K Gyires (2004) Neuropeptides and gastric mucosal homeostasis. *Curr Top Med Chem* **4**: 63–73.
9. A Zagon (2001) Does the vagus nerve mediate the sixth sense? *Trends Neurosci* **24**: 671–673.
10. P Holzer (2003) Afferent signalling of gastric acid challenge. *J Physiol Pharmacol* **54 (Suppl 4)**: 43–53.
11. PJ Hornby (2001) Receptors and transmission in the brain–gut axis. II. Excitatory amino acid receptors in the brain–gut axis. *Am J Physiol Gastrointest Liver Physiol* **280**: 1055–1060.

12. M Palkovits (1999) Interconnections between the neuroendocrine hypothalamus and the central autonomic system. Geoffrey Harris Memorial Lecture, Kitakyushu, Japan, October 1998. *Front Neuroendocrinol* **20**: 270–295.
13. V Kormos, B Gaszner (2013) Role of neuropeptides in anxiety, stress, and depression: From animals to humans. *Neuropeptides* **47**: 401–419.
14. JV Esplugues, MD Barrachina, B Beltran, S Calatayud, BJ Whittle, S Moncada (1996) Inhibition of gastric acid secretion by stress: A protective reflex mediated by cerebral nitric oxide. *Proc Natl Acad Sci USA* **93**: 14839–14844.
15. LP Filaretova, AA Filaretov, GB Makara (1998) Corticosterone increase inhibits stress-induced gastric erosions in rats. *Am J Physiol* **274**: 1024–1030.
16. AA Monnig, JE Prittie (2011) A review of stress-related mucosal disease. *J Vet Emerg Crit Care (San Antonio)* **21**: 484–495.
17. Y Tache (2012) Brainstem neuropeptides and vagal protection of the gastric mucosal against injury: Role of prostaglandins, nitric oxide and calcitonin-gene related peptide in capsaicin afferents. *Curr Med Chem* **19**: 35–42.
18. K Gyires, J Nemeth, ZS Zadori (2013) Gastric mucosal protection and central nervous system. *Curr Pharm Des* **19**: 34–39.
19. K Gyires, ZS Zadori (2014) Brain neuropeptides in gastric mucosal protection. *Curr Opin Pharmacol* **19**: 24–30.
20. ZS Zadori, VE Toth, A Feher, K Philipp, J Nemeth, K Gyires (2014) Evidence for the gastric cytoprotective effect of centrally injected agmatine. *Brain Res Bull* **108**: 51–59.
21. AJ Kastin, W Pan (2008) Peptides and hormesis. *Crit Rev Toxicol* **38**: 629–631.
22. Y Tache, RL Jr. Stephens, T Ishikawa (1989) Central nervous system action of TRH to influence gastrointestinal function and ulceration. *Ann N Y Acad Sci* **553**: 269–285.
23. K Gyires (2012) Analysis of the effect of different neuropeptides in gastric mucosal defense initiated centrally. In: L Filaretova & K Takeuchi (eds.), *Cell/Tissue Injury and Cytoprotection/Organoprotection in the Gastrointestinal Tract: Mechanisms, Prevention and Treatment*, Vol. 30: pp. 161–169. Frontiers of Gastrointestinal Research, Basel, Krager.
24. MW Pawlik, R Obuchowicz, J Biernat, W Szczepanski, R Pajdo, S Kwiecien, T Brzozowski, SJ Konturek, WW Pawlik (2011) Effects of peripherally and centrally applied ghrelin in the pathogenesis of ischemia-reperfusion induced injury of the small intestine. *J Physiol Pharmacol* **62**: 429–439.
25. YM Zhang, EQ Wei, X Hu, M Xu, Y Shi, JF Zhang (2008) Administration of angiotensin II in the paraventricular nucleus protects gastric mucosa from ischemia-reperfusion injury. *Brain Res* **1212**: 25–34.

26. PM Smith, V Mollaret, AV Ferguson (1998) Leptin acts in the rat hypothalamic paraventricular nucleus to induce gastric mucosal damage. *Am J Physiol* **275**: 2081–2084.
27. R Schuligoi, M Jocic, A Heinemann, E Schoninkle, MA Pabst, P Holzer (1998) Gastric acid-evoked c-fos messenger RNA expression in rat brainstem is signaled by capsaicin-resistant vagal afferents. *Gastroenterology* **115**: 649–660.
28. P Holzer, T Wultsch, M Edelsbrunner, M Mitrovic, A Shahbazian, E Painsipp, E Bock, MA Pabst (2007) Increase in gastric acid-induced afferent input to the brainstem in mice with gastritis. *Neuroscience* **145**: 1108–1119.
29. P Holzer, M Danzer, R Schicho, C Samberger, E Painsipp, IT Lippe (2004) Vagal afferent input from the acid-challenged rat stomach to the brainstem: Enhancement by interleukin-1beta. *Neuroscience* **129**: 439–445.
30. YY Zhang, GH Cao, WX Zhu, XY Cui, HB Ai (2009) Comparative study of c-Fos expression in rat dorsal vagal complex and nucleus ambiguus induced by different durations of restraint water-immersion stress. *Chin J Physiol* **52**: 143–150.
31. JE Mawdsley, DS Rampton (2005) Psychological stress in IBD: New insights into pathogenic and therapeutic implications. *Gut* **54**: 1481–1491.
32. K Bradford, W Shih, EJ Videlock, AP Presson, BD Naliboff, EA Mayer, L Chang (2012) Association between early adverse life events and irritable bowel syndrome. *Clin Gastroenterol Hepatol* **10**: 385–390.
33. G Engelmann, D Erhard, M Petersen, P Parzer, AA Schlarb, F Resch, R Brunner, GF Hoffmann, H Lenhartz, A Richterich (2015) Health-related quality of life in adolescents with inflammatory bowel disease depends on disease activity and psychiatric comorbidity. *Child Psychiatry Hum Dev* **46**: 300–307.
34. BR Filipovic, BF Filipovic (2014) Psychiatric comorbidity in the treatment of patients with inflammatory bowel disease. *World J Gastroenterol* **20**: 3552–3563.
35. P Persoons, S Vermeire, K Demyttenaere, B Fischler, J Vandenberghe, L Van Oudenhove, M Pierik, T Hlavaty, G Van Assche, M Noman, P Rutgeerts (2005) The impact of major depressive disorder on the short- and long-term outcome of Crohn's disease treatment with infliximab. *Aliment Pharmacol Ther* **22**: 101–110.
36. LM Kurina, MJ Goldacre, D Yeates, LE Gill (2001) Depression and anxiety in people with inflammatory bowel disease. *J Epidemiol Community Health* **55**: 716–720.
37. JE Ghia, P Blennerhassett, Y Deng, EF Verdu, WI Khan, SM Collins (2009) Reactivation of inflammatory bowel disease in a mouse model of depression. *Gastroenterology* **136**: 2280–2288.

38. JE Ghia, AJ Park, P Blennerhassett, WI Khan, SM Collins (2011) Adoptive transfer of macrophage from mice with depression-like behavior enhances susceptibility to colitis. *Inflamm Bowel Dis* **17**: 1474–1489.
39. G Matteoli, GE Boeckxstaens (2013) The vagal innervation of the gut and immune homeostasis. *Gut* **62**: 1214–1222.
40. Z Nahas, C Teneback, JH Chae, Q Mu, C Molnar, Kozel FA, J Walker, B Anderson, J Koola, S Kose, M Lomarev, DE Bohning, MS George (2007) Serial vagus nerve stimulation functional MRI in treatment-resistant depression. *Neuropsychopharmacology* **32**: 1649–1660.
41. JE Ghia, P Blennerhassett, H Kumar-Ondiveeran, EF Verdu, SM Collins (2006) The vagus nerve: A tonic inhibitory influence associated with inflammatory bowel disease in a murine model. *Gastroenterology* **131**: 1122–1130.
42. JE Ghia, P Blennerhassett, SM Collins (2008) Impaired parasympathetic function increases susceptibility to inflammatory bowel disease in a mouse model of depression. *J Clin Invest* **118**: 2209–2218.
43. C Tuglu, SH Kara, O Caliyurt, E Vardar, E Abay (2003) Increased serum tumor necrosis factor-alpha levels and treatment response in major depressive disorder. *Psychopharmacology* (*Berl*) **170**: 429–433.
44. W Hauser, G Moser, P Klose, A Mikocka-Walus (2014) Psychosocial issues in evidence-based guidelines on inflammatory bowel diseases: A review. *World J Gastroenterol* **20**: 3663–3671.
45. BL Bonaz, CN Bernstein (2013) Brain-gut interactions in inflammatory bowel disease. *Gastroenterology* **144**: 36–49.
46. M Gue, C Bonbonne, J Fioramonti, J More, C Del Rio-Lacheze, C Comera, L Buéno (1997) Stress-induced enhancement of colitis in rats: CRF and arginine vasopressin are not involved. *Am J Physiol* **272**: 84–91.
47. SM Collins, K McHugh, K Jacobson, I Khan, R Riddell, K Murase, HP Weingarten (1996) Previous inflammation alters the response of the rat colon to stress. *Gastroenterology* **111**: 1509–1515.
48. BS Qiu, BA Vallance, PA Blennerhassett, SM Collins (1995) The role of CD4+ lymphocytes in the susceptibility of mice to stress-induced reactivation of experimental colitis. *Nat Med* **5**: 1178–1182.
49. RH Straub, FS Dhabhar, JW Bijlsma, M Cutolo (2005) How psychological stress via hormones and nerve fibers may exacerbate rheumatoid arthritis. *Arthritis Rheum* **52**: 16–26.
50. B Brzozowski, A Mazur-Bialy, R Pajdo, S Kwiecien, J Bilski, M Zwolinska-Wcislo, T Mach, T Brzozowski (2016) Mechanisms by which stress affects the experimental and clinical inflammatory bowel disease (IBD). Role of brain–gut axis. *Curr Neuropharmacol.*

51. C Chen, DR Brown, Y Xie, BT Green, M Lyte (2003) Catecholamines modulate Escherichia coli O157:H7 adherence to murine cecal mucosa. *Shock* **20**: 183–188.
52. JD Galley, MC Nelson, Z Yu, SE Dowd, J Walter, PS Kumar, M Lyte, MT Bailey (2014) Exposure to a social stressor disrupts the community structure of the colonic mucosa-associated microbiota. *BMC Microbiol* **14**: 189.
53. P Holzer, AM Hassan, P Jain, F Reichmann, A Farzi (2015) Neuroimmune pharmacological approaches. *Curr Opin Pharmacol* **25**: 13–22.
54. F Reichmann, AM Hassan, A Farzi, P Jain, R Schuligoi, P Holzer (2015) Dextran sulfate sodium-induced colitis alters stress-associated behaviour and neuropeptide gene expression in the amygdala-hippocampus network of mice. *Sci Rep* **5**: 9970.
55. CB Saper, AA Romanovsky, TE Scammell (2012) Neural circuitry engaged by prostaglandins during the sickness syndrome. *Nat Neurosci* **15**: 1088–1095.
56. KD Nyuyki, QJ Pittman (2015) Toward a better understanding of the central consequences of intestinal inflammation. *Ann N Y Acad Sci* **1351**: 149–154.
57. S Nikolaus, J Bauditz, P Gionchetti, C Witt, H Lochs, S Schreiber (1998) Increased secretion of pro-inflammatory cytokines by circulating polymorphonuclear neutrophils and regulation by interleukin 10 during intestinal inflammation. *Gut* **42**: 470–476.
58. WA Banks, MA Erickson (2010) The blood–brain barrier and immune function and dysfunction. *Neurobiol Dis* **37**: 26–32.
59. JC Schiltz, PE Sawchenko (2002) Distinct brain vascular cell types manifest inducible cyclooxygenase expression as a function of the strength and nature of immune insults. *J Neurosci* **22**: 5606–5618.
60. F Sallusto, D Impellizzieri, C Basso, A Laroni, A Uccelli, A Lanzavecchia, B Engelhardt (2012) T-cell trafficking in the central nervous system. *Immunol Rev* **248**: 216–227.
61. R Dantzer (2009) Cytokine, sickness behavior, and depression. *Immunol Allergy Clin North Am* **29**: 247–264.
62. SB Beynon, FR Walker (2012) Microglial activation in the injured and healthy brain: What are we really talking about? Practical and theoretical issues associated with the measurement of changes in microglial morphology. *Neuroscience* **225**: 162–171.
63. H Anisman, Z Merali, MO Poulter, S Hayley (2005) Cytokines as a precipitant of depressive illness: Animal and human studies. *Curr Pharm Des* **11**: 963–972.
64. SS Yarandi, DA Peterson, GJ Treisman, TH Moran, PJ Pasricha (2016) Modulatory effects of gut microbiota on the central nervous system: How gut could play a role in neuropsychiatric health and diseases. *J Neurogastroenterol Motil* **22**: 201–212.

65. RM Stilling, TG Dinan, JF Cryan (2014) Microbial genes, brain & behaviour — epigenetic regulation of the gut–brain axis. *Genes Brain Behav* **13**: 69–86.
66. G De Palma, P Blennerhassett, J Lu, Y Deng, AJ Park, W Green, E Denou, MA Silva, A Santacruz, Y Sanz, MG Surette, EF Verdu, SM Collins (2015) Microbiota and host determinants of behavioural phenotype in maternally separated mice. *Nat Commun* **6**: 7735.
67. P Holzer, A Farzi (2014) Neuropeptides and the microbiota–gut–brain axis. *Adv Exp Med Biol* **817**: 195–219.
68. YK Mao, DL Kasper, B Wang, P Forsythe, J Bienenstock, WA Kunze (2013) Bacteroides fragilis polysaccharide A is necessary and sufficient for acute activation of intestinal sensory neurons. *Nat Commun* **4**: 1465.
69. M Lyte (2013) Microbial endocrinology in the microbiome–gut–brain axis: How bacterial production and utilization of neurochemicals influence behavior. *PLoS Pathog* **9**: 1003726.
70. KA Kim, W Gu, IA Lee, EH Joh, DH Kim (2012) High fat diet-induced gut microbiota exacerbates inflammation and obesity in mice via the TLR4 signaling pathway. *PLoS One* **7**: 47713.
71. M Carabotti, A Scirocco, MA Maselli, C Severi (2015) The gut–brain axis: Interactions between enteric microbiota, central and enteric nervous systems. *Ann Gastroenterol* **28**: 203–209.

Chapter 2

Nesfatin-1: The Novel Appetite Peptide with Therapeutic Efficacy to Prevent Acute Hemorrhagic Gastric Lesions and Accelerate Gastric Ulcer Healing

Aleksandra Szlachcic, Jolanta Majka, and Tomasz Brzozowski

Abstract

The recent identification of nucleobindin2 (NUCB2)/nesfatin-1 in the rat hypothalamus sheds more light to the understanding of control of food intake and energy expenditure. Interestingly, nesfatin-1 immunoreactivity co-localized in the same oxyntic endocrine X/A-like cells with another important peptide ghrelin, which has been found to exert protective activity in the stomach. Further studies revealed the NUBC2/nesfatin expression to the periphery with the several-fold higher mRNA expression in gastric mucosa than in the brain suggesting that this hormone is an important component of the brain–gut axis consisting of bidirectional communication between the central and the enteric nervous systems, linking the brain with peripheral gastrointestinal functions. This includes protection against various irritants resulting from the activation of local protective mechanisms that also accelerate healing processes. In this review, we focused on the possible involvement of nesfatin-1 in the mechanism of gastric integrity, gastroprotection, and ulcer healing. These protective and ulcer-healing actions of nesfatin-1 involve an increase in gastric microcirculation in cooperation with some protective factors, including endogenous prostaglandins, nitric oxide, and neuropeptides such as calcitonin gene-related peptide (CGRP) released from sensory afferent nerves and possibly acting via the activation of TRPV1 receptors. In addition, the crosstalk with the protective peptide ghrelin, the anti-inflammatory and anti-oxidizing activity of nesfatin-1 could contribute to the protective and ulcer-healing actions of this peptide in the stomach.

Introduction

Food intake is controlled by numerous peptides produced in cells located not only in various areas of the central nervous system (CNS), but also in peripheral tissues. Peptides controlling food intake interact with each other, and a mechanism of their action involves a direct effect on the hypothalamus and brain stem or an indirect effect on these centers through activation of vagal afferent nerves and neuropeptides released from their endings. The peptides known to trigger hunger are called orexigenic, but those responsible for feeling of satiety are named anorexigenic. Among anorexigenic factors is a hormone nesfatin-1, described for the first time by Oh-I *et al.* in 2006.

At the beginning of the 1990s, the nucleobindin or NEFA (DNA binding/EF-hand/acidic amino-acid-rich region), a peptide able to bind Ca^{2+} and DNA has been identified in human and mouse cells.[1,2] Following further research, the two types of nucleobindin: nucleobindin1 (NUCB1) and nucleobindin2 (NUCB2) have been discovered.[3] At its N-terminus, an NUCB2 molecule contains a signal peptide of 24 amino acids and a chain of 396 amino acids of a sequence responsible for this peptide's physiological significance and is well consistent in rodents and humans.[3,4] As a result of post-translational modifications of an NUCB2 molecule in the presence of prohormone convertase, (PC)-1/3, three compounds are formed: nesfatin-1 (1–82), nesfatin-2 (85–163), and nesfatin-3 (166–396).[5]

Within nesfatins, only nesfatin-1 exhibits biological activity, and its major physiological effect is to inhibit food intake as originally documented in rats after this peptide administration either peripherally or to cerebral ventricles.[4,6] The name of nesfatin-1 is an acronym of the phrase NUCB2-encoded satiety and fat influencing protein.[5] Nesfatin-1 is an 82 amino acid peptide whose molecular weight is 9.8 kDa. Furthermore, structural and functional analyses showed that only the mid segment of nesfatin-1 exerts biological activity.[6,7]

Originally, the mRNA expression for NUCB2 was exclusively identified by immunohistochemistry in groups of neurons in the hypothalamus and brain stem, including paraventricular nucleus (PVN), supraoptic nucleus, arcuate nucleus, lateral hypothalamic area, zone incerta, and nuclei of the solitary tract (NTS).[5] It is accepted that cells immunopositive for NUCB2/nesfatin-1 are also present in other areas of the hypothalamus, midbrain, and hindbrain, including dorsomedial hypothalamic nucleus, tuberal hypothalamic area, PVN, Edinger–Westphal nucleus, locus coeruleus, medullary raphe nuclei, and dorsal motor nucleus of the vagus nerve.[6,8–10] Furthermore, Stengel *et al.*[11] found neurons immunoreactive for nesfatin-1 in rat insular cortex, central amygdaloidal nucleus, ventrolateral medulla, and cerebellum, and the presence of nesfatin-1 immunoreactivity in sympathetic and parasympathetic preganglionic neurons of the spinal cord in thoracic, lumbar, and sacral sections.[11]

The analysis of nesfatin-1 immunoreactive content in neurons revealed that other neurotransmitters such as melanin-concentrating hormone (MCH), cocaine- and amphetamine-regulated transcript (CART), proopiomelanocortin (POMC), α-melanocyte-stimulating hormone (α-MSH), mammalian target of rapamycin (m-TOR), vasopressin, oxytocin, neuropeptide Y (NPY), somatostatin, growth hormone-releasing hormone (GHRH), thyrotrophic-releasing hormone (TRH), corticotropin-releasing factor (CRF), and neurotensin co-localize with this hormone,[6,8–10,12–14] Furthermore, in the neurons of nucleus Edinger–Westphal and medulla oblongata, nesfatin-1 co-localizes with acetylcholine and urocortin-1, and serotonin, respectively,[8,14] Since nesfatin-1 has been solely identified in cytoplasm of cerebral neuronal bodies and is absent in varices and axonal endings, it probably acts as an intracellular transmitter.[6,8,11,12] However, the neural bodies also exert secretory properties,[15,16] suggesting that nesfatin-1 acts as an extracellular transmitter. These suspicions have been confirmed by recent studies in rats, in which nesfatin-1 has been found in secretory granules of PVN neurons.[12]

Expression of NUCB2/nesfatin-1 in peripheral tissues

Majority of peptides participating in food intake control and detected in cerebral cells are also of peripheral origin, and their main source is in the gastrointestinal tract. This also applies to nesfatin-1 which can be released from cells other than cerebral neurons.

Molecular analyses including the determination of nesfatin-1 mRNA and protein by reverse transcription polymerase chain reaction (RT-PCR) and Western blotting, respectively, have shown that both NUCB2 mRNA and protein were highly expressed in the pancreas, stomach, and duodenum with a lower expression in the esophagus, liver, small intestine, and colon.[17] Furthermore, the expression of NUCB2 mRNA in gastric parietal cells is 20 times higher than that in cerebral neurons.[18] In rat stomachs, the presence of NUCB2/nesfatin-1 is found mainly in X/A-like endocrine cells. Interestingly, another orexigenic peptide ghrelin, involved in the control of food intake and appetite, has been identified in the same location as nesfatin-1. However, nesfatin-1 immunopositive cells were found in other subpopulations of cellular vesicles compared with ghrelin.[18]

Similarly, the presence of nesfatin-1 in human and rodent pancreas is considerably limited to β-pancreatic cells, but the location of this hormone seems to be unrelated to insulin.[19,20] This is supported by functional observation that levels of nesfatin-1 in normal rat islets β-cells showed only a slight increase following glucose challenge. This increase was notably smaller than that observed for insulin, which suggested that the release of nesfatin-1 into blood coincided with insulin release.[20] Nakata *et al.* have shown that nesfatin-1 enhanced glucose-induced insulin secretion by promoting Ca^{2+} influx through L-type channels independently of protein kinase A (PKA) and phospholipase A2 (PLA2).[21] But this effect was observed only in the presence of high concentration of glucose *in vitro.* This suggests an insulin tropic action of nesfatin-1.[21] Furthermore, the NUCB2 gene expression decreased in the pancreatic islets of patients with type 2 diabetes mellitus, but it has been enhanced under glucolipotoxic conditions, suggesting that nesfatin-1 may contribute to the regulation of β-cell secretion.[17]

The co-occurrence of nesfatin-1, ghrelin, or insulin in the major abdominal organs such as stomach and pancreas suggests that these peptides may cooperate on control of food intake and maintaining a glucose homeostasis. Furthermore, nesfatin-1 has been shown to pass the blood–brain barrier in both directions with lack of full saturation of this transport, thus indicating that nesfatin-1 originating from peripheral tissues also can participate in processes of food intake control.[22,23]

Ramanjaneya *et al.* confirmed that the expression and distribution of NUCB2 mRNA and nesfatin-1 protein were site-specific in murine and human adipose tissues and also showed that the expression of NUCB2 is significantly higher in subcutaneous adipose tissue than in visceral tissue.[24] It was also observed that nesfatin-1 secretion into conditioned media dramatically increased throughout the differentiation of preadipocytes 3T3-L1 in mature adipocytes suggesting that NUCB2 and nesfatin-1 may play an important role in adipocytes development and differentiation. Interestingly, the expression of other biologically active adipokines such as leptin, adiponectin, and apelin had increased during the process of differentiation and maturation of adipocytes implying that the increased expression of nesfatin-1 may result from maturation rather than being a cause of this process.[24,25]

The gastrointestinal tract, adipose tissue, and pancreas are not the only peripheral tissues in which the presence of NUCB2 and nesfatin-1 was detected. Also, Stengel *et al.* revealed the NUCB2 expression in the rat heart and found that it is 10-fold higher than that detected in extracts from the rat gastric mucosa.[18] Angelone *et al.* have indicated that nesfatin-1 directly affected heart myocardial performance, possibly involving particular guanylate cyclase (pGC)-linked natriuretic peptide receptor A (NPR-A), the pGC/PKG pathway, and extracellular signal-regulated kinases 1/2 (ERK 1/2).[26] This peptide protected the heart muscle against ischemia/reperfusion injury. Because of this protective action, they proposed that nesfatin-1 could be considered as neuroendocrine modulator and a hormone capable of preserving the cardiac function. Interestingly, the described hypertensive effect of nesfatin-1 was mediated by sympathetic nerves activity possibly also involving melanocortin-3/4 receptors.[27] Nesfatin-1 affected the isolated mesenteric artery in rats interfering with sodium nitroprusside-induced smooth muscle relaxation through its inhibitory effect of cyclic guanosine monophosphate (cGMP).[27] These results clearly suggest that nesfatin-1 plays an important role in the control and regulation of central and peripheral blood pressure.

In addition, the presence of NUCB2/nesfatin-1 protein in interstitial mature Leydig cells of rat, mouse, and human testes and the evidence that nesfatin-1 can influence the hypothalamic–pituitary–ovarian axis of goldfish suggest that nesfatin-1 could be implicated in the control of reproductive system.[28–30]

The role of nesfatin-1 in the regulation of food intake

The first described biological action of NUCB2/nesfatin-1 was the reduction of dark-phase food intake by this hormone. This effect of nesfatin-1 appeared within 1–6 hours upon its administration.[5] Administering nesfatin-1 in an analogous manner directly to PVN caused its first effects to appear within first 3 hours of it being administered, while its administration to the IV cerebral ventricle or the cisterna magna resulted in the immediate and prolonged inhibition of food intake during the night.[12,22] Diversified kinetics of the nesfatin-1 effect indicates different areas of nesfatin-1 action in the forebrain and the hindbrain.

Based on accumulated evidence, it is concluded that nesfatin-1 administered at small (picomolar) doses into the cerebrospinal fluid, similarly as it's administered into cerebral ventricles, the cisterna magna and PVN, causes the prolonged inhibition of food intake in the night time in rats with free access to food and to a smaller extent reduces food intake in rodents fasting during the night time. Nesfatin-1 administered to the III cerebral ventricle not only inhibits food intake but also causes body weight loss in rats, indicating its possible participation in processes concerning energy expenditure.[5]

As NUCB2/nesfatin-1 in cells are accompanied by other peptides engaged in food intake control, numerous studies were carried out aiming at establishing whether there is any cooperation between nesfatin-1 and those substances. On the basis of obtained results, numerous interactions were described, explaining the anorexigenic effect of nesfatin-1.

In *in vitro* studies, it was found out that nesfatin-1 directly, through the autocrine or intracrine pathway, inhibits neurons of the hypothalamic arcuate nucleus containing orexigenic NPY.[7] Furthermore, neurons of the hypothalamic arcuate nucleus immunopositive for phosphor-mTOR (pm-TOR) are also immunopositive for nesfatin-1. It is possible that nesfatin-1 participates in the reduction of the NPY mRNA expression through pm-TOR.[13,27] Contrary to that data it was found out that nesfatin-1 action is independent of the central effect of leptin. Moreover, leptin administered to cerebral ventricles does not affect the nesfatin-1-induced inhibition of food intake during the night.[5]

Another peptide cooperating with nesfatin-1 in food intake control is oxytocin which, when administered to the III cerebral ventricle, inhibits food intake through the leptin-independent path.[12] Nesfatin-1 administered to cerebral ventricles stimulates oxytocin-positive neurons in the PVN and as indicated in *in vitro* studies it stimulates its secretion.[12] Moreover, it was found that oxytocinergic pathways between the PVN and the nucleus of the solitary tract are involved in the anorexigenic effect of nesfatin-1.[12] Furthermore, it was discovered that by administering antagonists of oxytocin receptors to the III ventricle, the inhibiting effect of nesfatin-1 on food intake was abolished.[12]

Nesfatin-1 exerts its anorexigenic effect possibly through the path also related to CRF_2 receptors, and this is proved by similarities between results of its action and those of urocortin, the CRF_2 receptor antagonist.[7,27] Probably an interaction between nesfatin-1 and CRF_2 receptors concerns not only food intake control but also may occur during the body's reaction to stress. It was shown in rats that stress agents, such as infection or surgery, activated neurons immunopositive for nesfatin-1. In the case of a surgery, neurons located in the anterior parvicellular part of PVN, Edinger–Westphal nucleus, nuclei of catecholaminergic and serotoninergic paths were stimulated,[31] while infections stimulated neurons of the supraoptic nucleus, PVN, the arcuate nucleus, and NTS.[32] Similarly, when stress is of emotional character, the activity of immunopositive neurons increases in various areas of the hypothalamus and the hindbrain.[14,33] Nesfatin-1, administered intraventrically (i.c.) in doses larger than those inhibiting food intake in the night, influences emotional behaviors related to reaction to fear.[34] Furthermore, neurons immunoreactive for nesfatin-1 were found in the amygdales, which are responsible for behaviors caused by fear and anger, and that may suggest nesfatin-1 participation in those reactions.[11,35] Nesfatin-1 connection to cerebral structures involved in the body's reaction to stress agents of various origins may indicate its participation in stress-induced feeding disorders.

The NUCB2/nesfatin-1 expression in the hypothalamus shows diversification depending on a current metabolic status and that seems to confirm their physiological significance in food intake control. The expression of NUCB2 mRNA in the PVN decreases after 24 hours of fasting, similarly as in the supraoptic nucleus. It returns to normal after food intake.[5,10] A similar situation is observed for the activity of neurons immunopositive for nesfatin-1, which increases after feeding preceded by 24 hours of fasting.[22] This data indicates a relationship between the activity of these neurons and the satiation status, where a change in the NUCB2/nesfatin-1 expression depending on metabolic conditions is specific for the hypothalamus, but not for the Edinger–Westphal nucleus.[36] Moreover, it was demonstrated that the NUCB2 mRNA expression increased under the influence of anorexigenic compounds such as antagonists to $5\text{-HT}_{1B/2C}$ or α-MSH serotonin receptors.[5,37] The intraperitoneal administration of cholecystokinin (CCK) activates cells immunopositive for nesfatin-1 in the PVN and in the nucleus of the solitary tract, and that indicates the participation of nesfatin-1 of central origin in triggering the feeling of satiation caused by intestinal peptides.[22]

The emerging role of nesfatin-1 in the mechanism of gastric mucosal integrity and gastroprotection against damage induced by noxious agents

The gastric mucosa is a region of active proliferation of cell divisions that mainly occurs in the neck region of fundic glands. This contributes to the mechanism of maintenance of gastric mucosal integrity and enables a proper restitution and regeneration of gastric mucosa compromised by gastric irritants and damaging agents. Moreover, this process strengthens the gastric mucosa and helps this mucosa to withstand highly concentrated hydrochloric acid in the stomach without major damage to its wall.[38] Numerous factors contribute to protection of the gastric mucosa against damage and allowing for fast restitution and mucosal regeneration, including prostaglandins (PG) and growth factors, that is, epidermal growth factor (EGF), transforming growth factor-α (TGF-α), polyamines (spermine, putrescine), the vasoactive neuropeptides released from afferent sensory nerve endings such as CGRP, nitric oxide (NO) released from the vascular endothelial, and epithelial cells of the gut and afferent sensory nerve endings, including CCK and gastrin.[38–40] These factors have a direct protective effect by activating processes necessary to maintain the integrity of the gastric mucosa, mediating in a gastroprotective effect of other mechanisms, as well as cooperating in that area.

The anatomic distribution of cells in which the presence of NUCB2/nesfatin-1 was found, as well as the presence of other neurotransmitters in these cells, indicates that nesfatin-1 is not just another neuropeptide controlling food intake. Nesfatin-1 takes part in mechanisms related to urge and emotional and neuroendocrine reactions as well as those responsible for controlling internal organs' functions. The data obtained in experimental studies suggested that peptides regulating food intake including ghrelin, orexin A (OXA), and also newly discovered nesfatin-1, similar to leptin and PYY, participate in other physiological mechanisms. Namely, this hormonal participation includes processes related to the control of the secretory and motor activity of the gastrointestinal tract. As the research results indicate, they probably also participate in the protection of the gastric mucosa against damaging factors, the cell proliferation, and gastric tissue regeneration. Their gastroprotective activity seems to depend upon cooperation with other factors responsible for the protection of the gastric mucosa including sensory afferent fibers, PG synthesis pathway, and NO.

In experimental studies, it was found that the group of factors with protective and regenerating effects on the gastric mucosa needs to be expanded with peptides regulating food intake. These hormones were shown to act at the central level because they seem to be effective not only after systemic administration but also after single intracerebroventricular (i.c.v.) injection. For instance, the i.c.v. administration of leptin, an anorexigenic peptide produced by adipocytes and gastric epithelial cells, afforded protection against 75% ethanol-induced gastric lesions and those resulting from gastric ischemia followed by reperfusion.[41,42] It was documented that leptin's mimics gastroprotective effects of CCK accompanied by an increase in gastric blood flow (GBF). Therefore, leptin is possibly one of the factors enabling CCK to maintain the integrity of the gastric mucosa, especially, as CCK, similar to food, increases the plasma leptin levels.[43] Furthermore, the leptin's protective effect on the gastric mucosa can be mediated by NO production and the release of neuropeptide CGRP from afferent sensory nerve endings.[44] Previous studies revealed that leptin stimulates the proliferation of the gastric mucosa cells, which may confirm its contribution to gastroprotection and ulcer healing.[45] Also, peptide YY (PYY), belonging to appetite-inhibiting peptides, similar to leptin, participates in the regulation of the physiological function of the gastrointestinal tract. PYY found in numerous hormone-secreting cells in the intestine and pancreas, and in neurons of the gastrointestinal tract, when administered intravenously, has been shown to inhibit gastric acid secretion and gastric emptying in humans and to reduce pancreatic secretion in rats and dogs.[46,47] These findings support the notion that PYY is a physiological factor responsible for the inhibition of motility of the upper gastrointestinal tract after the meal has moved to its distal part.[47] Moreover, it was shown that the intravascular administration of PYY at doses corresponding to the increase in the serum PYY levels after the meal exhibits gastroprotective action against gastric mucosa injury induced by concentrated ethanol. This gastroprotective effect of PYY could be mediated by the central activation of the vagus nerves by this peptide, resulting in a peripheral release of vasoactive mediators CGRP and NO. However, the bilateral vagotomy failed to affect the gastroprotective effect of intravenously administered PYY, indicating that signals transmitted by vagal afferent and efferent fibers do not play a major role in this protection.[47]

We reported that ghrelin, OXA, and obestatin dose-dependently decrease the area of chronic gastric ulcers produced by the serosal application of acetic acid. Moreover, these peptides increased the blood flow at the margin of ulcers compared with the flow in contralateral non-ulcerated gastric mucosa. Both the decrease in ulcer size and the rise in GBF at the ulcer margin were significantly inhibited by indomethacin (a non-selective inhibitor of cyclooxygenase-1 (COX-1) and cyclooxygenase-2 (COX-2) activity) and rofecoxib (a selective COX-2 inhibitor) and, although to a lesser extent, by the SC-560 (a selective inhibitor of COX-1). The functional ablation of sensory nerves by capsaicin or inhibition of TRPV1 receptors by capsazepine also reduced the ulcer healing-activity of ghrelin, OXA, and obestatin. Furthermore, in animals with gastric ulcers treated with ghrelin or OXA, the gene expression of pro-inflammatory cytokines IL-1β and TNF-α was significantly reduced while the expression of mRNA for ghrelin, OXA, and COX-2 was significantly increased. These results indicate that ghrelin, OXA, and obestatin can accelerate ulcer healing and this effect is mediated by the mechanism involving endogenous PGs, neuropeptides released from sensory afferent fibers as well as inhibition of pro-inflammatory cytokines.[48]

Whether nesfatin-1 participates in the protection and repair processes of gastric mucosa remains to be studied, but so far the protective efficacy of nesfatin-1 has been documented in an experimental model of stress-induced gastric lesions by 3.5 hours of rats' immobilization and restraint in cold water.[37,49] Stress induced at these experimental conditions resulted in the formation of gastric erosions and microbleedings in oxyntic gastric mucosa followed by a significant fall in the GBF. The intraperitoneal administration of nesfatin-1 administered in graded doses ranging from 5 µg/kg to 40 µg/kg prior to the onset of stress, dose-dependently reduced gastric lesions. This effect was accompanied by the significant increase in the GBF as compared to respective values of mean number lesions and GBF observed in vehicle (saline, control)-pretreated rats. Moreover, the plasma level of nesfatin-1, which was not significantly affected in stressed animals pretreated with vehicle, showed the rise in those pretreated with nesfatin-1 dependent on the dose of the peptide being administered. The most pronounced protective and blood flow increasing effects were observed with nesfatin-1 applied at a dose of 40 µg/kg. However, this peptide was effective in smaller dosages because the dose of nesfatin-1 which inhibited macroscopic lesions induced by water restraint stress (WRS) by 50% averaged 20 µg/kg. This study documented that the number of bleeding stress-induced gastric erosions was significantly limited and the protective effect of nesfatin-1 was accompanied by an increase in the plasma level of that peptide (Figure 1).

Interestingly, nesfatin-1 was effective after it was administered into the right cerebral ventricle. This protective effect was accompanied, similar to the case of the intraperitoneal administration of nesfatin-1, by an increase in gastric mucosal blood flow and plasma NUCB2/nesfatin-1 concentrations (Figure 1). As mentioned above, the intraperitoneal administration of nesfatin-1 at a dose of 20 µg/kg was applied before exposure to stress resulted in gastroprotection as manifested by a significant decrease in the number of gastric lesions and an increase in gastric mucosal blood flow versus animals receiving vehicle and subsequently compromised by WRS. When rats exposed to stress were administered with non-selective or selective COX-1 and COX-2 inhibitors, the gastric lesions were exacerbated and the fall in blood flow was much greater than in those exposed only to the stress. The most severe changes in the number of WRS damages was evoked by indomethacin, the non-selective COX-1 and COX-2 inhibitor. In rats with a blocked activity of COX-1 and COX-2 enzymes resulting in a suppression of the endogenous prostaglandin E_2 (PGE_2) biosynthetic pathway, the nesfatin-1-induced protection and the increase in the GBF were significantly attenuated as compared with the number of gastric lesions and alterations in blood flow observed in animals receiving only nesfatin-1. On the other hand,

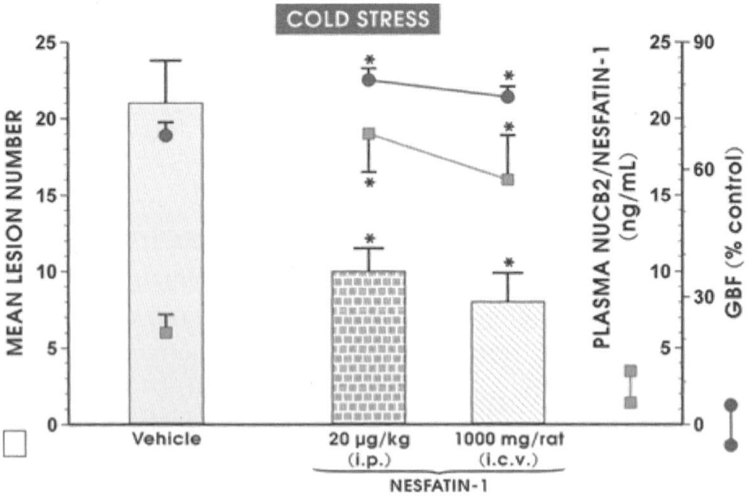

Figure 1. The efficacy of nesfatin-1 to protect the gastric mucosal lesions induced by cold stress in rats. The mean number of gastric lesions and the accompanying changes in the gastric blood flow (GBF) and plasma NUCB2/nesfatin-1 levels in rats pretreated with or without vehicle (saline) or nesfatin-1 administered either intraperitoneally (i.p.) in a dose of 20 µg/kg or centrally (i.c.v.) in a dose of 1000 ng/rat and 30 min later these animals were exposed to cold water immersion stress for 3.5 hours. Results are mean ±SEM of 6–8 rats. Asterisks indicate significant changes ($P < 0.05$) as compared to the value recorded in vehicle-saline-pretreated animals.

SC-560, a selective COX-1 inhibitor, and rofecoxib, a selective COX-2 inhibitor, also reversed the protective effect of nesfatin-1 against stress ulcerogenesis. This suggests that endogenous PG could mediate both gastroprotection and the accompanying hyperemia induced by nesfatin-1. This notion is supported by the observation that the protective function of nesfatin-1 at a "gastroprotective" dose of 20 µg/kg (i.p.) was restored when the exogenous PGE_2 at a dose of 5 µg/kg was administered in combination with nesfatin-1 in the presence of COX-1 and COX-2 inhibitors in animals compromised by stress. This evidence supports a conclusion that endogenous PG derived from COX-1 and COX-2 activity plays an important role in the mechanism of gastroprotection induced by nesfatin-1. Since endogenous PGs cooperate with NO in the mechanism of gastric integrity and cytoprotection, it was of interest to determine the involvement of NO in the gastroprotective activity of nesfatin-1. The NO-synthase (NOS) blocker, NG-nitro-L-arginine (L-NNA), augmented the damage caused by stress and further decreased the GBF as compared to vehicle-treated control rats exposed to WRS. Nesfatin-1 administered at a dose of 20 μg/kg, intraperitoneally, reduced not only the consequences of the damaging effect of the stress itself but also the consequences of the NOS inhibition by L-NNA preceding exposure to stress. L-Arginine, the substrate for NOS co-administered with L-NNA in the presence of nesfatin-1, completely reversed the increase in the lesion index and the decline in the GBF observed in rats compromised by stress. An analysis of NO levels in gastric juice in the above examination groups showed them to be the highest in the group that received nesfatin-1 and L-arginine before exposure to stress, and the lowest values in those animals in which exposure to stress was combined with the administration of L-NNA. At the molecular level, the mRNA expression for a constitutive NOS (cNOS) and the rise in the inducible isoform of NOS (iNOS) were observed in gastric mucosa following exposure to stress. Pretreatment with nesfatin-1 not only evidently enhanced the mRNA expression for cNOS but also produced a visible drop in the mRNA expression for iNOS. These data suggest that nesfatin-1, a peptide controlling food intake, participates in the mechanism of gastroprotection against gastric mucosal lesions caused by stress. Nesfatin-1 was also effective when administered to the right cerebral ventricle because its central administration led to the rise in the gastric mucosal blood flow and reduced the severity of damage in a dose-dependent fashion.

Previous studies revealed that peptides controlling food intake, such as leptin, ghrelin, orexin-A, or obestatin, can contribute to the mechanism ensuring the maintenance of gastric mucosa integrity. This protective action of food-intake-controlling peptides could be attributed to the vasoactive mediators, including endogenous PG, NO as well as neuropeptide CGRP released from afferent sensory nerve endings. This notion is supported by the fact that the pretreatment with nesfatin-1 together with selective or non-selective COX-1 and COX-2 inhibitors to animals exposed to the damaging effect of stress reduced gastric mucosal blood flow and intensified the damage in a dose-dependent fashion as compared to the control group in which only nesfatin-1 was used. This finding indicates that nesfatin-1 exerts protection against the damaging effect of stress through a common mechanism such as the activation of biosynthesis of endogenous PGs, similar to orexin-A, ghrelin, or other appetite-controlling peptides. However, arachidonic acid metabolites are not the sole factors through which nesfatin-1 attenuates the consequences of factors known to exhibit injurious action to the gastric mucosa. Another protective mechanism is NO because the administration of an NOS blocker not only aggravated the gastric lesions caused by stress but also reduced its protective action. When L-arginine, an NOS substrate, was additionally administered, the inhibitory effect of NOS blockers on nesfatin-1 induced protection and accompanying changes in luminal NO content and GBF were reversed. Moreover, an overexpression of cNOS mRNA and downregulation of iNOS mRNA were observed in the gastric mucosa when pretreated with nesfatin-1 before the exposure of animals to stress. This seems corroborative with the conclusion that endogenous PGs and NO play an important role in the mechanism of nesfatin-1-induced gastroprotection against stress ulcerogenesis.[50]

Thus, nesfatin-1 exhibits similar gastroprotective properties as ghrelin and OXA, both of which were shown to ameliorate the gastric mucosa damage caused by various ulcerogenic agents, including 100% ethanol, ischemia with successive reperfusion, cold stress, or aspirin.[50,51] In all cases, the reduction in the area of gastric lesions was accompanied by the statistically significant increase in GBF. Moreover, the expression of ghrelin mRNA was increased in gastric mucosa pretreated with nesfatin-1, suggesting the possible crosstalk between nesfatin-1 and ghrelin in the mechanism of gastroprotection against stress-induced gastric lesions. The mRNA signal for ghrelin was increased by a stressor versus intact gastric mucosa, suggesting the self-defense mobilization of mucosal "protective" ghrelin in the pathogenesis of stress ulceration. Interestingly, this signal for ghrelin mRNA was further augmented by pretreatment with nesfatin-1, indicating the possible "reciprocal" interaction of these two peptides known for their protective action against various stressors (Figure 2).

The gastroprotective effect of these peptides may depend upon to the activation of sensory afferent fibers, the endogenous PG pathway, and NO (Figure 3). This assumption is based on the fact that the functional ablation of sensory nerves by capsaicin, the administration of COX-1 and COX-2 inhibitors, or NO-synthase blockade by L-NAME or L-NNA increased the susceptibility of the gastric mucosa to damage by ulcerogenic stimuli and reduced the mucosal blood flow, even when ghrelin and OXA were administered.[52] Furthermore, ghrelin exhibited a protective effect on the gastric

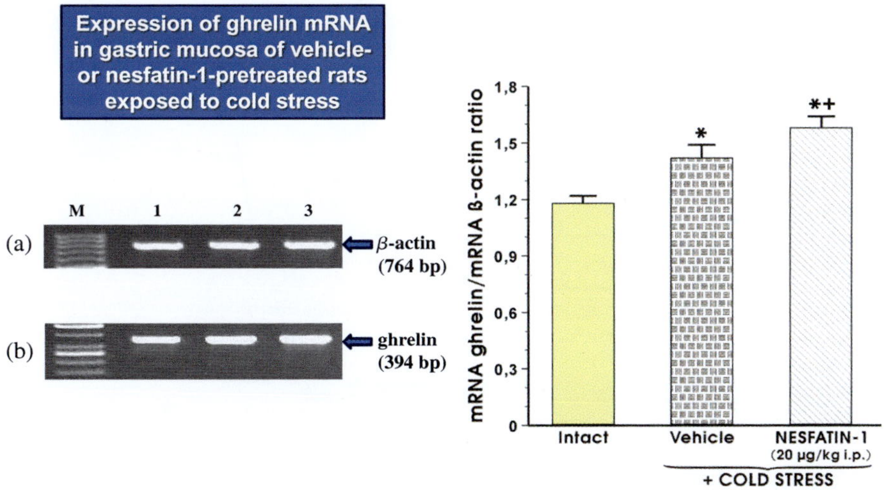

Figure 2. The crosstalk between two hormones regulating appetite nesfatin-1 and ghrelin in the mechanism of protection induced by exogenous nesfatin-1 against mucosal damage caused by cold stress. Determination of the ghrelin messenger RNA expression by RT-PCR (left panel, a and b) and the ratio of ghrelin mRNA over β-actin mRNA (right panel) in the intact gastric mucosa (lane 1) and in those pretreated i.p. with vehicle (saline) (lane 2) and nesfatin-1 (20 μg/kg i.p.) (lane 3) and exposed 30 min later to 3.5 hours of cold stress; M – DNA size marker. Mean ± SEM of three determinations in five rats per group. The asterisk indicates a significant change ($P < 0.05$) as compared with intact gastric mucosa. The asterisk and cross indicate a significant change ($P < 0.05$) as compared with vehicle.

mucosa after peripheral and central administration because when it was injected i.c.v., the damaged area of ethanol lesions was reduced in a dose-dependent manner.[53] One of the mediating agents of the ghrelin gastroprotective mechanism is probably NO, the source of which in this case remains unknown. NO is synthesized from L-arginine in neurons of the plexus wall of the visceral enteric nervous system, by the vascular endothelial cells and surface epithelial cells of the gastric mucosa.[53] Thus, it is not known whether ghrelin affords the protection of the gastric mucosa via the reflex or local mechanism, involving the mucosal blood flow, production of PG, and the enhancement of mucus and HCO_3^- secretion. Undoubtedly, the centrally administered ghrelin limits the damaging effects of stress with its effect related to the brain–gut axis, because sensory nerve deafferentation

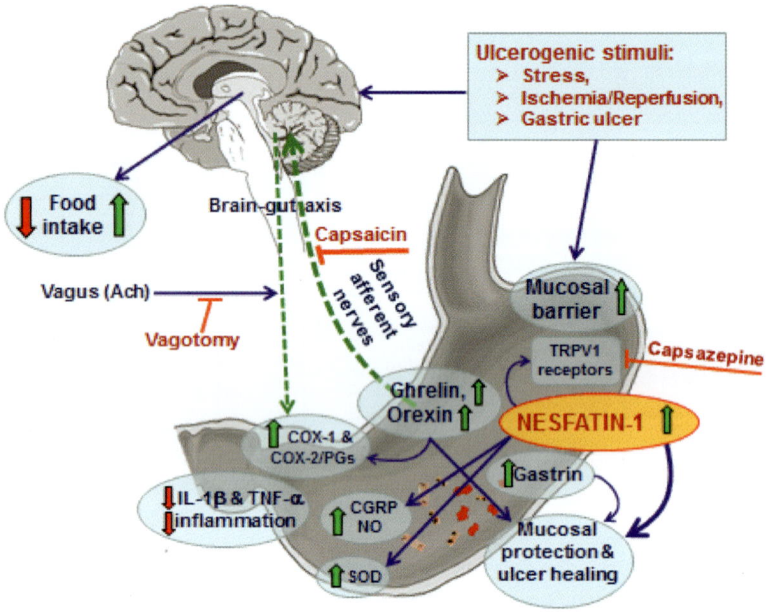

Figure 3. The proposed mechanisms of NUCB2/nesfatin-1 contribution to gastroprotection against acute gastric lesions and the healing of chronic ulcers. Nesfatin-1 plays an important role in the mechanism of gastroprotection against a variety of ulcerogenes and can accelerate ulcer healing via the activation of the brain–gut axis involving the protective pathways in the stomach including COX-1/COX-2-PG and NOS/NO systems, and sensory nerves releasing vasodilatory mediators such as CGRP acting through TRPV1 receptors. The nesfatin-1-induced decrease in the expression and release of pro-inflammatory cytokines (IL-1β and TNF-α) and an increase in the activity of SOD indicates that this peptide can strengthen the mucosal integrity due to its anti-inflammatory and anti-oxidizing properties.

by capsaicin impaired its gastroprotective properties.[51] The endogenous PG cannot be ruled out because the protective effect of ghrelin, OXA, and nesfatin-1 was restored when these peptides were administered together with exogenous PGE_2 in the presence of COX-1 and COX-2 inhibitors.[54]

Doubtlessly, ghrelin, OXA, and nesfatin-1 participation in gastroprotection and healing of chronic gastric ulcers is related to sensory afferent fibers, and this is proved by the reduction in the ulcer-healing dynamics following damaging of these fibers with capsaicin, as well as after blocking vanilloid receptors with capsazepine (Figure 3). Additionally, it was found that the administration of endogenous CGRP, released from sensory nerve endings mimicking physiological conditions, restores the regenerative effect of OXA or nesfatin-1. In the case of capsaicin denervation, the administration of OXA or nesfatin-1 combined with CGRP reduces the ulcer area and increases blood flow at the ulcer niche periphery in a manner comparable to the control group with the sensory fibers intact. Furthermore, OXA and nesfatin-1 participate in acetic ulcers healing by interacting with the NO synthesis pathway. The administration of the NOS blocker, L-NNA, increased the damaging effect of concentrated acetic acid despite the administration of OXA or nesfatin-1, whereas exogenous L-arginine, NO-synthase substrate, facilitated the restoration of OXA and nesfatin-1 effects, and this has been documented by the reduced ulcer area and gastric hyperemia.[55]

Involvement of nesfatin-1 and other appetite-controlling hormones the mechanism of gastric ulcer healing: A possible translation to the human peptic ulcer disease?

Under physiological conditions, the gastric mucosa is continuously exposed to a potential deleterious action of hydrochloric acid, microbial agents, such as *Helicobacter pylori* infection, ingested food products, including spices and drugs, such as non-steroidal anti-inflammatory drugs (NSAIDs), and, therefore, it developed a number of mechanisms facilitating the maintenance of its integrity and protection against damage. Effectiveness of protective and regenerative mediators in the gastric mucosa is reduced during diabetic conditions, and this has been confirmed by studies using the experimental model of diabetes induction in rodents with streptozotocin. Exposure of animals to cold stress, ischemia with successive reperfusion, or administration of NSAIDs is exacerbation of gastric damage by these ulcerogenes in the case of comorbid diabetes.[56,57] The gastric mucosa is more susceptible to damage caused by these ulcerogenes possibly during diabetes because of the following reasons: (1) weakening of the antioxidative system in the gastric mucosa, (2) reduction in duodenal HCO_3^- and mucus secretion, (3) limited basic fibroblast growth factor (bFGF) synthesis in the gastric mucosa, (4) inhibition of angiogenesis, and (5) dysfunction of sensory afferent fibers.[50,51,58] Diabetes not only weakens protective mechanisms in the gastric mucosa, but also reduces the dynamics of chronic gastric ulcers healing and causes frequent complications in the ulcer disease in the form of gastrointestinal bleeding.[59] Impaired healing of chronic gastric ulcers during diabetes is certainly a multifactor phenomenon, and this is confirmed by numerous studies. During diabetes, a decrease in the VEGF expression at the ulcer niche periphery was observed, and it is known to be an important cytokine regulating all stages of angiogenesis related to gastric ulcers healing.[51–53] Moreover, impaired gastric ulcers healing during diabetes may result from the increased production of pro-inflammatory cytokines IL-1β and TNF-α, responsible for triggering the inflammatory reaction, and forming of lesions and inducing carcinogenesis in many tissues, including the gastric mucosa. Brzozowski *et al.* proposed that the increase in the expression and release of pro-inflammatory cytokines IL-1β and TNF-α not only led to the intensification of the ulcerogenic effects of ischemia with successive reperfusion but also were responsible for the delay in the healing rate for ulcers caused by *Helicobacter pylori*.[54] The blood flow rate is extremely important during the regeneration of the gastric mucosa, as it ensures an adequate supply of oxygen and nutrients and removes toxic metabolites from the ulcer area. According to studies by Tashima *et al.*[55] the reduced blood flow in the ulcer area is probably related to the functional impairment of sensory afferent fibers, playing a crucial role in mucosal defense and regenerative mechanisms in the gastric mucosa.[55] Another mechanism certainly related to the reduced healing rate during diabetes is the impairment of the endogenous PG synthesis, as the fall in PGE_2 synthesis at the acetic ulcer periphery during diabetes was recently evidenced.[55] The administration of rofecoxib or aspirin, while suppressing PGE_2 biosynthesis, delayed ulcer healing in rats with diabetes and without diabetes, but, for instance, the prolongation of ulcer healing by COX-2 inhibitors was much more pronounced in rats with experimental diabetes than that in non-diabetic animals.[55]

The factors contributing to the acceleration of healing of chronic gastric ulcers may include peptides regulating food intake, such as nesfatin-1 and OXA, which increase the regeneration processes' activity also during diabetic conditions. The intraperitoneal administration of nesfatin-1 or OXA significantly reduced the area of pre-existing gastric ulcers and increased GBF at the ulcer margin, despite the co-occurring diabetes. The simultaneous administration of OXA and its receptor antagonist did not affect the healing process activity during diabetes. Probably the effect of nesfatin-1 and OXA is related to their anti-oxidative properties because in animals with diabetes and gastric ulcers, an increase in the superoxide dismutase (SOD) mRNA expression was observed when these peptides were administered. Additionally, both nesfatin-1 and OXA attenuated the expression of mRNA for pro-inflammatory cytokine HIF-1α, but this was not a strongly pronounced effect because an overexpression of HIF-1α mRNA still persisted during diabetic conditions despite the daily treatment with these peptides throughout the period of 9 or 15 days.[60]

In summary: (1) ghrelin, OXA, and nesfatin-1 participate in the healing of chronic pre-existing gastric ulcers, and this is reflected by the reduced ulcer area and increased blood flow at the ulcer margin; (2) ghrelin, OXA, and nesfatin-1 accelerate the mucosal regeneration processes due to the activation of the vasoactive NO/NOS system and sensory afferent nerve endings, releasing CGRP; (3) OXA and nesfatin-1 can accelerate the healing of chronic gastric ulcers and cause an increase in blood flow at the ulcer margin despite diabetic comorbidity, and (4) the mechanism of the beneficial action of these peptides potentially important for diabetic patients may involve the increase in the expression of anti-oxidative enzyme SOD and the downregulation of the mRNA expression for the pro-inflammatory factor HIF-1α.

References

1. Y Kanai, S Tanuma (1992) Purification of a novel B cell growth and differentiation factor associated with lupus syndrome. *Immunol Lett* **32**: 43–48.
2. S Barnikol-Watanabe, NA Gross, H Götz, T Henkel, A Karabinos, H Kratzin, HU Barnikol, N Hilschmann (1994) Human protein NEFA, a novel DNA binding/EF-hand/leucine zipper protein. Molecular cloning and sequence analysis of the cDNA, isolation and characterization of the protein. *Biol Chem Hoppe Seyler* **375**: 497–512.
3. K Miura, K Titani, Y Kurosawa, Y Kanai (1992) Molecular cloning of nucleobindin, a novel DNA-binding protein that contains both a signal peptide and a leucine zipper structure. *Biochem Biophys Res Commune* **187**: 375–380.
4. S Oh-I, H Shimizu, T Satoh, S Okada, S Adachi, K Inoue, H Eguchi, M Yamamoto, T Imaki, K Hashimoto, T Tsuchiya, T Monden, K Horiguchi, M Yamada, M Mori (2006) Identification of nesfatin-1 as a satiety molecule in the hypothalamus. *Nature* **443**: 709–712.

5. H Shimizu, S Oh-I, K Hashimoto, M Nakata, S Yamamoto, N Yoshida, H Eguchi, I Kato, K Inoue, T Satoh, S Okada, M Yamada, T Yada, M Mori (2009) Peripheral administration of nesfatin-1 reduces food intake in mice: The leptin-independent mechanism. *Endocrinology* **150**: 662–671.
6. KS Foo, H Brismar, C Broberger (2008) Distribution and neuropeptide coexistence of nucleobindin-2 mRNA/nesfatin-like immunoreactivity in the rat CNS. *Neuroscience* **156**: 563–579.
7. A Stengel, M Goebel, L Wang, J Rivier, P Kobelt, H Mönnikes, NW Lambrecht, Y Taché (2009) Central nesfatin-1 reduces dark-phase food intake and gastric emptying in rats: Differential role of corticotropin-releasing factor 2 receptor. *Endocrinology* **150**: 4911–4919.
8. GC Brailoiu, SL Dun, E Brailoiu, S Inan, J Yang, JK Chang, NJ Dun (2007) Nesfatin-1: Distribution and interaction with a G protein-coupled receptor in the rat brain. *Endocrinology* **148**: 5088–5094.
9. P Fort, D Salvert, L Hanriot, S Jego, H Shimizu, K Hashimoto, M Mori, PH Luppi (2008) The satiety molecule nesfatin-1 is co-expressed with melanin concentrating hormone in tuberal hypothalamic neurons of the rat. *Neuroscience* **155**: 174–181.
10. D Kohno, M Nakata, Y Maejima, H Shimizu, U Sedbazar, N Yoshida, K Dezaki, T Onaka, M Mori, T Yada (2008) Nesfatin-1 neurons in paraventricular and supraoptic nuclei of the rat hypothalamus coexpress oxytocin and vasopressin and are activated by refeeding. *Endocrinology* **149**: 1295–1301.
11. M Goebel, A Stengel, L Wang, NWG Lambrecht, Y Tache (2009) Nesfatin-1 immunoreactivity in rat brain and spinal cord autonomic nuclei. *Neurosci Lett* **452**: 241–246.
12. Y Maejima, U Sedbazar, S Suyama, D Kohno, T Onaka, E Takano, N Yoshida, M Koike, Y Uchiyama, K Fujiwara, T Yashiro, TL Horvath, MO Dietrich, S Tanaka, K Dezaki, S Oh-I, K Hashimoto, H Shimizu, M Nakata, M Mori, T Yada (2009) Nesfatin-1-regulated oxytocinergic signaling in the paraventricular nucleus causes anorexia through a leptin-independent melanocortin pathway. *Cell Metab* **10**: 355–365.
13. T Inhoff, A Stengel, L Peter, M Goebel, Y Tache, N Bannert, B Wiedenmann, BF Klapp, H Mónnikes, P Kobelt (2010) Novel insight in distribution of nesfastin-1 and phosphor-mTOR in the arcuate nucleus of the hypothalamus of rats. *Peptide* **31**: 257–262.
14. B Okere, L Xu, EW Roubos, D Sonetti, T Kozicz (2010) Restraint stress alters the secretory activity of neurons co-expressing urocortin-1, cocaine- and amphetamine-regulated transcript peptide and nesfatin-1 in the mouse Edinger–Westphal nucleus. *Brain Res* **1317C**: 92–99.

15. G Bustos, J Abarca, J Campusano, V Bustos, V Noriega, E Aliaga (2004) Functional interactions between somatodendritic dopamine release, glutamate receptors and brain-derived neurotrophic factor expression in mesencephalic structures of the brain. *Brain Res* **47**: 126–144.
16. R Landgraf, ID Neumann (2004) Vasopressin and oxytocin release within the brain: A dynamic concept of multiple and variable modes of neuropeptide communication. *Front Neuroendocrinol* **25**: 150–176.
17. C Xun, L Xiao-Min, Z Li-Hong (2013) Recent progress in research on the distribution and function of NUCB2/Nesfatin-1 in peripheral tissues. *Endocr J* **60**: 1021–1027.
18. A Stengel, M Goebel, I Yakubov, L Wang, D Witcher, T Coskun, Y Taché, G Sachs, NW Lambrecht (2009) Identification and characterization of nesfatin-1 immunoreactivity in endocrine cell types of the rat gastric oxyntic mucosa. *Endocrinology* **150**: 232–238.
19. R Gonzalez, A Tiwari, S Unniappan (2009) Pancreatic beta cells colocalize insulin and pronesfatin immunoreactivity in rodents. *Biochem Biophys Res Commun* **381**: 643–648.
20. KS Foo, H Brauner, CG Ostenson, C Broberger (2010) Nucleobindin-2/nesfatin in the endocrine pancreas: Distribution and relationship to glycaemic state. *J Endocrinol* **204**: 255–263.
21. M Nakata, K Manaka, S Yamamoto, M Mori, T Yada (2011) Nesfatin-1 enhances glucose-induced insulin secretion by promoting Ca^{2+} influx through L-type channels in mouse islet beta-cells. *Endocr J* **58**: 305–313.
22. W Pan, H Hsuchou, AJ Kastin (2007) Nesfatin-1 crosses the blood–brain barrier without saturation. *Peptides* **28**: 2223–2228.
23. TO Price, WK Samson, ML Niehoff, WA Banks (2007) Permeability of the blood–brain barrier to a novel satiety molecule nesfatin-1. *Peptides* **28**: 2372–2381.
24. M Ramanjaneya, J Chen, JE Brown, G Tripathi, M Hallschmid, S Patel, W Kern, EW Hillhouse, H Lehnert, BK Tan, HS Randeva (2010) Identification of nesfatin-1 in human and murine adipose tissue: A novel depot-specific adipokine with increased levels in obesity. *Endocrinology* **151**: 3169–3180.
25. Y Gui, JV Silha, S Mishra, LJ Murphy (2003) Changes in adipokine expression during food deprivation in the mouse and the relationship to fasting-induced insulin resistance. *Can J Physiol Pharm* **81**: 979–985.
26. T Angelone, E Filice, T Pasqua, N Amodio, M Galluccio, G Montesanti, AM Quintieri, MC Cerra (2013) Nesfatin as a novel cardiac peptide: Identification, functional characterization, and protection against ischemia/reperfusion injury. *Cell Mol Life Sci* **70**: 495–509.

27. GL Yosten, WK Samson (2009) Nesfatin-1 exerts cardiovascular actions in brain: Possible interaction with the central melanocortin system. *Am J Physiol Regul Integr Comp Physiol* **297**: R330–R336.
28. R Gonzales, E Shepperd, V Thiruppugazh, S Lohan, CL Grey, JP Chang, S Unniappan (2012) Nesfatin-1 regulates the hypothalamo-pituitary-ovarian axis of fish. *Biol Reprod* **87**: 1–11.
29. H Yamawaki, M Takahashi, M Mukohda, T Morita, M Okada, Y Hara (2012) A novel adipocytokine, nesfatin-1 modulates peripheral arterial contractility and blood pressure in rats. *Biochem Biophys Res Commun* **418**: 676–681.
30. D Garcia-Galiano, R Pineda, T Ilhan, JM Castellano, F Ruiz-Pino, MA Sanchez-Garrido, MJ Vazquez, S Sangiao-Alvarellos, A Romero-Ruiz, L Pinilla, C Dieguez, F Gaytan, M Tena-Sempere (2012) Cellular distribution, regulated expression, and functional role of the anorexigenic peptide NUCB2/nesfatin-1, in the testis. *Endocrinology* **153**: 1959–1971.
31. CJ Price, WK Samn, AV Fergon (2008) Nesfatin-1 inhibits NPY neurons in arcuate nucleus. *Brain Res* **1230**: 99–106.
32. H Shimizu, H Arima, Y Ozawa, M Watanabe, R Banno, Y Sugimura, N Ozaki, H Nagasaki, Y Oiso (2010) Glucocorticoids increase NPY gene expression in the arcuate nucleus by inhibiting mTOR signaling in rat hypothalamic organotypic cultures. *Peptides* **31**: 145–149.
33. EP Zorrilla, Y Taché, GF Koob (2003) Nibbling at CRF receptor control of feeding and gastrocolonic motility. *Trends Pharmacol Sci* **24**: 421–427.
34. EM Fekete, K Inoue, Y Zhao, JE Rivier, WW Vale, A Szücs, GF Koob, EP Zorrilla (2007) Delayed satiety-like actions and altered feeding microstructure by a selective type 2 corticotropin-releasing factor agonist in rats: Intra-hypothalamic urocortin 3 administration reduces food intake by prolonging the post-meal interval. *Neuropsychopharmacology* **32**: 1052–1068.
35. A Stengel, M Goebel, L Wang, Y Taché (2010) Abdominal surgery activates nesfatin-1 immunoreactive brain nuclei in rats. *Peptides* **31**: 263–270.
36. MS Bonnet, E Pecchi, J Trouslard, A Jean, M Dallaporta, JD Troadec (2009) Central nesfatin-1-expressing neurons are sensitive to peripheral inflammatory stimulus. *J Neuroinflammation* **6**: 27.
37. M Goebel, A Stengel, L Wang, Y Taché (2009) Restraint stress activates nesfatin-1-immunoreactive brain nuclei in rats. *Brain Res* **1300**: 114–124.
38. SJ Konturek (2001) Choroba wrzodowa. Fizjopatologia i leczenie. *Przew Lek* **1–2**: 98–107.
39. SJ Konturek, I Piastucki, T Brzozowski, T Radecki, A Dembińska-Kieć, A Żmuda, R Gryglewski (1981) Role of prostaglandins in the formation of aspirin induced ulcers. *Gastroenterology* **80**: 4–9.

40. SJ Konturek, T Brzozowski, J Majka, A Dembiński, A Slomiany, BL Slomiany (1992) Transforming growth factor and epidermal growth factor in protection and healing of gastric mucosal injury. *Scand J Gastroenterol* **27**: 649–655.
41. BJR Whittle, J Lopez-Bolmonte, S Moncada (1990) Regulation of gastric mucosal integrity by endogenous nitric oxide: Interactions with prostanoids and sensory neuropeptides in the rat. *Br J Pharmacol* **99**: 607–611.
42. A Bado, S Levasseur, S Attoub, S Kermorgant, JP Laigneau, MN Bortoluzzi, L Moizo, T Lehy, M Guerre-Millo, Y Le Marchand-Brustel, MJ Lewin (1998) The stomach is a source of leptin. *Nature* **394**: 790–793.
43. ML Hakansson, H Brown, N Ghilardi, RC Skoda, B Meister (1998) Leptin receptor immunoreactivity in chemically defined target neurons of the hypothalamus. *J Neurosci* **18**: 559–572.
44. T Brzozowski, PC Konturek, R Pajdo, S Kwiecień, A Ptak, Z Śliwowski, D Drozdowicz, M Pawlik, SJ Konturek, EG Hahn (2001) Brain–gut axis gastroprotection by leptin and cholecystokinin against ischemia-reperfusion induced gastric lesions. *J Physiol Pharmacol* **52**: 583–602.
45. T Brzozowski, PC Konturek, SJ Konturek, R Pajdo, A Duda, P Pierzchalski, W Bielanski, EG Hahn (1999) Leptin in gastroprotection induced by cholecystokinin or by a meal. Role of vagal and sensory nerves and nitric oxide. *Eur J Pharmacol* **374**: 263–276.
46. R Schneider, SR Bornstein, GP Chrousos, S Boxberger, G Ehninger, M Breidert (2001) Leptin mediates a proliferative response in human gastric mucosa cells with functional receptor. *Horm Metab Res* **33**: 1–6.
47. JM Lundberg, K Tatemoto, L Terenius, PM Hellström, V Mutt, T Hökfelt, B Hamberger (1982) Localization of peptide YY (PYY) in gastrointestinal endocrine cells and effects on intestinal blood flow and motility. *Proc Natl Acad Sci USA* **79**: 4471–4475.
48. K Kawakubo, H Yang, Y Tache (2002) Gastric protective effects of peripheral PYY through PYY preferring receptors in anesthetized rats. *Am J Physiol Gastrointest Liv Physiol* **283**: 1035–1041.
49. Z Merali, C Cayer, P Kent, H Anisman (2008) Nesfatin-1 increases anxiety-and fear-related behaviors in the rat. *Psychopharmacology* **201**: 115–123.
50. A Szlachcic, Z Sliwowski, G Krzysiek-Mączka, J Majka, M Surmiak, R Pajdo, D Drozdowicz, SJ Konturek, T Brzozowski (2013) New satiety hormone nesfatin-1 protects gastric mucosa against stress-induced injury: Mechanistic roles of prostaglandins, nitric oxide, sensory nerves and vanilloid receptors. *Peptides* **49 C**: 9–20.
51. K Takeuchi, K Takehara, K Tajima, S Kato, T Hirata (1997) Impaired healing of gastric lesions in streptozotocin-induced diabetic rats: Effect of basic fibroblast growth factor. *J Pharmacol Exp Ther* **281**: 200–207.

52. S Szabo, A Vincze, Z Sandor, M Jadus, Z Gombos, A Pedram, E Levin, J Hagar, G Iaquinto (1998) Vascular approach to gastro-duodenal ulceration. *Dig Dis Sci* **43**: 40S–45S.
53. Y Matsui, K Mitsuyama, N Tomiyasu, A Toyomaga, M Sata (2002) Efficacy of vascular endothelial growth factor in the treatment of experimental gastric injury. *Digestion* **66**: 99–105.
54. IA Harsch, T Brzozowski, K Bazela, SJ Konturek, V Kukharsky, T Pawlik, E Pawlowski, EG Hahn, PC Konturek (2003) Impaired gastric ulcer healing in diabetic rats: Role of heat shock protein, growth factors, prostaglandins and proinflammatory cytokines. *Eur J Pharmacol* **481**: 249–260.
55. K Tashima, R Korolkiewicz, M Kubomi, K Takeuchi (1998) Increased susceptibility of gastric mucosa to ulcerogenic stimulation in diabetic rats role of capsaicin-sensitive sensory fibers. *Br J Pharmacol* **124**: 1359–1402.
56. K Tashima, A Fujita, K Takeuchi (2000) Aggravation of ischemia/reperfusion-induced gastric lesions in streptozotocin-diabetic rats. *Life Sci* **67**: 1707–1718.
57. R Korolkiewicz, K Tashima, M Kubomi, S Kato, K Takeuchi (1999) Increased susceptibility of diabetic rat gastric mucosa to food deprivation during cold stress. *Digestion* **60**: 528–537.
58. E Goldin, E Ardite, JI Elizalde, A Odriozola, J Panes, JM Pique, JC Fernandez-Checa (1997) Gastric mucosal damages in experimental diabetes in rats: Role of endogenous glutathione. *Gastroenterology* **112**: 855–863.
59. M Pietzsch, S Theuer, G Haase, F Plath, M Kayser, AK Riethling (2002) Results of systematic screening for serious gastrointestinal bleeding associated with NSAIDs in Rostock Hospitals. *Int J Pharmacol Ther* **40**: 111–115.
60. A Szlachcic, J Majka, M Strzałka, J Szmyd, R Pajdo, A Ptak-Belowska, S Kwiecień, T Brzozowski (2013) Experimental healing of pre-existing gastric ulcers induced by hormones controlling food intake ghrelin, orexin-A, nesfatin-1 is impaired under diabetic conditions. A key to understand the diabetic gastropathy? *J Physiol Pharmacol* **64**: 625–637.

Chapter 3

Chemoprophylaxis in Inflammatory Bowel Diseases

Nikola Mitrev, Aladdin Alswaifi, and Rupert W. Leong

Abstract

Inflammatory bowel disease (IBD) increases the lifetime risk of colorectal cancer (CRC). Given the mortality, morbidity, and health costs associated with CRC in IBD, various chemoprophylactic agents have been investigated as adjuncts to surveillance colonoscopies. As molecular mechanisms of carcinogenesis differ between sporadic and colitis-associated dysplasia, agents that reduce sporadic CRC risk cannot be assumed to have the same effect on IBD-associated CRC. The excess risk of dysplasia in IBD is secondary to colonic inflammation, and anti-inflammatory agents have been proposed to be chemoprophylactic, including 5-aminosalicylates, thiopurines, corticosteroids, and anti-tumor necrosis factor-α agents. Certain agents, such as 5-aminosalicylates and ursodeoxycholic acid, appear to have chemoprophylactic properties beyond control of inflammation. Control of colonic inflammation and mucosal healing is the key to reducing dysplasia risk in IBD. Patients who never achieve mucosal healing would benefit from a chemoprophylactic agent as adjunct to surveillance colonoscopies. Currently, apart from 5-aminosalicylates and ursodeoxycholic acid, the lack of evidence limits most agents from being recommended.

Introduction

Inflammatory bowel disease (IBD) increases the lifetime risk of developing colorectal cancer (CRC). Dysplasia risk is proportional to the duration of IBD and the extent of colonic involvement among other risk factors.[1,2] The cumulative incidence of CRC in left-sided colitis or pancolitis is estimated to be 2% by 10 years, 8% by 20 years, and 18% by 30 years.[2] More recent population-based studies suggest lower CRC rates of 1 in 14 after 30 years of IBD.[3,4] Other risk factors for CRC in IBD include a family history of CRC and concurrent diagnosis of primary sclerosing cholangitis (PSC).[1] Studies indicate the risk of CRC to be slightly less with Crohn's disease (CD) as compared to ulcerative colitis (UC) with the same extent of colonic involvement.[5] IBD patients with macroscopically and microscopically normal colon have higher CRC risk comparable to the general population, indicating colitis to be the driver of carcinogenesis.[6] Current guidelines recommend regular screening colonoscopies for all patients with IBD of at least 8 years duration, apart from those with only UC proctitis or Crohn's colitis involving less than a third of the colon length.[5]

A number of mechanisms have been proposed by which IBD leads to the formation of cancer (see Figure 1). Inflammation results in increased cell turnover, increasing the risk of DNA mutation and neoplastic transformation.[7] Tumor suppressor genes including those involved in DNA mismatch repair undergo promoter hypermethylation and downregulation in inflammatory tissues, resulting in genetic instability.[8] Overexpressed genes in inflammation may act as proto-oncogenes to promote carcinogenesis, including nuclear factor-κB (NF-κB) and toll-like receptor 4 (TLR4).[9,10] Inflammatory cells produce various angiogenic factors, including prostaglandin E_2, which promote tumor growth.[11] Owing to the production of reactive oxygen species (ROS) and reactive nitrogen species (RNS) by macrophages and neutrophils, cells in inflamed tissues are also exposed to increased oxidative stress, which itself is damaging to macromolecules such as protein and DNA, resulting in the deactivation of proteins that monitor DNA integrity as well as the direct mutation of tumor suppressor genes and proto-oncogenes, respectively.[12,13]

Some molecular differences have been demonstrated between pathogenesis of inflammatory and sporadic CRC. Mutations in the p53 gene tend to occur early in colitis-associated dysplasia pathogenesis, in contrast to

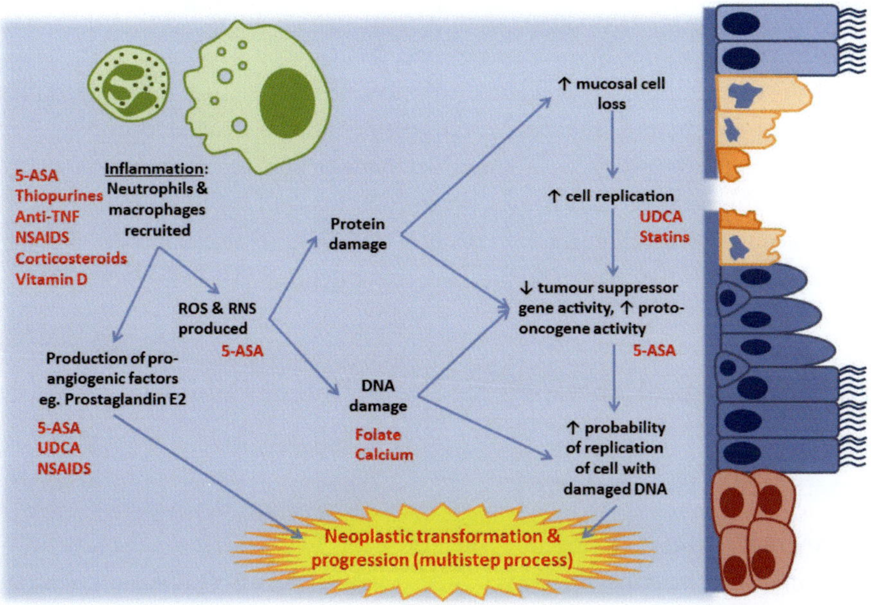

Figure 1. Mechanism of carcinogenesis in inflamed colonic mucosa. Within the inflamed colonic mucosa in inflammatory IBD, recruited macrophages and neutrophils produce ROS and RNS. ROS and RNS in turn damage macromolecules including DNA and protein which results in cell death and increased cell turnover. Damage to DNA, protein, and the requirement for increased cell replication to replace the lost cells results in increase in proto-oncogene expression and reduced expression of tumor suppressor genes, such as those involved in apoptosis and ensuring DNA fidelity. The effect of this is to increase the probability that cells with DNA mutations would continue to enter the cell cycle rather than undergo apoptosis, thereby contributing to the multistep process of neoplastic transformation. In addition, inflammatory cells produce angiogenic factors to further promote tumor growth and development. The proposed site of action of various medications proposed to reduce risk of colorectal cancer has been indicated in red.

Abbreviations: 5-aminosalicylates (5-ASA), anti-tumor necrosis factor drugs (Anti-TNF), ursodeoxycholic acid (UDCA).

sporadic CRC, in which they are found late.[14] Due to these differences, chemoprotective therapies in sporadic CRC cannot be assumed to have the same protective effect in colitis-associated dysplasia.

In recent years, human and animal studies of chemoprophylactic therapies have been conducted against colitis-associated dysplasia. An effective chemoprophylactic agent may complement regular surveillance colonoscopies, given the morbidity, mortality, and health cost associated with CRC. Data on the ability of surveillance colonoscopies to reduce CRC mortality have been conflicting, sparking even greater interest in chemoprophylactic therapies.[15] Medications with potential benefit include 5-aminosalicylates (5-ASA), thiopurines, anti-tumor necrosis factor-α (TNF-α) agents, aspirin, non-steroidal anti-inflammatory drugs (NSAIDs), corticosteroids, ursodeoxycholic acid (UDCA), statins, folate, and calcium.

Potential Medical Therapies for Prevention of Colorectal Cancer in Inflammatory Bowel Disease

5-Aminosalicylates (5-ASA)

5-ASA are traditional first-line therapies for UC and have topical anti-inflammatory effects on the bowel. 5-ASA have also been studied as potential chemoprophylacitc drugs in preventing colitis-associated dysplasia. In fact, the reducing incidence of CRC in UC patients has been attributed in part to increase in surveillance colonoscopies and 5-ASA use.[16,17]

Potential mechanisms for the antineoplastic effects of 5-ASA have been proposed. 5-ASA inhibit cyclooxygenase-2 (COX)-2 and lipoxygenase, thereby reducing the formation of pro-inflammatory and pro-angiogenic factors, with prostaglandin E_2 being one such factor implicated in tumor development.[11,18] 5-ASA are also scavengers of reactive oxygen and nitrogen species which are overproduced in inflamed tissues and responsible for DNA damage and neoplastic transformation.[19] Animal studies have demonstrated that the antineoplastic effects of 5-ASA are largely mediated via inducing the expression of the peroxisome proliferator-activated receptor-gamma (PPARγ).[20,21] The administration of a PPARγ antagonist inhibited the anti-neoplastic effects of 5-ASA on HT-29 cells, and in PPARγ knockout cells, the antineoplastic effects of 5-ASA were blunted. Similarly, with *in vivo* studies of 5-ASA in a mouse model of colitis-associated dysplasia, only wild-type mice derived benefit from 5-ASA, whereas PPARγ knockout mice did not. PPARγ acts to reduce the pro-inflammatory cytokine expression and mediators that promote cell cycling and hence neoplastic transformation. This accounts for their anti-inflammatory and chemoprotective effects.

A meta-analysis published by Zhao *et al.* in 2014 concluded that there is a benefit of 5-ASA in UC-related CRC.[22] This meta-analysis comprised of 20,193 subjects from 17 studies and showed that 5-ASA use was associated with the reduced risk of CRC (odds ratio [OR]: 0.63, 95% confidence interval [CI]: 0.48–0.84). A greater risk reduction was demonstrated when 5-ASA were used at higher doses, defined as sulfasalazine ≥2.0 g/day or mesalazine ≥1.2 g/day (OR: 0.51, 95% CI: 0.35–0.75). Interestingly, no CRC risk reduction was demonstrated with the use of 5-ASA in patients with extensive colitis (OR: 1.00, 95% CI: 0.53–1.89), indicating possible saturating effects of inability to overcome ongoing carcinogenic pathways with more severe diseases. Furthermore, the regular use of 5-ASA has been shown to reduce rates of CRC in UC to a greater extent as compared to the irregular use.[23]

It remains unclear what duration of 5-ASA use is required to reduce the risk of colitis-associated dysplasia, and whether there is a linear relationship between the duration of use and the CRC risk reduction or if benefit plateaus. Studies included in the above meta-analysis have defined the minimal use of 5-ASA for inclusion, from at least 2 months to at least 2 years of use, with no subgroup analysis based on the duration of use.

Pooled results of UC and CD patients have been less clear, with a meta-analysis by Nguyen *et al.* demonstrating no CRC risk reduction in patients with IBD using 5-ASA (adjusted odds ratio [aOR]: 0.95, 95% CI: 0.66–1.38).[24] However, CD involving only one segment of the colorectum does not result in the increased risk of CRC compared to the general population.[5] In a study of 1,000 patients with CD followed up for 20 years, of the 7 patients that developed CRC all had colonic involvement and the mean disease duration of 22 years (range 7–40 years).[25] Hence, when pooling results from all IBD patients treated with 5-ASA, patients with CD treated with 5-ASA who do not have significant colitis may potentially dilute the beneficial effect of 5-ASA in reducing CRC as compared to patients that have colitis-associated dysplasia and other risk factors for CRC. This may explain the different results of meta-analysis assessing the CRC risk reduction with 5-ASA in UC patients versus IBD patients. Indeed, the four studies included in the meta-analysis by Nguyen *et al.* demonstrated a moderate amount of heterogeneity, and it was proposed by the authors that an explanation of this may be the varying proportions of UC versus CD patients in each of the studies.[24] The latest American Gastroenterological Association (AGA) position statement is that there is moderate evidence of the CRC-preventative benefits of 5-ASA in IBD, but it does not go so far as to recommend a dose or a patient subgroup for chemoprophylaxis.[26] The European Crohn's and Colitis Organization (ECCO) recommends a minimal dose of 1.2 g/day of 5-ASA to reduce the risk of CRC in patients with IBD at increased risk, including those with UC and PSC, family history of CRC, or with an extent and duration of colonic involvement that results in elevated risk of CRC.[27] It is recommended that 5-ASA is commenced at diagnosis and adherence to therapy be emphasized given the high rates of treatment non-compliance.[28,29]

Thiopurines

Thiopurines, including azathioprine and 6-mercaptopurine, are frequently used as maintenance therapy in IBD. Azathioprine and its active metabolite 6-mercaptopurine are eventually metabolized to 6-thioguanine nucleotides (6-TGN), which are incorporated into the DNA of replicating lymphocytes as purine analogs, causing DNA breaks and eventual immunosuppression. In addition, 6-thioguanine-triphosphate (6-TGTP), one of the 6-TGNs, induces T-cell apoptosis by inhibiting Rac1 upon CD28 costimulation.[30]

Thiopurines are believed to protect against CRC via reduction in colonic inflammation, rather than a specific anticancer effect.[31] Thiopurines have not been shown to reduce sporadic CRC risk among patients treated for indications other than IBD, such as transplant patients.[32]

Studies of the protective effects of thiopurines on CRC in patients with IBD have yielded conflicting results. A meta-analysis of 9 case-control and 10 cohort studies demonstrated that thiopurine use in IBD was associated with significantly reduced colitis-associated dysplasia risk (relative risk [RR]: 0.71, 95% CI: 0.54–0.94, $P = 0.017$).[33] A recent study of IBD-associated dysplasia in UC based on the Spanish nationwide database indicated a statistically significant protective effect of thiopurines on the incidence of IBD-associated dysplasia (OR: 0.21, 95% CI: 0.06–0.74, $P = 0.015$).[34] A French prospective cohort study by Beaugerie *et al.*, of 19,484 patients demonstrated thiopurines protect from high-grade dysplasia and CRC among IBD patients with extensive colitis, defined as colitis involving at least 50% of the colon (adjusted hazard ratio [aHR]: 0.28, 95% CI: 0.1–0.9, $P = 0.03$).[35] Contrary to this, a meta-analysis of 15 studies by Jess *et al.*, which included the study by Beaugerie *et al.*, indicated no benefit of thiopurines in preventing CRC among IBD patients (OR: 0.87, 95% CI: 0.71–1.06).[36]

High heterogeneity in studied populations may explain the different conclusions from the above studies.[31] As thiopurines only reduce the incidence of colitis-associated dysplasia, the overrepresentation of IBD patients not at significant risk of colitis-associated dysplasia in a particular cohort, such as CD patients without colitis or UC patients with only proctitis, will dilute the beneficial effects of thiopurines on inflammation-associated dysplasia. Alternatively, the studies of populations with an increased risk of inflammation-related dysplasia, where there is an overrepresentation of patients with pan-colitis, may demonstrate a beneficial effect of thiopurines on reducing dysplasia. More than 80% of patients selected from the Spanish national database study were enrolled in a CRC screening program and were at a higher risk of inflammation-related dysplasia, explaining the beneficial effects of thiopurines in reducing dysplasia observed in this study.

Thiopurine use in IBD has been associated with more serious side effects than 5-ASA use, including an increased risk of hematological malignancies and non-melanoma skin cancers.[1] They may be less likely to be used for chemoprophylaxis alone but may be used as maintenance therapies. Current guidelines from both the ECCO and the AGA do not recommend the routine use of thiopurines for chemoprevention due to insufficient evidence.[26,27]

Anti-tumor necrosis factor-α (anti-TNF-α) therapy

TNF-α is a key mediator in the immune system and a crucial mediator of inflammation in IBD. Although TNF-α acts to enhance the immune response directed against cancer cells, through the stimulation of tumor proliferation, invasion, metastasis, and angiogenesis, it also paradoxically enhances the development of inflammation-mediated cancers.[37] Animal model data also suggest that TNF-α-driven inflammation may contribute to dysplasia.[38] In a mouse model of colitis-associated dysplasia, mice were administered azoxymethane (AOM) and dextran sulfate sodium (DSS) to induce colonic inflammation and dysplasia. These mice had elevated levels of TNF-α as well as increased infiltrating lymphocytes in the lamina propria of their intestines containing the major receptor for TNF-α, p55 (TNF-Rp55). Interestingly, TNF-Rp55 knockout mice administered with the same AOM and DSS regimen did not demonstrate the same extent of tumor formation. Furthermore, treatment with etanercept, a TNF-α–IgG fusion peptide which has been shown to bind and inhibit TNF-α, resulted in less intestinal inflammation and tumor formation in the wild-type mouse model for inflammation-induced intestinal cancer.[38]

Human studies of the chemoprophylactic effects of anti-TNF-α therapy have yielded conflicting results.[39] A study involving the Danish National Patients Registry, comprising of 46,780 patients, did not demonstrate a convincing difference in rates of CRC between IBD patients exposed to the anti-TNF-α therapy and IBD patients not exposed to anti-TNF-α therapy (RR: 0.83, 95% CI: 0.46–1.48).[40] However, a subsequent Dutch case-control study demonstrated that the use of anti-TNF-α therapy in IBD was associated with the reduced risk of CRC (OR: 0.09, 95% CI: 0.01–0.68, $P < 0.02$).[41] This study compared 173 cases with 393 controls. Current guidelines make no recommendation in terms of the use of anti-TNF-α agents in reducing colitis-associated dysplasia.[26,27]

Ursodeoxycolic acid (UDCA)

PSC is a chronic inflammatory disorder of the bile ducts, which in 60–80% of cases occurs together with IBD and is also associated with a fourfold increase in CRC as compared to IBD alone.[15,42] UDCA is a hydrophilic bile acid used in the treatment of PSC. Animal studies have indicated that UDCA inhibits CRC formation in a rat model of AOM-induced CRC.[43] A number of mechanisms have been implicated to account for this. UDCA reduces the levels of tumor promoting-deoxycholic acid (DCA), a secondary bile acid which has been shown to stimulate cell proliferation, apoptosis, and CRC formation in animal models.[44] UDCA also downregulates the COX-2 expression, with a subsequent reduction of pro-inflammatory and pro-angiogenic cytokines that promote tumor growth and development.[45]

There has been conflicting evidence on the effects of UDCA on the risk of CRC in IBD. In a cross-sectional study by Tung *et al.* in 2001 including 59 patients with UC and PSC who were undergoing colonoscopic surveillance for colonic dysplasia, the use of UDCA was associated with a significantly reduced rate of colorectal dysplasia (OR: 0.18, 95% CI: 0.05–0.6, P = 0.005).[46] A prior randomized control trial of UDCA in UC and PSC, comprising of 52 participants followed up for 355 person-years, revealed a protective effect of UDCA versus placebo for developing dysplasia or CRC (RR: 0.26, 95% CI: 0.06–0.92, P = 0.034).[47] However, two other studies have demonstrated no benefit.[48,49] Eaton *et al.* analyzed colonoscopy and pathology reports from a prior randomized placebo-controlled double-blinded trial of high-dose UDCA, involving 56 subjects with UC and PSC. Patients randomized to high-dose UDCA had a significantly increased risk of dysplasia (low or high grade) or CRC (hazard ratio [HR]: 4.44, 95% CI: 1.30–20.10, P = 0.02). These conflicting results may be explained by a dual effect of UDCA on the development of CRC, with lower doses offering protection and higher doses increasing risk.

Studies suggest that UDCA may also have a protective effect on sporadic CRC rather than just colitis-associated dysplasia. A double-blinded, placebo-controlled trial of 1,285 subjects over 3 years demonstrated a non-statistically significant 12% reduction in adenoma recurrence.[50] However, patients randomized to UDCA had a statistically significant reduction in recurrence of adenomas with high-grade dysplasia (aOR: 0.61, 95% CI: 0.39–0.96, P = 0.03). Subsequent analysis of the above results yielded a statistically significant reduction in CRC risk with the use of UDCA in men (OR: 0.62, 95% CI: 0.43–0.89), while an unexpected statistically significant increase in CRC risk in a subset of women, including those below 65 years of age (OR: 3.24, 95% CI: 1.10–9.56), body mass index (BMI) ≥30 kg/m^2 (OR: 5.45, 95% CI: 1.42–20.9) or high dietary fat intake ≥56.2 g/day (OR: 3.48, 95% CI: 1.35–8.95).[51]

Current recommendations from both the ECCO and the AGA are to give UDCA chemoprevention only to patients with IBD that have PSC.[26,27]

Folate

Folate supplementation is another chemoprophylactic approach that has been studied in IBD. Folate deficiency has been associated with an increased risk of sporadic CRC development by several studies.[52,53] Furthermore, folate deficiency, particularly in the setting of hyperhomocysteinemia, has been strongly associated with the development of CRC in UC.[54]

Folate has an important role in DNA methylation and nucleotide synthesis.[55] It is postulated that folate may exert its chemoprotective effect via ensuring normal DNA methylation and a steady state of DNA precursors, thereby influencing the expression of tumor suppressor genes and proto-oncogenes and reducing DNA replication errors respectively.[56] Folate deficiency has been shown to reduce p53 tumor suppressor gene expression in the colonic mucosa of rats, and also to lead to an increased incidence of p53-mutated CRCs in humans.[57,58] Folate supplementation has been shown to significantly reduce cellular proliferation kinetics in the rectal mucosa of patients with long-standing UC, which further accounts for its chemoprotective effects.[59]

Patients with IBD are at risk of folate deficiency due to anorexia, reduced absorption, and increased intestinal losses as a result of active disease and also antagonism by sulfasalazine.[15,55] The prevalence of folate deficiency is 28.8% among CD patients, 8.8% among UC patients, and 3% among controls. Although folate deficiency has been clearly linked to sporadic CRC development in several studies, folate supplementation has failed to demonstrate the reduction in sporadic CRC risk.[15,52,53] However, folate supplementation may have a different effect on CRC in patients with IBD. Most studies on folate supplementation in IBD have shown a trend toward reduced dysplasia risk. A case-control study in 2010 by Tang *et al.* showed a higher use of folate supplementation in UC patients without CRC as compared to those with CRC (absolute risk 40.0% vs. 16.7%, $P = 0.002$).[60] However, this study evaluated the impact of folate supplement use on CRC only as a secondary outcome. At present, there is insufficient evidence to recommend universal folate supplementation in IBD patients as a chemoprophylactic measure.[15,26]

Aspirin and NSAIDs

The benefits of aspirin, NSAIDs, and COX-2 selective inhibitors in reducing the risk of CRC have been well established in sporadic and familial CRC, with studies demonstrating an RR of 40–50%.[61,62] Animal studies have demonstrated a reduced rate of carcinogen-induced CRC formation with NSAIDs in rodent models.[61] Approximately, 50% of sporadic colorectal adenomas and 80% of sporadic CRCs have been demonstrated to have upregulated levels of COX-2 mRNA.[61] NSAIDs are postulated to be chemoprotective via their inhibition of COX, which in turn leads to less conversion of arachidonic acid to prostaglandins and leukotrienes with angiogenic and tumor promoting-properties.[11]

The benefit of COX inhibition in colitis-associated dysplasia, however, is less clear.[62] One case-control study found a statistically significant protective effect of both aspirin use and NSAID use in terms of CRC prevention in patients with IBD.[15,63] However, data were in the form of a questionnaire on two consecutive visits and the above result may be significantly influenced by recall bias. Indeed, this protective effect of either NSAIDs or aspirin has not been replicated in another six studies that have assessed the chemoprotective effect of either aspirin or NSAIDs.[15] At this stage, there are no recommendations for the routine use of NSAIDs and aspirin purely for CRC prevention in IBD patients.

Corticosteroids

As inflammation is the main driver of colorectal dysplasia in IBD, it is expected that corticosteroids with their anti-inflammatory effects would reduce colitis-associated dysplasia incidence. However, studies of corticosteroids on the risk of CRC in IBD have yielded conflicting results, ranging from statistically significant benefit to harm.[15] But there is an inherit problem with case-control and cohort studies as an important confounder is the severity of inflammation. Extended periods of steroid use are likely associated with uncontrolled inflammation, the main driver of CRC in IBD. This is potentially the reason why in some cohort studies a positive association has been found between corticosteroid use and dysplasia risk.

According to the latest position statement from the AGA, the use of corticosteroids for CRC prevention in IBD is a grade D recommendation, as certainty of net harm is high.[26] Even despite the lack of consistent evidence of benefit on colitis-associated dysplasia with corticosteroids, many side effects warrant against their long-term use purely as chemoprophylactic agents.

Calcium and vitamin D

Low dairy intake has been associated with sporadic CRC and supplementation has been shown to reduce colorectal adenoma recurrence in randomized control trials.[64,65] It has been postulated that calcium may bind carcinogenic bile acids as a potential chemoprotective mechanism.[15] However, among the three case-control and cohort studies that have assessed the impact of calcium on colitis-associated dysplasia, none of them have demonstrated a statistically significant result when adjusted for confounders.[15]

Similarly, low vitamin D levels have been positively correlated with the risk of sporadic CRC.[66] Randomized control trials and cohort studies of vitamin D supplementation on sporadic CRC risk have yielded conflicting results.[67,68] Vitamin D may exert its anticancer effects through several mechanisms, including altering immune function and promoting cellular differentiation, inhibiting cellular proliferation, inducing apoptosis, and inhibiting angiogenesis.[66,69] Vitamin D deficiency has been shown to increase severity of IBD in human trials and supplementation has been shown to reduce activity.[70] Also, mouse models of colitis-driven CRC have indicated that high-dose vitamin D supplementation reduces colonic inflammation and CRC formation.[71] However, to date there have been no human studies that assess the impact of vitamin D levels or vitamin D supplementation on colitis-associated dysplasia.

The latest position statement from the AGA is that currently there is insufficient evidence to recommend calcium or vitamin supplementation to prevent colitis-associated dysplasia.[26]

Statins

Statins have been proposed as CRC preventing agents, with early cardiovascular disease trials with pravastatin demonstrating a trend toward reduced incidence that was, however, non-statistically significant.[72] Statins reduce cholesterol synthesis by inhibiting the enzyme 3-hydroxy-3-methyl-glutaryl-CoA reductase (HMG-CoA reductase).[73] HMG-CoA reductase expression is elevated in cancer cells, and is believed to have a role in growth control. Statins also induce apoptosis in cancer cell lines *in vitro*.

Although there have been no separate trials to assess the effect of statins on colitis-associated dysplasia, in two cohort studies of effects of statins on CRC risk, a subgroup analysis of CRC among patients with IBD was performed.[73,74] In both of these studies, statin use was associated with a statistically significant risk reduction of colitis-associated dysplasia. However, at this stage more robust evidence is needed on the impact of statins on colitis-associated dysplasia risk before recommendations for widespread use can be made.[26]

Limitations of Current Evidence

There are a range of issues with the currently available evidence on chemoprophylactic medical therapies for colitis-associated dysplasia. Apart from one randomized control trial involving UDCA, the remainder of the human data comes from either cohort or case-control studies. A potential confounder resulting in an overall no significant chemoprophylactic benefit from many of the above studied medical therapies, including 5-ASA and thiopurines, is that patients with more severe colitis activity are likely to be on higher doses of 5-ASA and immunosuppressant medication. Dysplasia risk is proportional to severity of colitis, which may confound trial results. However, randomized control trials in this instance would be inherently difficult to perform given the need for long-term follow-up and large sample sizes.[15]

Animal data are useful in exploring mechanisms of chemoprevention and discovering potential targets for future research in humans; however, it is unclear to what extent this can be applied to humans. For instance, many rodent models of IBD use chemically induced colitis.

Most of the above cohort and case-control studies do not have inclusion and exclusion criteria that select for a subpopulation of IBD patients that are at an increased risk of CRC as compared to the general population. IBD is a heterogeneous disorder, and only UC and CD patients with significant colonic involvement are at increased risk of CRC.[5] Studies that include CD patients without significant colonic involvement and UC patients with only proctitis may dilute potential beneficial effect of a studied medical therapy.

Conclusion

Although several potential chemoprophylactic agents have been proposed in colitis-associated dysplasia, current recommendations only support the use of 5-ASA and UDCA, the later only in the setting of IBD and concurrent PSC.[26]

Control of inflammation is likely the key in reducing colitis-associated dysplasia risk in IBD. Once inflammation has been controlled, it is unclear if any medical therapy can offer additional dysplasia prophylaxis in IBD. Indeed, UC patients with endoscopic remission and a macroscopically normal looking colon on colonoscopy are not at the increased risk of CRC as compared to the general population.[6] Mucosal healing, therefore, is an appropriate aim for treatment and part of the "treat-to-target" strategy in IBD. In patients who maintain mucosal healing, colorectal dysplasia risk reduction strategies should mirror that of the general population, directed against sporadic dysplasia.

A challenge remains with patients with areas of active colitis despite maximal therapy; however, not severe enough to warrant a colectomy. Currently, 5-ASA are the only medical therapy with sufficient evidence in preventing colitis-associated dysplasia that appears to have a specific chemoprophylactic effect outside of simply suppressing inflammation. In these cases, a step-up strategy toward more efficacious treatment should be adopted. Further studies that focus on PPARγ agonists and COX-2 inhibitors are also required.

References

1. V Annese, L Beaugerie, L Egan, *et al.* (2015) European evidence-based consensus: Inflammatory bowel disease and malignancies. *J Crohns Colitis* **9**: 945–965.
2. JA Eaden, KR Abrams, JF Mayberry (2001) The risk of colorectal cancer in ulcerative colitis: A meta-analysis. *Gut* **48**: 526–535.
3. CP Selinger, J Andrews, OF Dent, I Norton, B Jones, C McDonald, J Cowlishaw, G Barr, W Selby, RW Leong (2013) Cause-specific mortality and 30-year relative survival of Crohn's disease and ulcerative colitis. *Inflamm Bowel Dis* **19**: 1880–1888.
4. CP Selinger, JM Andrews, A Titman, I Norton, BD Jones, C McDonald, G Barr, W Selby, RW Leong (2014) Long-term follow-up reveals low incidence of colorectal cancer, but frequent need for resection, among Australian patients with inflammatory bowel disease. *Clin Gastroenterol Hepatol* **12**: 644–650.
5. V Annese, M Daperno, MD Rutter, A Amiot, P Bossuyt, J East, M Ferrante, M Gotz, KH Katsanos, R Kiesslich, I Ordas, A Repici, B Rosa, S Sebastian, T Kucharzik, R Eliakim (2013) European evidence based consensus for endoscopy in inflammatory bowel disease. *J Crohns Colitis* **7**: 982–1018.
6. MD Rutter, BP Saunders, KH Wilkinson, S Rumbles, G Schofield, MA Kamm, CB Williams, AB Price, IC Talbot, A Forbes (2004) Cancer surveillance in longstanding ulcerative colitis: Endoscopic appearances help predict cancer risk. *Gut* **53**: 1813–1816.

7. SH Itzkowitz, X Yio (2004) Inflammation and cancer IV. Colorectal cancer in inflammatory bowel disease: The role of inflammation. *Am J Physiol Gastrointest Liver Physiol* **287**: G7–17.
8. AS Fleisher, M Esteller, N Harpaz, A Leytin, A Rashid, Y Xu, J Liang, OC Stine, J Yin, TT Zou, JM Abtaham, D Kong, KT Wilson, SP James, JG Herman, SJ Meltzer (2000) Microsatellite instability in inflammatory bowel disease-associated neoplastic lesions is associated with hypermethylation and diminished expression of the DNA mismatch repair gene, hMLH1. *Cancer Res* **60**: 4864–4868.
9. M Fukata, A Chen, AS Vamadevan, J Cohen, K Breglio, S Krishnareddy, D Hsu, R Xu, N Harpaz, AJ Dannenberg, K Subbaramaiah, HS Cooper, SH Itzkowitz, MT Abreu (2007) Toll-like receptor-4 promotes the development of colitis-associated colorectal tumors. *Gastroenterology* **133**: 1869–1881.
10. AJ Schottelius, H Dinter (2006) Cytokines, NF-kappaB, microenvironment, intestinal inflammation and cancer. *Cancer Treat Res* **130**: 67–87.
11. D Wang, RN DuBois (2004) Cyclooxygenase 2-derived prostaglandin E2 regulates the angiogenic switch. *Proc Natl Acad Sci USA* **101**: 415–416.
12. CL Chang, G Marra, DP Chauhan, HT Ha, DK Chang, L Ricciardiello, JM Carethers, CR Boland (2002) Oxidative stress inactivates the human DNA mismatch repair system. *Am J Physiol Cell Physiol* **283**: C148–154.
13. H Kimura, R Hokari, S Miura, T Shigematsu, M Hirokawa, Y Akiba, I Kurose, H Higuchi, H Fujimori, Y Tsuzuki, H Serizawa, H Ishii (1998) Increased expression of an inducible isoform of nitric oxide synthase and the formation of peroxynitrite in colonic mucosa of patients with active ulcerative colitis. *Gut* **42**: 180–187.
14. K Shigaki, H Mitomi, T Fujimori, K Ichokawa, S Tomita, J Imura, S Fujii, M Itabashi, S Kameoka, R Sahara, S Takenoshita (2013) Immunohistochemical analysis of chromogranin A and p53 expressions in ulcerative colitis-associated neoplasia: Neuroendocrine differentiation as an early event in the colitis-neoplasia sequence. *Hum Pathol* **44**: 2393–2399.
15. V Subramanian, RF Logan. (2011) Chemoprevention of colorectal cancer in inflammatory bowel disease. *Best Pract Res Clin Gastroenterol* **25**: 593–606.
16. PL Lakatos, L Lakatos (2008) Risk for colorectal cancer in ulcerative colitis: Changes, causes and management strategies. *World J Gastroenterol* **14**: 3937–3947.
17. CH Choi, MD Rutter, A Askari, GH Lee, J Warusavitarne, M Moorghen, S Thomas-Gibson, BP Saunders, TA Graham, AL Hart (2015) Forty-year analysis of colonoscopic surveillance program for neoplasia in ulcerative colitis: An updated overview. *Am J Gastroenterol* **110**: 1022–1034.

18. P Sharon, M Ligumsky, D Rachmilewitz, U Zor (1978) Role of prostaglandins in ulcerative colitis. Enhanced production during active disease and inhibition by sulfasalazine. *Gastroenterology* **75**: 638–640.
19. I Ahnfelt-Ronne, OH Nielsen, A Christensen, E Langholz, V Binder, P Riis (1990) Clinical evidence supporting the radical scavenger mechanism of 5-aminosalicylic acid. *Gastroenterology* **98**: 1162–1169.
20. C Rousseaux, N El-Jamal, M Fumery, C Dubuquoy, O Romano, D Chatelain, A Langlois, B Bertin, D Buod, JF Colombel, A Cortot, P Desreumax, L Dubuqouy (2013) The 5-aminosalicylic acid antineoplastic effect in the intestine is mediated by PPARgamma. *Carcinogenesis* **34**: 2580–2586.
21. C Rousseaux, B Lefebvre, L Dubuquoy, P Lefebvre, O Romano, J Auwerx, D Metzger, W Wahli, B Desvergne, BC Naccari, P Chavatte, A Farce, P Bulois, A Cortot, JF Colombel, P Desreumaux (2005) Intestinal antiinflammatory effect of 5-aminosalicylic acid is dependent on peroxisome proliferator-activated receptor-gamma. *J Exp Med* **201**: 1205–1215.
22. LN Zhao, JY Li, T Yu, GC Chen, YH Yuan, QK Chen (2014) 5-Aminosalicylates reduce the risk of colorectal neoplasia in patients with ulcerative colitis: An updated meta-analysis. *PLoS One* **9**: e94208.
23. TP van Staa, T Card, RF Logan, HG Leufkens (2005) 5-Aminosalicylate use and colorectal cancer risk in inflammatory bowel disease: A large epidemiological study. *Gut* **54**: 1573–1578.
24. GC Nguyen, A Gulamhusein, CN Bernstein (2012) 5-aminosalicylic acid is not protective against colorectal cancer in inflammatory bowel disease: A meta-analysis of non-referral populations. *Am J Gastroenterol* **107**: 1298–1304.
25. HJ Freeman (2002) Tabulation of myeloid, lymphoid and intestinal malignancies in Crohn's disease. *Can J Gastroenterol* **16**: 779–784.
26. FA Farraye, RD Odze, J Eaden, SH Itzkowitz, RP McCabe, T Dassopoulos, JD Lewis, TA Ullman, T James, R McLeod, LJ Burgart, J Allen, JV Brill (2010) AGA medical position statement on the diagnosis and management of colorectal neoplasia in inflammatory bowel disease. *Gastroenterology* **138**: 738–745.
27. M Harbord, R Eliakim, F Magro, V Annese, F Carbonnel, A Strum, P Gionchetti (2014) European Crohn's and Colitis Organisation e-Guide: Aminosalicylates. http://www.e-guide.ecco-ibd.eu/ interventions-therapeutic/aminosalicylates#ulcerative-colitis. Accessed February 21, 2016.
28. CP Selinger, J Eaden, DB Jones, P Katelaris, G Chapman, C McDonald, P Smith, S Lal, RW Leong, J McLaughlin, A Robinson (2013) Modifiable factors associated with nonadherence to maintenance medication for inflammatory bowel disease. *Inflamm Bowel Dis* **19**: 2199–2206.

29. CP Selinger, A Kemp, RW Leong (2014) Persistence to oral 5-aminosalicylate therapy for inflammatory bowel disease in Australia. *Expert Rev Gastroenterol Hepatol* **8**: 329–334.
30. LJ Derijks, LP Gilissen, PM Hooymans, DW Hommes (2006) Review article: Thiopurines in inflammatory bowel disease. *Aliment Pharmacol Ther* **24**: 715–729.
31. L Beaugerie (2015) Do thiopurines really decrease the risk of colorectal cancer in ulcerative colitis? The light is coming from concept-based subgroup analyses. *J Crohns Colitis* **9**: 1061–1062.
32. A Gutierrez-Dalmau, JM Campistol (2007) Immunosuppressive therapy and malignancy in organ transplant recipients: A systematic review. *Drugs* **67**: 1167–1198.
33. J Gong, L Zhu, Z Guo, Y Li, W Zhu, N Li, J Li (2013) Use of thiopurines and risk of colorectal neoplasia in patients with inflammatory bowel diseases: A meta-analysis. *PLoS One* **8**: e81487.
34. J Gordillo, E Cabre, E Garcia-Planella, E Ricart, Y Ber-Nieto, L Marquez, F Bodriguez-Moranta, A Ponferrada, I Vera, JP Gisbert, J Barrio, M Esteve, O Merino, F Munoz, E Domenech (2015) Thiopurine therapy reduces the incidence of colorectal neoplasia in patients with ulcerative colitis. Data from the ENEIDA Registry. *J Crohns Colitis* **9**: 1063–1070.
35. L Beaugerie, M Svrcek, P Seksik, AM Bouvier, T Simon, M Allez, H Brixi, JM Gornet, R Altwegg, P Beau, B Duclos, A Bourreille, J Faivre, L Peyrin-Biroulet, JF Flejou, F Carrat (2013) Risk of colorectal high-grade dysplasia and cancer in a prospective observational cohort of patients with inflammatory bowel disease. *Gastroenterology* **145**: 166–175.
36. T Jess, A Lopez, M Andersson, L Beaugerie, L Peyrin-Biroulet (2014) Thiopurines and risk of colorectal neoplasia in patients with inflammatory bowel disease: A meta-analysis. *Clin Gastroenterol Hepatol* **12**: 1793–1800.
37. X Wang, Y Lin (2008) Tumor necrosis factor and cancer, buddies or foes? *Acta Pharmacol Sin* **29**: 1275–1288.
38. BK Popivanova, K Kitamura, Y Wu, *et al.* (2008) Blocking TNF-alpha in mice reduces colorectal carcinogenesis associated with chronic colitis. *J Clin Invest* **118**: 560–570.
39. CG Chapman, DT Rubin (2014) The potential for medical therapy to reduce the risk of colorectal cancer and optimize surveillance in inflammatory bowel disease. *Gastrointest Endosc Clin N Am* **24**: 353–365.
40. N Nyboe Andersen, B Pasternak, S Basit, M Andersson, H Svanstrom, S Caspersen, P Munkholm, A Hviid, T Jess (2014) Association between tumor necrosis factor-alpha antagonists and risk of cancer in patients with inflammatory bowel disease. *JAMA* **311**: 2406–2413.

41. JE Baars, CW Looman, EW Steyerberg, R Beukers, AC Tan, BL Weusten, EJ Kuipers, CJ van der Woude (2011) The risk of inflammatory bowel disease-related colorectal carcinoma is limited: Results from a nationwide nested case-control study. *Am J Gastroenterol* **106**: 319–328.
42. RE Rossi, D Conte, S Massironi (2016) Primary sclerosing cholangitis associated with inflammatory bowel disease: An update. *Eur J Gastroenterol Hepatol* **28**: 123–131.
43. DL Earnest, H Holubec, RK Wali, CS Jolley, M Bissonette, AK Bhattacharyya, H Roy, S Khare, TA Brasitus (1994) Chemoprevention of azoxymethane-induced colonic carcinogenesis by supplemental dietary ursodeoxycholic acid. *Cancer Res* **54**: 5071–5074.
44. JD Martinez, ED Stratagoules, JM LaRue, AA Powell, PR Gause, MT Craven, CM Payne, MB Powell, EW Gerner, DL Earnest (1998) Different bile acids exhibit distinct biological effects: The tumor promoter deoxycholic acid induces apoptosis and the chemopreventive agent ursodeoxycholic acid inhibits cell proliferation. *Nutr Cancer* **31**: 111–118.
45. S Khare, R Mustafi, S Cerda, W Yuan, S Jagadeeswaran, U Dougherty, M Tretiakova, A Samarel, G Cohen, J Wang, C Moore, R Wali, C Holgren, L Joseph, A Fichera, YC Li, M Bissonnette (2008) Ursodeoxycholic acid suppresses Cox-2 expression in colon cancer: Roles of Ras, p38, and CCAAT/enhancer-binding protein. *Nutr Cancer* **60**: 389–400.
46. BY Tung, MJ Emond, RC Haggitt, MP Bronner, MB Kimmey, KV Kowdley, TA Brantnall (2001) Ursodiol use is associated with lower prevalence of colonic neoplasia in patients with ulcerative colitis and primary sclerosing cholangitis. *Ann Intern Med* **134**: 89–95.
47. DS Pardi, EV Loftus Jr., WK Kremers, J Keach, KD Lindor (2003) Ursodeoxycholic acid as a chemopreventive agent in patients with ulcerative colitis and primary sclerosing cholangitis. *Gastroenterology* **124**: 889–893.
48. JE Eaton, MG Silveira, DS Pardi, E Sinakos, KV Kowdley, VA Luketic, ME Harrison, T McCashland, AS Befeler, D Harnois, R Jorgensen, J Petz, KD Lindor (2011) High-dose ursodeoxycholic acid is associated with the development of colorectal neoplasia in patients with ulcerative colitis and primary sclerosing cholangitis. *Am J Gastroenterol* **106**: 1638–1645.
49. JM Wolf, LA Rybicki, BA Lashner (2005) The impact of ursodeoxycholic acid on cancer, dysplasia and mortality in ulcerative colitis patients with primary sclerosing cholangitis. *Aliment Pharmacol Ther* **22**: 783–788.
50. DS Alberts, ME Martinez, LM Hess, JG Einspahr, SB Green, AK Bhattacharyya, J Guillen, M Krutzsch, AK Batta, G Salen, L Fales, K Koonce, D Parish, M Clouser, D Roe, P Lance (2005) Phase III trial of ursodeoxycholic acid to prevent colorectal adenoma recurrence. *J Natl Cancer Inst* **97**: 846–853.

51. PA Thompson, BC Wertheim, DJ Roe, EL Ashbeck, ET Jacobs, P Lance, ME Martinez, DS Alberts (2009) Gender modifies the effect of ursodeoxycholic acid in a randomized controlled trial in colorectal adenoma patients. *Cancer Prev Res (Phila)* **2**: 1023–1030.
52. JL Freudenheim, S Graham, JR Marshall, BP Haughey, S Cholewinski, G Wilkinson (1991) Folate intake and carcinogenesis of the colon and rectum. *Int J Epidemiol* **20**: 368–374.
53. T Qin, M Du, H Du, Y Shu, M Wang, L Zhu (2015) Folic acid supplements and colorectal cancer risk: Meta-analysis of randomized controlled trials. *Sci Rep* **5**: 12044.
54. JM Phelip, V Ducros, JL Faucheron, B Flourie, X Roblin (2008) Association of hyperhomocysteinemia and folate deficiency with colon tumors in patients with inflammatory bowel disease. *Inflamm Bowel Dis* **14**: 242–248.
55. C Hwang, V Ross, U Mahadevan (2012) Micronutrient deficiencies in inflammatory bowel disease: From A to zinc. *Inflamm Bowel Dis* **18**: 1961–1981.
56. G Biasco, MC Di Marco (2005) Folate and prevention of colorectal cancer in ulcerative colitis. *Eur J Cancer Prev* **14**: 395–398.
57. ES Schernhammer, S Ogino, CS Fuchs (2008) Folate and vitamin B6 intake and risk of colon cancer in relation to p53 expression. *Gastroenterology* **135**: 770–780.
58. KJ Sohn, JM Stempak, S Reid, S Shirwadkar, JB Mason, YI Kim (2003) The effect of dietary folate on genomic and p53-specific DNA methylation in rat colon. *Carcinogenesis* **24**: 81–90.
59. G Biasco, U Zannoni, GM Paganelli, R Santucci, P Gionchetti, G Rivolta, R Miniero, L Pironi, C Calabrese, G Di Febo, M Miglioli (1997) Folic acid supplementation and cell kinetics of rectal mucosa in patients with ulcerative colitis. *Cancer Epidemiol Biomarkers Prev* **6**: 469–471.
60. J Tang, O Sharif, C Pai, AL Silverman (2010) Mesalamine protects against colorectal cancer in inflammatory bowel disease. *Dig Dis Sci* **55**: 1696–1703.
61. L Moreira, A Castells (2011) Cyclooxygenase as a target for colorectal cancer chemoprevention. *Curr Drug Targets* **12**: 1888–1894.
62. B Rigas, GJ Tsioulias (2015) The evolving role of nonsteroidal anti-inflammatory drugs in colon cancer prevention: A cause for optimism. *J Pharmacol Exp Ther* **353**: 2–8.
63. FS Velayos, EV Loftus Jr., T Jess, WS Harmsen, J Bida, AR Zinsmeister, WJ Tremaine, WJ Sandborn (2006) Predictive and protective factors associated with colorectal cancer in ulcerative colitis: A case-control study. *Gastroenterology* **130**: 1941–1949.

64. A Shaukat, N Scouras, HJ Schunemann (2005) Role of supplemental calcium in the recurrence of colorectal adenomas: A metaanalysis of randomized controlled trials. *Am J Gastroenterol* **100**: 390–394.
65. D Aune, R Lau, DS Chan, R Vieira, DC Greenwood, E Kampman, T Norat (2012) Dairy products and colorectal cancer risk: A systematic review and meta-analysis of cohort studies. *Ann Oncol* **23**: 37–45.
66. JC Fleet, M DeSmet, R Johnson, Y Li (2012) Vitamin D and cancer: A review of molecular mechanisms. *Biochem J* **441**: 61–76.
67. JA Baron, EL Barry, LA Mott, JR Rees, RS Sandler, DC Snover, RM Bostick, A Ivanova, BF Cole, DJ Ahnen, GJ Beck, RS Bresalier, CA Burke, TR Church, M Cruz-Correa, JC Figueiredo, M Goodman, AS Kim, GJ Robertson, R Rothstein, A Shaukat, ME Seabrook, RW Summers (2015) A trial of calcium and vitamin D for the prevention of colorectal adenomas. *New Engl J Med* **373**: 1519–1530.
68. M Chung, J Lee, T Terasawa, J Lau, TA Trikalinos (2011) Vitamin D with or without calcium supplementation for prevention of cancer and fractures: An updated meta-analysis for the U.S. Preventive Services Task Force. *Ann Intern Med* **155**: 827–838.
69. GH Cai, MX Li, L Lu, RL Yi Chan, JH Wang, CH Cho (2015) The current role and therapeutic targets of vitamin D in gastrointestinal inflammation and cancer. *Curr Pharm Des* **21**: 2917–2923.
70. VP Mouli, AN Ananthakrishnan (2014) Review article: Vitamin D and inflammatory bowel diseases. *Aliment Pharmacol Ther* **39**: 125–136.
71. S Meeker, A Seamons, J Paik, PM Treuting, T Brabb, WM Grady, L Maggio-Price (2014) Increased dietary vitamin D suppresses MAPK signaling, colitis, and colon cancer. *Cancer Res* **74**: 4398–4408.
72. FM Sacks, MA Pfeffer, LA Moye, JL Rouleau, JD Rutherford, TG Cole, L Brown, JW Warnica, JM Arnold, CC Wun, BR Davis, E Braunwald (1996) The effect of pravastatin on coronary events after myocardial infarction in patients with average cholesterol levels. Cholesterol and Recurrent Events Trial investigators. *New Engl J Med* **335**: 1001–1009.
73. JN Poynter, SB Gruber, PD Higgins, R Almog, JD Bonner, HS Rennert, M Low, JK Greenson, G Rennart (2005) Statins and the risk of colorectal cancer. *New Engl J Med* **352**: 2184–2192.
74. NJ Samadder, B Mukherjee, SC Huang, J Ahn, HS Rennert, JK Greenson, G Rennert, SB Gruber (2011) Risk of colorectal cancer in self-reported inflammatory bowel disease and modification of risk by statin and NSAID use. *Cancer* **117**: 1640–1648.

Chapter 4

Targeting the Nuclear Receptor HNF4α as a Potential Therapy for Gut Inflammation and Cancer

Jean-Philippe Babeu and François Boudreau

Abstract

Nuclear receptors are modulatable regulators influenced by the binding of specific ligands that in turn will dictate their capacities to control gene transcription. The hepatocyte nuclear factor-4α (HNF4α) belongs to this class of transcription factors and is expressed in the epithelium of several tissues of endoderm origin. HNF4α functions have been associated with many cellular and developmental processes, including morphogenesis, cellular proliferation, cellular differentiation, metabolism, and inflammation. It is thus not surprising that HNF4α has been linked to several pathologies, including diabetes, cancer, and chronic inflammation. This chapter will review the overall structure of HNF4α and its multiple isoforms that are produced within the cell. An overlook of documented roles for HNF4α in cancer and inflammation will be provided, with a focus on the gastrointestinal system. The nature of the multiple molecular mechanisms that has been reported to influence the HNF4α expression and activity will also be covered. Finally, the potential of targeting this unique class of nuclear receptors as therapeutic means will be discussed.

Introduction

Most of all characteristics and biological functions of a cell are encoded in its genome. The genes contain under their specific deoxyribonucleic acid (DNA) sequences all the necessary information to allow the synthesis of ribonucleic acids (RNAs), which in turn will be decoded as proteins in order to ensure the diverse biological functions of the various cells that constitute a specific tissue. However, this information contained in the genome must be closely controlled, so that the cells of an entire organism can express only the genes that are required for their specific functions. The tight regulation of the entire set of RNA molecules produced within a cell, the so-called transcriptome, is thus of a crucial importance to the cell function. It now becomes well accepted that significant alterations in the cell transcriptome can be associated with diverse pathologies, including chronic inflammation and cancer. Although very complex, the mechanisms that dictate gene expression and transcriptome composition within the cell rely on a subtype of cellular proteins referred to as transcription factors. These proteins control gene expression by their capacity to interact directly on specific sequence sets of the genome for which their nature will dictate what specific transcription factor will interact with them. This direct interaction of the transcription factor with the chromatin influences the recruitment of multiple protein complexes to activate or inhibit gene transcription and, by extension, specify cellular behavior. There is a growing interest in targeting transcription factors as a means for cancer therapy.[1] One particular class of transcription factors that has been the subject of most druggable strategies is the nuclear receptors, mainly because of their ability to naturally interact with ligands, often metabolites, that influence their transcriptional activities. In this chapter, a structural overview of the nuclear receptors, with a focus on hepatocyte nuclear factor-4α (HNF4α), will be provided. Cellular functions of HNF4α and its isoforms will be discussed and integrated in the context of cancer. The nature of multiple mechanisms known to control HNF4α activity will be covered and discussed as potential strategies for therapeutic usage against gut inflammation and cancer.

Nuclear Receptors as Subtypes of Transcriptional Regulators

Transcription factors are divided into various classes of proteins according to their structure and their type of DNA-binding domains (DBDs). Among

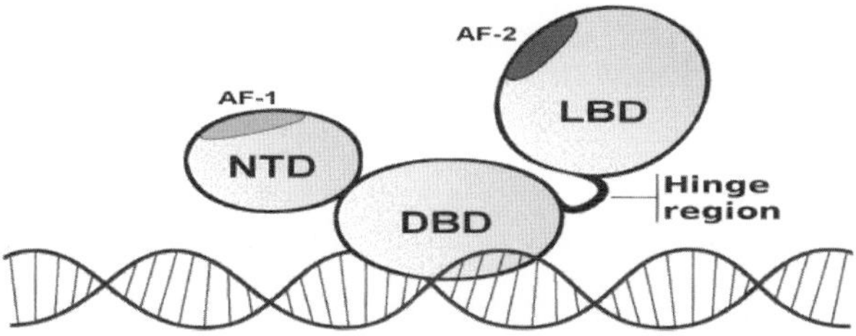

Figure 1. Nuclear receptors and their structural features. The nuclear receptors share a conserved flexible structure that contains four major domains. The NTD contains the activating region AF-1 that allows interactions with cofactors. The DBD is highly conserved and contains two zinc finger motifs that allow interaction with DNA. The hinge region links the DBD to the LBD that is localized at the C-terminal region. The LBD contains a hydrophobic pocket responsible for ligand binding as well as a second activating region AF-2 that also allows interactions with cofactors.

these classes are the nuclear receptors that are functionally involved in a large number of cellular processes, including metabolism, development, reproduction, proliferation, and inflammation.[2,3] The nuclear receptors share a common structure and are characterized by their flexible activation via their interaction with a ligand. Their structure is divided into four main domains: the N-terminal domain (NTD), the DBD, the hinge region, and the ligand-binding domain (LBD; Figure 1).

The NTD contains the transcriptional activating function (AF-1) of nuclear receptors, and this motif is independent of ligand interaction. However, AF-1 allows synergic activation with a second activating region (AF-2) that is classically located in the LBD of the nuclear receptors.[3] The NTD varies in terms of size which gives rise to the specificity of action for each member that belongs to the large nuclear receptors family. The DBD represents the region that is the most preserved one among nuclear receptor members. It contains two zinc finger motifs, allowing the recognition and interaction of the nuclear receptors with their respective specific DNA elements. In addition, the DBD second zinc finger motif facilitates dimerization between nuclear receptors. The hinge region, for which its flexible nature allows connecting the DBD with the LBD, contains a nuclear location signal and is the target of numerous posttranslational modifications. Finally, the LBD contains a hydrophobic pocket responsible for ligand binding that then engenders a conformation change, allowing cofactors to interact with the AF-2 and stimulate gene transcription. For a subclass of nuclear receptors, the absence of ligand will lead to corepressors recruitment and to block gene transcription. Besides its transactivation activity, the LBD region is also involved in nuclear receptors dimerization, an essential step for the recruitment of many nuclear receptors to their specific DNA elements.[2,3]

Nuclear receptors are expressed in a wide range of tissues and cellular types. While some are ubiquitous, others are restricted to precise cellular types where they can regulate specific transcriptional networks. In the gastrointestinal epithelium, several transcription factors have been identified to collaborate together for the establishment and maintenance of a cell-specific transcriptional program. Among these, the nuclear receptor HNF4α turned out to be particularly important for the development and the homeostasis of the digestive tract.

The nuclear receptor HNF4α

HNF4α was first identified as a protein binding to the promoter of genes specifically expressed in the liver. However, it became rapidly obvious that this nuclear receptor was not exclusive to this tissue. The HNF4α expression can be detected in the epithelia of the stomach, small intestine, colon, liver, pancreas, kidneys, and the epididymis.[4] HNF4α has become an epithelial transcription factor that is today considered as a key regulator of the transcriptome in the liver, the pancreas, and the gut.[5–9]

Structural characteristics of HNF4α

HNF4α belongs to the superfamily of the nuclear receptors based on its overall structural organization. HNF4α contains one or two AF regions, depending on the nature of the isoforms studied. The AF-2 region is located in the LBD region, while the AF-1 region is located in the NTD region.[10] The HNF4α DBD region contains two zinc fingers involved in HNF4α homodimerization and DNA recognition.[11] Besides the AF-2 region, the LBD harbors a ligand-binding pocket, also involved in receptor dimerization.[11] HNF4α also displays a long C-terminal region for which the function is not well understood. Some studies have suggested that this region could be involved in the regulation of its overall transcriptional activity.[10,12]

In order to regulate the transcription of its target genes, HNF4α binds to a responsive element constituted by a repetition of the sequence AGGTCA separated by some nucleotides to constitute a DR1 type sequence. It is, however, recognized that HNF4α can also bind to variants of this consensus sequence; this would explain why HNF4α is able to bind to a very large number of sites in the genome.[13] To interact with DNA, HNF4α needs to homodimerize in order to allow every partner to interact with one of the repetitions of the DR1 site. However, HNF4α distinguishes itself from other nuclear receptors because of its lack of potential to form heterodimers, even though its structure shares important similarities with other nuclear receptors such as Retinoid X receptor alpha (RXRα).[11]

What also distinguishes HNF4α from other nuclear receptors is that its endogenous activity appears to be independent from ligand–LBD interactions.[14] Although originally identified as an orphan nuclear receptor, several follow-up studies suggested that 14–18 carbon fatty acids could interact within the HNF4α ligand-binding pocket. Controversy remains, however, as for the identity and the real contribution of these ligands to HNF4α activity since a vast majority of transcriptional studies were done with recombinant proteins produced in bacteria, excluding the possibility of endogenous interactions with such lipids.[14,15] Furthermore, crystallography experiments suggest that the presence of a fatty acid in the LBD is not required for HNF4α to adopt a closed and active structure on the DNA, but rather the interaction of a cofactor would allow HNF4α to keep its active conformation for this to occur.[16] Nevertheless, several studies indicated that HNF4α transcriptional activity can be efficiently modulated by agonists or antagonists.[17–20] The potential of regulating HNF4α activity by synthetic compounds represents an interesting therapeutic asset, given HNF4α involvement in several pathologies, including diabetes, hemophilia, inflammatory bowel diseases, and cancer.

HNF4α consists of several isoforms

HNF4α is located on chromosome 20, contains 13 exons, and is characterized by the presence of two distinct and functional promoters. The regulatory combination of alternative splicing and usage of these promoters allows the synthesis of nine different HNF4α isoforms (Figure 2). Two main classes of

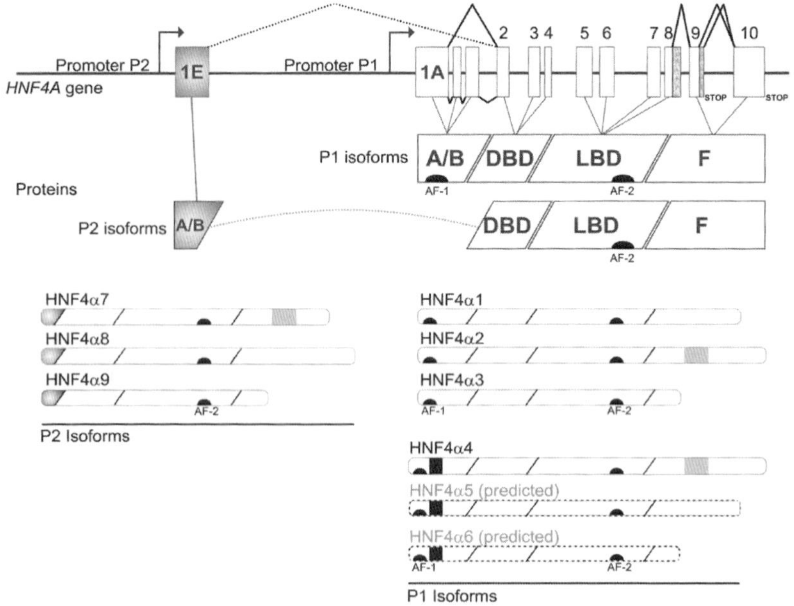

Figure 2. HNF4α isoforms. The *HNF4α* gene allows the production of nine distinct isoforms with the combination of alternative splicing and the use of two independent promoters. HNF4α isoforms are divided into two main classes according to the promoter that is used for their production. The P1 isoforms class contains isoforms α1–α6 that are produced from the P1 proximal promoter. The P2 isoforms class contains isoforms α7–α9 that are produced from the distal P2 promoter. Isoforms from each class are distinct from the result of alternative splicing. 3′ alternative splicing affects all isoforms from each class, whereas 5′ alternative splicing only affects P1 isoforms with the result of leading to a unique NTD for the P1 isoforms. This domain contains the activating region AF-1 that is not present in the P2 isoforms.

HNF4α isoforms are classified according to the nature of the promoter responsible for their initial transcription. The P1 class of isoforms (HNF4α1 to HNF4α6) harbors all the isoforms transcribed from the proximal promoter, while the P2 class of isoforms (HNF4α7 to HNF4α9) contains those transcribed from the distal promoter. Alternative splicing modifies the C-terminal region for some of these isoforms by allowing the inclusion of 10 additional amino acids or by creating a codon stop that results in premature translational ending. In the case of P1 isoforms, alternative splicing results in the incorporation of 30 additional amino acids at the NTD region. The major structural distinction between P1 and P2 classes of isoforms is thus located at the NTD and results from the usage of different exons during splicing events. This leads to the production of P1 isoforms containing the

AF-1 region within the NTD and P2 isoforms having a shorter and different NTD that is devoid of AF-1.

The overall cellular impact generated by the alternative splicing of *HNF4α* and the production of multiple isoforms is not known. Many nuclear receptors undergo similar alternative splicing events, suggesting a regulatory phenomenon of functional importance for these regulators in general. Experiments based on the activation of genes reporters showed that, in general, P1 isoforms represent better positive modulators of transcription than P2 isoforms.[21] This difference was accounted to the absence of the AF-1 in P2 isoforms, a region known to allow the synergistic activation of target gene promoters in combination with the AF-2 region, as well as to allow physical interactions with cofactors and general transcription factors. Nevertheless, both P1 and P2 isoforms share the same DBD that allows specific interaction with DNA. They also contain the AF-2 region that recruits cofactors for transcription. It would then be tempting to conclude that these isoforms share similar cellular functions based on their similar capacity to be recruited on the chromatin via the exact same DNA element, as well as to similarly recruit the same cofactors via interaction with the AF-2 region.[22] However, there are several arguments suggesting that P1 and P2 isoforms could functionally display different cellular roles. Firstly, the expression of P1 and P2 isoforms varies according to specific organs and developmental stage. In an adult, only P1 isoforms are expressed in the liver and kidneys, while both stomach and pancreas solely express P2 isoforms. The adult small intestine and colon are the only organs where both classes of isoforms are simultaneously expressed. During mouse fetal development, the liver expresses both classes of isoforms, while the expression of P2 isoforms declines at birth to completely vanish in adulthood.[23] Secondly, HNF4α conditional deletion in the mouse pancreas (P2-only isoforms) as compared to the liver (P1-only isoforms) differently affects biological processes in these tissues. Indeed, the conditional deletion of HNF4α in hepatocytes leads to abnormal cellular differentiation that results in premature death,[24] while the specific deletion of HNF4α into pancreatic islets stimulates cellular proliferation without significantly affecting cellular differentiation.[25,26] Thirdly, transgenic mice expressing P2-only isoforms display dyslipidemia, while mice expressing P1-only isoforms show some glucose intolerance.[27] Thus, although some redundancy of functions exists between P1 and P2 isoforms, it becomes clear that specific roles for each of these classes of isoforms must exist in the organism. The nature of these differences remains, however, to be clarified.

Cellular functions of HNF4α

HNF4α regulates a large number of genes that collectively regulate several cellular functions, including morphogenesis, tissue development, cellular proliferation, cellular differentiation, metabolism, and inflammation. HNF4α regulates a subset of genes that control embryonic development, more specifically during the liver and gut morphogenesis. Indeed, the disruption of HNF4α in mice resulted in impaired visceral endoderm gastrulation, leading to embryonic death around day 7.5 postcoitus.[28] To further study the function of HNF4α beyond this developmental stage, conditional-deletion strategies were developed. The conditional deletion of HNF4α in the mouse embryonic liver resulted in the loss of the architecture of this organ, as exemplified by incomplete hepatocyte differentiation and liver organization.[24] The conditional deletion of HNF4α in the mouse embryonic colon led to crypts architecture loss, altered cellular proliferation, incomplete goblet cell differentiation, and impaired expression of numerous genes associated to colonic functions.[9]

At the adult stage, HNF4α is involved in regulating cellular differentiation and metabolism. Numerous studies carried out with hepatic or intestinal epithelial cell lineages demonstrated that HNF4α regulates cellular differentiation.[29,30] Moreover, the HNF4α exogenous expression in fibroblasts allows the initiation of an epithelial differentiation program,[24] which can be managed toward an intestinal phenotype when combined with the intestinal epithelial transcription factors, CDX-2 and GATA-4.[7] HNF4α role in lipid metabolism was highlighted by its conditional deletion in the mouse adult liver. Contrary to the embryonic observations, the overall liver structure of these animals remained unaltered, but lipid metabolism was found to be profoundly altered with dyslipidemia and death up to 4 weeks following liver specific HNF4α deletion.[31] HNF4α is also suspected to regulate intestinal lipid metabolism through the direct regulation of apolipoproteins,[32] as well as several other genes intimately involved in this process.[6] HNF4α also regulates carbohydrate metabolism by activating the expression of several genes that encode key regulatory enzymes in gluconeogenesis.[33] Mutations within *HNF4α* are associated with the MODY1 form of maturity onset diabetes of the young, supporting again its role in glucose metabolism.[25]

Several experimental pieces of evidence support a functional role of HNF4α in the regulation of liver and gut inflammation. In the liver, HNF4α regulates a large number of genes associated with the acute phase response during inflammation[34] and is part of a retroinhibition loop of the IL-6/STAT3 inflammatory signaling pathway.[35] In the mouse colonic epithelium, HNF4α conditional deletion resulted in long-term spontaneous inflammation with similar features observed in human intestinal inflammatory diseases.[8] This phenotype correlates well with the decrease of the HNF4α expression as observed in human gut samples derived from ulcerative colitis and Crohn's disease.[8,36] Interestingly, HNF4α was identified as one of the susceptibility genes associated with ulcerative colitis.[37]

Finally, HNF4α influences cell proliferation by regulating and interacting with several cell cycle regulators. On the one hand, the forced expression of HNF4α in embryonic kidney cells is able to induce a gene network linked to the inhibition of cell proliferation.[38] Under the same cellular context, HNF4α can regulate the expression of the cell cycle inhibitor p21 to inhibit cell proliferation and induce differentiation.[39] HNF4α also binds to the Wnt/β-catenin transcriptional effector TCF4 to functionally reduce intestinal epithelial cells growth.[40] On the other hand, HNF4α acts differently in the pancreatic cellular context where its expression is required to support islet beta cell proliferation during metabolic stress.[41] On a mechanistic view, HNF4α pancreatic conditional deletion reduced the ST5 expression, an upstream activator of the Extracellular signal-regulated kinase/Mitogen-activated protein kinase (ERK/MAPK) pathway that is essential for cell proliferation.[41] In support of this apparent opposite role for HNF4α in controlling cell proliferation, the overexpression of the HNF4α8 P2 isoform stimulated the reentrance of pancreatic beta cells into the cellular cycle.[26]

Thus, HNF4α regulates several biological processes among various epithelial tissue sources. The molecular mechanisms and biological impacts by which HNF4α controls these processes appear to be variable according to the cellular context and this might be dependent on the nature of the specific HNF4α isoforms involved.

HNF4α's involvement in cancer

HNF4α regulates cellular proliferation, differentiation, and metabolism that are all closely related with carcinogenesis. Several studies have linked HNF4α

functions with the initiation and progression of cancer and this, in the context of several epithelial derived tissues. However, most of the studies so far have been done in the context of liver cancer.

HNF4α and liver cancer

HNF4α is expressed in hepatocytes where it regulates the metabolism of carbohydrates, lipids, and xenobiotic in differentiated cells. During mouse embryonic development, the liver expresses both classes of HNF4α isoforms with a strong ascendancy for P2 isoforms. At birth, the HNF4α P2 isoform expression declines progressively, while the HNF4α P1 isoform expression increases to become the only isoforms expressed in the adult liver.[23,42,43] During the premature phases of liver carcinogenesis, there is a switch of expression between HNF4α isoforms, where P2 becomes more abundant as it is observed during early liver development. However, the global HNF4α expression gradually decreases during carcinogenesis progression to become almost undetectable in most advanced disease stages, when hepatocytes dedifferentiate.[43,44]

Several experimental facts support the concept that HNF4α acts as a tumor suppressor gene in the liver. Firstly, HNF4α instructs hepatocytes to stop proliferation and initiate differentiation. Indeed, HNF4α conditional deletion in the mouse liver resulted in the reactivation of hepatocyte proliferation with the induction of numerous mitogenic signals.[45] Furthermore, the forced expression of HNF4α in hepatocarcinoma cells reduced their proliferative potential and stimulated differentiation,[46] two cellular processes associated with tumor regression. Secondly, HNF4α protects rodents against hepatic carcinogenesis induced by diethylnitrosamine treatment.[47] Thirdly, HNF4α can prevent epithelial–mesenchymal transition by interfering with Snail and Slug transcription factors.[48] Finally, HNF4α restrains a microRNA (miRNA)-inflammatory loop circuit that normally activates IL-6/STAT3 and NF-κB pathways that are functionally involved in hepatocellular transformation and progression to carcinogenesis.[35]

HNF4α and gastric cancer

The stomach epithelium exclusively expresses HNF4α P2 isoforms.[4] While the exact roles for HNF4α in this tissue are not well defined, its expression in gastric cancerous cells is required to support their proliferation.[49] As a mechanistic clue of how HNF4α acts in this context, it was reported that HNF4α allows the transactivation of the "myc" gene promoter by the recruitment of the transcription factor FOXO6.[50] This dependence in HNF4α to sustain cancerous cell growth correlates with the maintenance of the P2 isoform expression in the gastric primary tumors as well as their metastases in breasts.[4,51] However, a subclass of tumors correlating with the status of intestinal metaplasia was reported to express HNF4α P1 isoforms.[52] This association suggests that the switch in the isoform expression could be functionally involved in driving aberrant intestinal-specific phenotype in the stomach.

HNF4α and colorectal cancer

In contrast to its role in colorectal cancer, HNF4α is thought to act as a suppressor of tumor in liver cancer. The adult small intestine and colon are the only organs expressing simultaneously both classes of HNF4α isoforms.[4] The HNF4α expression is detectable in all epithelial cells of the gut, as supported by immunolocalization studies.[4,7,9] Several mouse conditional-deletion models supported a role for HNF4α during colon morphogenesis in the embryo, and during inflammation in the adult.[8,9,36] Several experimental observations suggested a functional role for HNF4α during colorectal cancer. Firstly, several studies demonstrated that the HNF4α expression changes in colorectal tumors. Indeed, the HNF4α P1 isoform expression decreases in colon tumors[12] in spite of a global HNF4α expression level being increased in the majority of the cases.[4,53,54] This global induction of expression correlates well with the observed chromosome 20q amplification that contains the *HNF4A* locus in human colorectal cancer.[55] In addition, the HNF4α expression appears to be required for the proliferation and survival of cultured colorectal cancer cell lines.[20,53,55] Besides these studies performed in the context of cultured cells, *in vivo* experimental observations supported a tumor-promoting role for HNF4α during intestinal tumorigenesis. HNF4α conditional deletion in *Apc*^{Min} mice, a model that spontaneously develops intestinal adenoma, resulted in a significant reduction of the number of polyps in these mice.[53] Whether the global role of HNF4α on cancer from different tissue sources is variable in the function of the cellular context or the nature of specific HNF4α isoforms involved is currently unclear and will remain to be carefully examined. Interestingly, a recent report has suggested that HNF4α isoforms could exert differential effects on tumor growth in the context of colorectal cancer cells.[56]

Regulation of HNF4α activity

In contrast to most nuclear receptors, HNF4α activity does not require ligand interaction for its function in regulating gene transcription. It is perhaps why numerous mechanisms at the transcriptional, posttranscriptional, and post-translational levels can regulate HNF4α in response to cellular environmental cues as observed during inflammation,[57] development,[23] carcinogenesis,[4] and nutrition.[58,59]

HNF4α isoforms are initially transcribed from the usage of two alternative promoters (Figure 2). Several transcription factors have been identified to regulate these specific promoters, and the nature of these regulators probably differs between mouse and human species.[60] In the human embryonic liver, P1 transcriptional regulation results from the synergistic cooperation between GATA-6, HNF3, and HNF1β, while in the adult liver, this regulation depends on HNF6, HNF1α, CCAAT/Enhancer Binding Protein (C/EBP), and the glucocorticoid receptor.[60] Retinoid acid can also induce P1 promoter activity from displacing the chicken ovalbumin upstream promoter-transcription factor 2 (COUP-TFII) transcriptional repressor in replacement of Retinoid X receptor/Retinoid acid receptor alpha (RXR/RARα) on one specific overlapping DNA element of the P1 promoter.[60] In addition, P1 isoforms are able to retroinhibit the transcriptional activity of their own promoter by interacting with the Sp1 transcription factor that binds to a specific DNA element of the P1 promoter.[61] As for the P2 promoter, two independent studies highlighted the presence of a crucial regulating region upstream to the transcription start site. This region allows the activation of the promoter by a synergic transcriptional cooperation between HNF1α, HNF1β, HNF6, and Onecut-2 (OC-2).[42] In the context of the pancreas, a tissue that exclusively expresses HNF4α P2 isoforms, pancreatic and duodenal homebox 1 (PDX1) was shown to transcriptionally regulate the P2 promoter via a conserved DNA element that is often mutated in MODY2.[62] In the mouse liver, P2 promoter activity can be repressed by HNF4α P1 isoforms, explaining why the P2 isoform expression level decreases coincidently with the induction of the P1 isoform expression.[42] The transcriptional regulation of HNF4α-specific promoters can also be dependent on the cellular and environmental context. For instance, inflammatory signals such as TNF-α can repress the HNF4α P1 promoter via the recruitment of the NF-κB transcription factor.[63] Also, the rifampicin antibiotic stimulates migration of hepatic cancerous cells by repressing HNF4α P1 promoter via the activation of the nuclear receptor PXR.[64] The HNF4α P1 promoter is also repressed by Snail and Slug transcription factors during TGF-β-induced hepatocyte epithelial–mesenchyme transition.[48]

There are several reports supporting miRNAs-dependent posttranscriptional downregulation of the HNF4α expression. Among these are miR-21,[65] miR-24,[66] miR-34a,[66] miR-34c-5p,[67] and miR-449a.[68] Once again, this type of regulation appears to be dependent on the cellular context. For example, the induction of miR-24 and miR-34a and coincident downmodulation of the HNF4α expression occur following hepatocytes exposure to cellular stresses.[66] In addition, miR-24 can prevent HNF4α to negatively feed back on the IL-6/STAT3 pathway that is essential for hepatocyte transformation and liver carcinogenesis.[35]

Finally, HNF4α can be regulated by numerous posttranslational modifications. These modifications can affect HNF4α overall activity, DNA-binding capacity, cellular localization, protein stability, and protein–protein interactions. Phosphorylation has been reported as one of the most frequent posttranslational modifications of HNF4α. Several kinases were identified to phosphorylate HNF4α.[12,57] However, most of these studies did not address whether these phosphorylation pathways were targeting specific HNF4α isoforms. One exception is the reported role for Src in phosphorylating HNF4α P1-only isoforms, a process that appeared to correlate with the degradation of these P1 isoforms in the context of colorectal cancer.[12] Acetylation of HNF4α by the acetyltransferase CREB-binding protein (CBP) was reported to promote nuclear retention and the increased affinity of HNF4α for DNA.[69] Finally, HNF4α polySUMOylation was reported to not only stimulate its degradation but also positively regulate its transactivation potential during hepatocyte differentiation.[70]

Concluding Remarks

In sum, HNF4α nuclear receptor activity is regulated at several levels, starting at the transcriptional level that dictates what class of isoforms will be produced within the cell, at the posttranscriptional level via the specific action of a subset of miRNAs, and at the posttranslational level with multiple possible covalent enzymatic modifications. In addition, HNF4α nuclear receptor activity is modulatable by pharmacological agents that can either stimulate or repress its transcriptional potential and then influence a defined subset of target genes. There are thus vast possibilities and strategies to be explored by the research community in order to design molecules that ultimately could specifically regulate cellular HNF4α activity in the context of intestinal diseases. HNF4α, globally, regulates many crucial functions among several tissues of the organism. This limits the design and the administration of a drug that could widely act on all HNF4α isoforms in a systemic manner. For instance, designing an antagonist that would limit HNF4α-increased activity in colon tumors could also interfere with HNF4α P1 isoforms in the liver, for which their activities are crucial for the functionality of this tissue. In the context of chronic gut inflammatory diseases where a decrease of the HNF4α expression is observed, an opposite strategy aiming to increase HNF4α activity would have to be considered. HNF4α P1 and P2 isoforms appear to be differentially expressed among the different tissues that harbor HNF4α-crucial dependence for their functions. Because targeting HNF4α nuclear receptor represents an exciting perspective for gut inflammation and cancer therapy, future challenges will reside in defining the exact profile of HNF4α P1 and P2 isoforms during gut pathologies as well as their specific functions in these contexts. This could then become the reference for exploring the nature of the molecular mechanisms involved into the specific regulation of given isoforms found to be highly relevant in the context of these gut diseases.

References

1. C Yan, PJ Higgins (2013) Drugging the undruggable: Transcription therapy for cancer. *Biochim Biophys Acta* **1835**: 76–85.
2. C Helsen, F Claessens (2014) Looking at nuclear receptors from a new angle. *Mol Cell Endocrinol* **382**: 97–106.
3. SE Mullican, JR Dispirito, MA Lazar (2013) The orphan nuclear receptors at their 25-year reunion. *J Mol Endocrinol* **51**: T115–T140.
4. T Tanaka, S Jiang, H Hotta, K Takano, H Iwanari, K Sumi, K Daigo, R Ohashi, M Sugai, C Ikegame, H Umezu, Y Hirayama, Y Midorikawa, Y Hippo, A Watanabe, Y Uchiyama, G Hasegawa, P Reid, H Aburatani, T Hamakubo,

J Sakai, M Naito, T Kodama (2006) Dysregulated expression of P1 and P2 promoter-driven hepatocyte nuclear factor-4α in the pathogenesis of human cancer. *J Pathol* **208**: 662–672.

5. DT Odom, N Zizlsperger, DB Gordon, GW Bell, NJ Rinaldi, HL Murray, TL Volkert, J Schreiber, PA Rolfe, DK Gifford, E Fraenkel, GI Bell, RA Young (2004) Control of pancreas and liver gene expression by HNF transcription factors. *Science* **303**: 1378–1381.
6. A Stegmann, M Hansen, Y Wang, JB Larsen, LR Lund, L Ritie, JK Nicholson, B Quistorff, P Simon-Assmann, JT Troelsen, J Olsen (2006) Metabolome, transcriptome, and bioinformatic cis-element analyses point to HNF-4 as a central regulator of gene expression during enterocyte differentiation. *Physiol Genomics* **27**: 141–155.
7. JP Babeu, M Darsigny, CR Lussier, F Boudreau (2009) Hepatocyte nuclear factor 4α contributes to an intestinal epithelial phenotype in vitro and plays a partial role in mouse intestinal epithelium differentiation. *Am J Physiol Gastrointest Liver Physiol* **297**: G124–G134.
8. M Darsigny, JP Babeu, AA Dupuis, EE Furth, EG Seidman, E Levy, EF Verdu, FP Gendron, F Boudreau (2009) Loss of hepatocyte-nuclear-factor-4α affects colonic ion transport and causes chronic inflammation resembling inflammatory bowel disease in mice. *PloS one* **4**: e7609–e7609.
9. WD Garrison, MA Battle, C Yang, KH Kaestner, FM Sladek, SA Duncan (2006) Hepatocyte nuclear factor 4α is essential for embryonic development of the mouse colon. *Gastroenterology* **130**: 1207–1220.
10. M Hadzopoulou-Cladaras, E Kistanova, C Evagelopoulou, S Zeng, C Cladaras, JA Ladias (1997) Functional domains of the nuclear receptor hepatocyte nuclear factor 4. *J Biol Chem* **272**: 539–550.
11. G Jiang, FM Sladek (1997) The DNA binding domain of hepatocyte nuclear factor 4 mediates cooperative, specific binding to DNA and heterodimerization with the retinoid X receptor α. *J Biol Chem* **272**: 1218–1225.
12. K Chellappa, L Jankova, JM Schnabl, S Pan, Y Brelivet, CLS Fung, C Chan, OF Dent, SJ Clarke, GR Robertson, FM Sladek (2012) Src tyrosine kinase phosphorylation of nuclear receptor HNF4 correlates with isoform-specific loss of HNF4 in human colon cancer. *Proc Natl Acad Sci USA* **109**: 2302–2307.
13. E Bolotin, K Chellappa, W Hwang-Verslues, JM Schnabl, C Yang, FM Sladek (2011) Nuclear receptor HNF4α binding sequences are widespread in Alu repeats. *BMC Genomics* **12**: 560–560.

14. X Yuan, TC Ta, M Lin, JR Evans, Y Dong, E Bolotin, MA Sherman, BM Forman, FM Sladek (2009) Identification of an endogenous ligand bound to a native orphan nuclear receptor. *PloS one* **4**: e5609–e5609.
15. V Chandra, P Huang, N Potluri, D Wu, Y Kim, F Rastinejad (2013) Multidomain integration in the structure of the HNF-4α nuclear receptor complex. *Nature* **495**: 394–398.
16. K Duda, YI Chi, SE Shoelson (2004) Structural basis for HNF-4α activation by ligand and coactivator binding. *J Biol Chem* **279**: 23311–23316.
17. A Kiselyuk, SHH Lee, S Farber-Katz, M Zhang, S Athavankar, T Cohen, AB Pinkerton, M Ye, P Bushway, AD Richardson, HA Hostetler, M Rodriguez-Lee, L Huang, B Spangler, L Smith, J Higginbotham, J Cashman, H Freeze, P Itkin-Ansari, MI Dawson, F Schroeder, Y Cang, M Mercola, F Levine (2012) HNF4α antagonists discovered by a high-throughput screen for modulators of the human insulin promoter. *Chem Biol* **19**: 806–818.
18. SH Lee, R Piran, E Keinan, A Pinkerton, F Levine (2013) Induction of beta-cell replication by a synthetic HNF4α antagonist. *Stem Cells* **31**: 2396–2407.
19. S-H Lee, S Athavankar, T Cohen, R Piran, A Kiselyuk, and F Levine (2013) Identification of Alverine and Benfluorex as HNF4α activators. *ACS Chem Biol* **8**: 1730–1736.
20. B Schwartz, A Algamas-Dimantov, R Hertz, J Nataf, A Kerman, I Peri, J Bar-Tana (2009) Inhibition of colorectal cancer by targeting hepatocyte nuclear factor-4α. *Int J Cancer* **124**: 1081–1089.
21. ME Torres-Padilla, MC Weiss (2003) Effects of interactions of hepatocyte nuclear factor 4α isoforms with coactivators and corepressors are promoter-specific. *FEBS Lett* **539**: 19–23.
22. E Bolotin, H Liao, TC Ta, C Yang, W Hwang-Verslues, JR Evans, T Jiang, FM Sladek (2010) Integrated approach for the identification of human hepatocyte nuclear factor 4α target genes using protein binding microarrays. *Hepatology* **51**: 642–653.
23. ME Torres-Padilla, C Fougere-Deschatrette, MC Weiss (2001) Expression of HNF4α isoforms in mouse liver development is regulated by sequential promoter usage and constitutive 3' end splicing. *Mech Dev* **109**: 183–193.
24. F Parviz, C Matullo, WD Garrison, L Savatski, JW Adamson, G Ning, KH Kaestner, JM Rossi, KS Zaret, SA Duncan (2003) Hepatocyte nuclear factor 4α controls the development of a hepatic epithelium and liver morphogenesis. *Nat Genet* **34**: 292–296.
25. RK Gupta, MZ Vatamaniuk, CS Lee, RC Flaschen, JT Fulmer, FM Matschinsky, SA Duncan, KH Kaestner (2005) The MODY1 gene HNF-4α regulates selected genes involved in insulin secretion. *J Clin Invest* **115**: 1006–1015.

26. S Rieck, J Zhang, Z Li, C Liu, A Naji, KK Takane, NM Fiaschi-Taesch, AF Stewart, JA Kushner, KH Kaestner (2012) Overexpression of hepatocyte nuclear factor-4α initiates cell cycle entry, but is not sufficient to promote beta-cell expansion in human islets. *Mol Endocrinol* **26**: 1590–1602.
27. N Briançon, MC Weiss, N Briancon, MC Weiss (2006) In vivo role of the HNF4α AF-1 activation domain revealed by exon swapping. *EMBO J* **25**: 1253–1262.
28. WS Chen, K Manova, DC Weinstein, SA Duncan, AS Plump, VR Prezioso, RF Bachvarova, JE Darnell (1994) Disruption of the HNF-4 gene, expressed in visceral endoderm, leads to cell death in embryonic ectoderm and impaired gastrulation of mouse embryos. *Genes Dev* **8**: 2466–2477.
29. H Chiba, N Sakai, M Murata, M Osanai, T Ninomiya, T Kojima, N Sawada (2006) The nuclear receptor hepatocyte nuclear factor 4α acts as a morphogen to induce the formation of microvilli. *J Cell Biol* **175**: 971–980.
30. CR Lussier, JP Babeu, BA Auclair, N Perreault, F Boudreau (2008) Hepatocyte nuclear factor-4α promotes differentiation of intestinal epithelial cells in a coculture system. *Am J Physiol Gastrointest Liver Physiol* **294**: G418–G428.
31. GP Hayhurst, YH Lee, G Lambert, M Ward, FJ Gonzalez, JM Ward (2001) Hepatocyte nuclear factor 4α (nuclear receptor 2A1) is essential for maintenance of hepatic gene expression and lipid homeostasis hepatocyte nuclear factor 4 (nuclear receptor 2A1) is essential for maintenance of hepatic gene expression and lipid H. *Mol Cell Biol* **21**: 1393–1403.
32. A Archer, D Sauvaget, V Chauffeton, PE Bouchet, J Chambaz, M Pincon-Raymond, P Cardot, A Ribeiro, M Lacasa (2005) Intestinal apolipoprotein A-IV gene transcription is controlled by two hormone-responsive elements: A role for hepatic nuclear factor-4 isoforms. *Mol Endocrinol* **19**: 2320–2334.
33. JI Sakamaki, H Daitoku, Y Kaneko, A Hagiwara, K Ueno, A Fukamizu (2012) GSK3β regulates gluconeogenic gene expression through HNF4α and FOXO1. *J Recept Signal Transduct* **32**: 96–101.
34. Z Wang, PA Burke (2007) Effects of hepatocyte nuclear factor-4α on the regulation of the hepatic acute phase response. *J Mol Biol* **371**: 323–335.
35. M Hatziapostolou, C Polytarchou, E Aggelidou, A Drakaki, GA Poultsides, SA Jaeger, H Ogata, M Karin, K Struhl, M Hadzopoulou-Cladaras, D Iliopoulos (2011) An HNF4α-miRNA inflammatory feedback circuit regulates hepatocellular oncogenesis. *Cell* **147**: 1233–1247.
36. SHH Ahn, YM Shah, J Inoue, K Morimura, I Kim, S Yim, G Lambert, R Kurotani, K Nagashima, FJ Gonzalez, Y Inoue (2008) Hepatocyte nuclear factor 4α in the intestinal epithelial cells protects against inflammatory bowel disease. *Inflamm Bowel Dis* **14**: 908–920.

37. UKIBDG Consortium, JC Barrett, JC Lee, CW Lees, NJ Prescott, CA Anderson, A Phillips, E Wesley, K Parnell, H Zhang, H Drummond, ER Nimmo, D Massey, K Blaszczyk, T Elliott, L Cotterill, H Dallal, AJ Lobo, C Mowat, JD Sanderson, DP Jewell, WG Newman, C Edwards, T Ahmad, JC Mansfield, J Satsangi, M Parkes, CG Mathew, WTCC Consortium, P Donnelly, L Peltonen, JM Blackwell, E Bramon, MA Brown, JP Casas, A Corvin, N Craddock, P Deloukas, A Duncanson, J Jankowski, HS Markus, CG Mathew, MI McCarthy, CN Palmer, R Plomin, A Rautanen, SJ Sawcer, N Samani, RC Trembath, AC Viswanathan, N Wood, CC Spencer, JC Barrett, C Bellenguez, D Davison, C Freeman, A Strange, P Donnelly, C Langford, SE Hunt, S Edkins, R Gwilliam, H Blackburn, SJ Bumpstead, S Dronov, M Gillman, E Gray, N Hammond, A Jayakumar, OT McCann, J Liddle, ML Perez, SC Potter, R Ravindrarajah, M Ricketts, M Waller, P Weston, S Widaa, P Whittaker, P Deloukas, L Peltonen, CG Mathew, JM Blackwell, MA Brown, A Corvin, MI McCarthy, CC Spencer, AP Attwood, J Stephens, J Sambrook, WH Ouwehand, WL McArdle, SM Ring, DP Strachan (2009) Genome-wide association study of ulcerative colitis identifies three new susceptibility loci, including the HNF4A region. *Nat Genet* **41**: 1330–1334.
38. K Grigo, A Wirsing, B Lucas, L Klein-Hitpass, GU Ryffel (2008) HNF4α orchestrates a set of 14 genes to down-regulate cell proliferation in kidney cells. *Biol Chem* **389**: 179–187.
39. H Chiba, T Itoh, S Satohisa, N Sakai, H Noguchi, M Osanai, T Kojima, N Sawada (2005) Activation of p21CIP1/WAF1 gene expression and inhibition of cell proliferation by overexpression of hepatocyte nuclear factor-4α. *Exp Cell Res* **302**: 11–21.
40. ALL Cattin, J Le Beyec, F Barreau, S Saint-Just, A Houllier, FJ Gonzalez, S Robine, M Pincon-Raymond, P Cardot, M Lacasa, A Ribeiro, M Pinçon-Raymond, P Cardot, M Lacasa, A Ribeiro (2009) Hepatocyte nuclear factor 4α, a key factor for homeostasis, cell architecture, and barrier function of the adult intestinal epithelium. *Mol Cell Biol* **29**: 6294–6308.
41. RK Gupta, N Gao, RK Gorski, P White, OT Hardy, K Rafiq, JE Brestelli, G Chen, CJ Stoeckert, KH Kaestner (2007) Expansion of adult beta-cell mass in response to increased metabolic demand is dependent on HNF-4α. *Genes Dev* **21**: 756–769.
42. N Briançon, A Bailly, F Clotman, P Jacquemin, FP Lemaigre, MC Weiss (2004) Expression of the α7 isoform of hepatocyte nuclear factor (HNF) 4 is activated by HNF6/OC-2 and HNF1 and repressed by HNF4α1 in the liver. *J Biol Chem* **279**: 33398–33408.

43. NL Lazarevich, DA Shavochkina, DI Fleishman, IF Kustova, OV Morozova, ES Chuchuev, YI Patyutko (2010) Deregulation of hepatocyte nuclear factor 4 (HNF4) as a marker of epithelial tumors progression. *Exp Oncol* **32**: 167–171.
44. BF Ning, J Ding, C Yin, W Zhong, K Wu, X Zeng, W Yang, YX Chen, JP Zhang, X Zhang, HY Wang, WF Xie (2010) Hepatocyte nuclear factor 4α suppresses the development of hepatocellular carcinoma. *Cancer Res* **70**: 7640–7651.
45. JA Bonzo, CH Ferry, T Matsubara, JH Kim, FJ Gonzalez (2012) Suppression of hepatocyte proliferation by hepatocyte nuclear factor 4α in adult mice. *J Biol Chem* **287**: 7345–7356.
46. C Yin, Y Lin, X Zhang, YX Chen, X Zeng, HY Yue, JL Hou, X Deng, JP Zhang, ZG Han, WF Xie (2008) Differentiation therapy of hepatocellular carcinoma in mice with recombinant adenovirus carrying hepatocyte nuclear factor-4α gene. *Hepatology* **48**: 1528–1539.
47. C Walesky, G Edwards, P Borude, S Gunewardena, M O'Neil, B Yoo, U Apte (2013) Hepatocyte nuclear factor 4α deletion promotes diethylnitrosamine-induced hepatocellular carcinoma in rodents. *Hepatology* **57**: 2480–2490.
48. M Yang, SN Li, KM Anjum, LX Gui, SS Zhu, J Liu, JK Chen, QF Liu, GD Ye, WJ Wang, JF Wu, WY Cai, GB Sun, YJ Liu, RF Liu, ZM Zhang, BA Li (2013) A double-negative feedback loop between Wnt-beta-catenin signaling and HNF4α regulates epithelial-mesenchymal transition in hepatocellular carcinoma. *J Cell Sci* **126**: 5692–5703.
49. HR Chang, S Nam, MC Kook, KT Kim, X Liu, H Yao, HR Jung, R Lemos, HH Seo, HS Park, Y Gim, D Hong, I Huh, YW Kim, D Tan, CG Liu, G Powis, T Park, H Liang, YH Kim (2016) HNF4α is a therapeutic target that links AMPK to WNT signalling in early-stage gastric cancer. *Gut* **65**: 19–32.
50. L Qinyu, C Long, D Zhen-Dong, S Min-Min, W Wei-Ze, Y Wei-Ping, P Cheng-Hong (2013) FOXO6 promotes gastric cancer cell tumorigenicity via upregulation of C-myc. *FEBS Lett* **587**: 2105–2111.
51. T Koyama, S Sekine, H Taniguchi, H Tsuda, M Ikegami, H Hano, R Kushima (2011) Hepatocyte nuclear factor 4A expression discriminates gastric involvement by metastatic breast carcinomas from primary gastric adenocarcinomas. *Hum Pathol* **42**: 1777–1784.
52. K Takano, G Hasegawa, S Jiang, I Kurosaki, K Hatakeyama, H Iwanari, T Tanaka, T Hamakubo, T Kodama, M Naito (2009) Immunohistochemical staining for P1 and P2 promoter-driven hepatocyte nuclear factor-4α may complement mucin phenotype of differentiated-type early gastric carcinoma. *Pathol Int* **59**: 462–470.
53. M Darsigny, JP Babeu, EG Seidman, FP Gendron, E Levy, J Carrier, N Perreault, F Boudreau (2010) Hepatocyte nuclear factor-4α promotes gut

neoplasia in mice and protects against the production of reactive oxygen species. *Cancer Res* **70**: 9423–9433.

54. T Oshima, T Kawasaki, R Ohashi, G Hasegawa, S Jiang, H Umezu, Y Aoyagi, H Iwanari, T Tanaka, T Hamakubo, T Kodama, M Naito (2007) Downregulated P1 promoter-driven hepatocyte nuclear factor-4α expression in human colorectal carcinoma is a new prognostic factor against liver metastasis. *Pathol Int* **57**: 82–90.
55. B Zhang, J Wang, X Wang, J Zhu, Q Liu, Z Shi, MC Chambers, LJ Zimmerman, KF Shaddox, S Kim, SR Davies, S Wang, P Wang, CR Kinsinger, RC Rivers, H Rodriguez, RR Townsend, MJC Ellis, SA Carr, DL Tabb, RJ Coffey, RJC Slebos, DC Liebler (2014) Proteogenomic characterization of human colon and rectal cancer. *Nature* **513**: 382–387.
56. LM Vuong, K Chellappa, JM Dhahbi, JR Deans, B Fang, E Bolotin, NV Titova, NP Hoverter, SR Spindler, ML Waterman, FM Sladek (2015) Differential effects of hepatocyte nuclear factor 4α isoforms on tumor growth and T-cell factor 4/ap-1 interactions in human colorectal cancer cells. *Mol Cell Biol* **35**: 3471–3490.
57. JP Babeu, F Boudreau (2014) Hepatocyte nuclear factor 4-α involvement in liver and intestinal inflammatory networks. *World J Gastroenterol* **20**: 22–30.
58. CG Dietrich, IV Martin, AC Porn, S Voigt, C Gartung, C Trautwein, A Geier (2007) Fasting induces basolateral uptake transporters of the SLC family in the liver via HNF4α and PGC1α. *Am J Physiol Gastrointest Liver Physiol* **293**: G585–G590.
59. EA Hanniman, G Lambert, Y Inoue, FJ Gonzalez, CJ Sinal (2006) Apolipoprotein A-IV is regulated by nutritional and metabolic stress: Involvement of glucocorticoids, HNF-4α, and PGC-1α. *J Lipid Res* **47**: 2503–2514.
60. P Hatzis, I Talianidis (2001) Regulatory mechanisms controlling human hepatocyte nuclear factor 4α gene expression. *Mol Cell Biol* **21**: 7320–7330.
61. J Magenheim, R Hertz, I Berman, J Nousbeck, J Bar-Tana (2005) Negative autoregulation of HNF-4α gene expression by HNF-4α1. *Biochem J* **388**: 325–332.
62. H Thomas, K Jaschkowitz, M Bulman, TM Frayling, SM Mitchell, S Roosen, A Lingott-Frieg, CJ Tack, S Ellard, GU Ryffel, AT Hattersley (2001) A distant upstream promoter of the HNF-4α gene connects the transcription factors involved in maturity-onset diabetes of the young. *Hum Mol Genet* **10**: 2089–2097.
63. R Simo, A Barbosa-Desongles, C Saez-Lopez, A Lecube, C Hernandez, DM Selva (2012) Molecular mechanism of TNFα-induced down-regulation of SHBG expression. *Mol Endocrinol* **26**: 438–446.

64. S Kodama, Y Yamazaki, M Negishi (2015) Pregnane X receptor represses HNF4α gene to induce insulin-like growth factor-binding protein IGFBP1 that alters morphology of and migrates HepG2 cells. *Mol Pharmacol* **88**: 746–757.
65. BF Ning, J Ding, J Liu, C Yin, WP Xu, WM Cong, Q Zhang, F Chen, T Han, X Deng, PQ Wang, CF Jiang, JP Zhang, X Zhang, HY Wang, WF Xie (2014) Hepatocyte nuclear factor 4α-nuclear factor-kappaB feedback circuit modulates liver cancer progression. *Hepatology* **60**: 1607–1619.
66. S Takagi, M Nakajima, K Kida, Y Yamaura, T Fukami, T Yokoi (2010) MicroRNAs regulate human hepatocyte nuclear factor 4α, modulating the expression of metabolic enzymes and cell cycle. *J Biol Chem* **285**: 4415–4422.
67. Z Wang, PA Burke (2013) The role of microRNAs in hepatocyte nuclear factor-4α expression and transactivation. *Biochim Biophys Acta* **1829**: 436–442.
68. A Ramamoorthy, L Li, A Gaedigk, LD Bradford, EA Benson, DA Flockhart, TC Skaar (2012) In silico and in vitro identification of microRNAs that regulate hepatic nuclear factor 4α expression. *Drug Metab Dispos* **40**: 726–733.
69. E Soutoglou, N Katrakili, I Talianidis (2000) Acetylation regulates transcription factor activity at multiple levels. *Mol Cell* **5**: 745–751.
70. W Zhou, Z Hannoun, E Jaffray, CN Medine, JR Black, S Greenhough, L Zhu, JA Ross, S Forbes, I Wilmut, JP Iredale, RT Hay, DC Hay (2012) SUMOylation of HNF4 regulates protein stability and hepatocyte function. *J Cell Sci* **125**: 3630–3635.

Chapter 5

Established Therapies and New Therapeutic Strategies in Alcoholic Liver Disease

Helmut Karl Seitz and Sebastian Mueller

Abstract

Chronic heavy alcohol consumption accounts for more than 200 diseases and/or symptoms. Among them alcoholic liver disease (ALD) is of special importance since it is frequent and often life threatening. In Europe, alcohol consumption has increased as compared to the rest of the world, and so has ALD. It has been estimated that about 500,000 people die every year in Europe due to ALD. ALD consists of alcoholic fatty liver (AFL), alcoholic steatohepatitis, alcoholic cirrhosis, and hepatocellular cancer. Alcoholic hepatitis (AH) is a clinical syndrome with jaundice, liver failure, and high mortality. The natural course of the ALD is modulated by genetics, gender, other types of liver diseases, toxic, drugs, and other factors. Therapy of ALD is mostly limited to alcohol abstinence, which may be difficult to achieve in an alcoholic. Thus, in these patients, cognitive behavior therapy can be combined with anticraving medication. The therapy of AH with its poor prognosis is limited. Although a great variety of therapeutic approaches have been made, the cornerstones of AH therapy consist still of intensive care combined with steroids, hyperalimentation, and eventually N-acetylcysteine. At present, an intensive debate whether liver transplantation should be performed in AH is ongoing. New therapeutic strategies aim to targets which have been identified as pathogenetic factors in ALD. This includes endotoxins, certain cytokines and chemokines, and inhibition of oxidative stress. Also, anticraving substances such as nalmefene may improve liver function since less alcohol is consumed. Furthermore betaine which stimulates methyl transfer and inhibits apoptosis has been investigated. Stimulating hepatic regeneration by the use of a granulocyte colony stimulating factor, as well as mesenchymal stem cell and bone marrow transplantation showed promising results. However, new therapeutic strategies are urgently needed, especially for AH.

Introduction

Alcoholic liver disease (ALD) is the leading liver disease in Europe, while in the United States, non-alcoholic fatty liver disease (NAFLD) seems to rank first. In 2012, alcohol consumption was responsible for 3.3 million deaths or 5.9% of all global deaths (7.6% males and 4.0% females). Alcohol is also responsible for 5.1% of the global burden of disease. Harmful consumption of alcohol rose from the eighth to the fifth leading cause of death and disability, between 1990 and 2010.[1,2]

In Europe, alcohol consumption per capita per year is approximately 11 liters which resembles 24 grams of pure alcohol per day.[1] The attributable burden in Europe with 6.5% of all deaths and 11.6% of disease associated loss of years (DALYs) attributable to alcohol is the highest proportion of total ill health and premature deaths in all the World Health Organization (WHO) regions.[2] The alcohol-attributable fraction for all deaths in all the WHO regions is 13.3%, by far the highest, as estimated by WHO regions in 2012 (compared to the United States with 4.7% and South East Asia with 4.6%).[1]

Alcohol-attributable deaths are primarily due to cardiovascular diseases and diabetes (33.4%), cancers (12.5%), unintentional injuries (17.1%), and gastrointestinal (GI) diseases (16.2%).[1,2]

Chronic alcohol consumption is responsible for more than 200 symptoms and/or diseases. GI diseases consist primarily of GI cancer (upper GI tract cancer, colon cancer, and hepatocellular cancer [HCC], and pancreatic cancer), pancreatitis, and ALD. Among them ALD is of considerable importance. In Europe, it was calculated that one million people die from cirrhosis of the liver with half a million due to alcoholic liver cirrhosis.[3] This is 0.9%

of all deaths and 10.4% of alcohol-attributable deaths. One-third of cirrhosis liver transplantations in Europe are due to alcohol. In some parts of Europe, alcohol consumption is still increasing. For example, in the United Kingdom, an approximately 500% increase in ALD in 2009 was observed as compared to 1970.[4]

In general, the pattern of drinking has been changed. Binge drinking (consumption of more than 60 grams or more of pure alcohol on at least one single occasion at least monthly) became more dominant, at least in some parts of Europe (UK). The costs of alcohol misuse are enormous. For example, in 2003, 155 billion Euros equivalent to 1.3–3.3% of gross domestic product (GDP) were spent in the European Union for alcohol-associated health problems.[1]

On the basis of these facts, the WHO has announced a European action plan to reduce the harmful use of alcohol in 2012–2020. The main action areas are the increase in taxation and the reduction in the physical availability of alcohol. Targeted policies such as a minimum unit pricing which has a greater impact on hazardous and harmful drinkers, contribute to reducing health inequalities. Thus, on the one side, great efforts are being made for the prevention and early detection of alcohol-associated disorders, especially ALD; on the other side, however, new strategies in the treatment of ALD are needed since medical treatment is disappointing and abstinence, sometimes difficult to achieve, and liver transplantation are the only options with success.

In the present overview, ALDs including their risk factors are briefly described, and established therapies as well as new therapeutic approaches are discussed. Most of these approaches are still based on animal experiments, while some have already entered clinical trials.

Natural History of ALD

The sequence of ALD is reflected in Figure 1. When sufficient amounts of alcohol hit the liver, almost everybody develops alcoholic fatty liver (AFL). The amount of alcohol producing fatty liver may vary. However, in general, alcohol doses exceeding 30 grams per day in men and half of this in women may be sufficient to generate fatty liver. If alcohol consumption is continued, only some of these individuals proceed into advanced ALD. The mechanisms

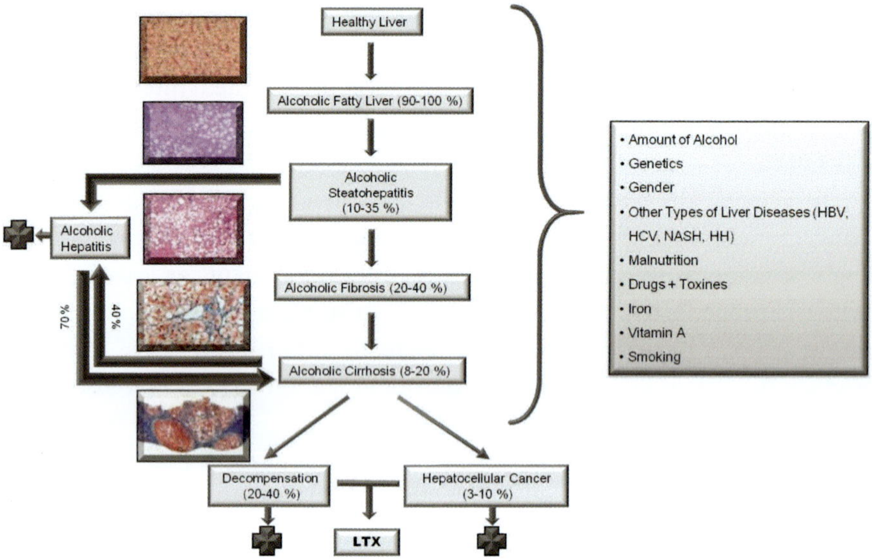

Figure 1. Natural course of alcoholic liver disease. Chronic alcohol consumption of more than 30 grams per day leads to alcoholic fatty liver. When alcohol consumption is continued up to 30%, alcoholic steatohepatitis and finally fibrosis of the liver develop. However, only 8–20% of all heavy drinkers present alcoholic cirrhosis of the liver. Forty percent of patients with cirrhosis also develop alcoholic hepatitis, a clinical syndrome with poor prognosis. On the other hand, patients with alcoholic hepatitis end in 70% in hepatic cirrhosis, and patients with alcoholic cirrhosis of the liver may decompensate and die of end stage liver disease when transplantation cannot be performed. They may also develop HCC. Since only a small percentage of heavy drinkers develop cirrhosis, other factors, in addition to the amount of alcohol consumed, may modify the sequence of the disease. These factors include genetics, gender (females are more sensitive towards the toxic action of ethanol), the presence of other types of liver disease, malnutrition as well as obesity, the concomitant exposure toward hepatotoxic drugs or xenobiotics, iron overload, vitamin A intake, and smoking.

of why a high percentage of patients with AFL do not proceed further are not clear. Some of these factors are shown in Figure 1 and will be discussed further.[5,6]

About 10–35% of patients with AFL develop alcoholic steatohepatitis (ASH).[7] ASH is characterized by signs of inflammation, such as cellular ballooning, infiltration with granulocytes, and sometimes the occurrence of Mallory-Denk bodies (MDBs). ASH is associated with an increase in the activity of serum transaminases. Most of the patients with ASH recover under alcohol abstinence. Some of the patients develop alcoholic hepatitis (AH), a clinical syndrome with jaundice and hepatic failure, leading to a high mortality rate. If they survive, approximately 70% go into cirrhosis of the liver. Mild-to-moderate ASH may be associated with an increase in fibrogenesis, leading to hepatic fibrosis and some of them advance to alcoholic liver cirrhosis. However, the percentage is relatively small with approximately 8–20%. In alcoholic cirrhosis, AH may also develop when alcohol consumption is continued with an extremely poor prognosis. Patients with alcoholic cirrhosis of the liver may die due to hepatic decompensation or the development of HCC. Liver transplantation is then the only therapeutic option with good results. In Germany, approximately 25% of all transplanted livers are due to end-stage ALD.[5,6]

A factor which modulates the natural course of ALD is the amount of alcohol consumed over time. The more alcohol consumed, the higher the risk for ALD. Since only up to 20% of heavy drinkers develop ALD, genetic factors may be involved in the pathogenesis of ALD.[7] Indeed, the PNPLA3 gene has been detected as a risk factor not only in ALD,[8] but also in NAFLD. It is polymorphic and codes for a hydrolase involved in fatty acid metabolism. At present, various genome-wide association studies (GWAS) are under investigation,[9,10] and such a study has recently identified further genes involved in the pathogenesis of ALD.[9]

Various clinical studies have shown that females are especially prone to ALD. Women generally need half the amount of alcohol in half the time to develop advanced ALD as compared to men.[5] Furthermore, hepatic iron is another risk factor in the pathogenesis of ALD. Therefore, patients with hereditary hemochromatosis have an enhanced risk for cirrhosis and HCC when they consume alcohol.[11]

Other types of liver diseases are a risk factor when alcohol is consumed. For example, the risk to develop hepatic fibrosis and cirrhosis in hepatitis C is significantly increased when alcohol is consumed, even in small amounts, such as 10 grams per day.[12] The risk to develop HCC in hepatitis B is dramatically elevated in the presence of continuous alcohol ingestion.[13] Patients with NAFLD who advance to non-alcoholic steatohepatitis (NASH) have an increased risk for HCC. This is especially true when they consume alcohol even at social levels.[14]

Finally, the exposure to certain xenobiotics, toxins, and drugs may increase the risk for ALD. This is true especially for methotrexate, acetaminophen, isoniacide, cocaine, and cannabis.[15,16] One has to also consider substances at the working place, such as solvents and chemicals in the cleaning industry.[15]

Established Therapy in ALD

The established therapy in ALD consists of abstinence in all types and severities of ALD. For AH, additional therapeutic approaches have been evaluated. Therapy at present consists of hyperalimentation as well as the administration of steroids, and eventually N-acetylcysteine. In alcoholic cirrhosis, similar to the cirrhosis of other origin, cirrhotic complications are treated. These include the treatment of ascites, hepatorenal syndrome (HRS), esophageal variceal bleeding, hepatic encephalopathy, and HCC. In end-stage ALD, liver transplantation is a promising option under certain conditions such as abstinence for more than six months.[6,17]

Abstinence

Abstinence for alcoholic fatty liver

The reversibility of AFL within 3–8 weeks is well known. This was among others shown in a careful study of 59 male patients with alcohol dependency.[18] AFL was diagnosed sonographically with digital registration and computer-based analysis. Of the 59 patients, 31% had a severe, 32% had a moderate, and 37% had a mild steatosis. Under alcohol abstinence, within 79 ± 26 days, a significant improvement of the fatty liver in 63% of the patients was observed. In summary, more than 50% of the patients' health with documented hepatic steatosis improved within three months. This improvement was associated with a significant decrease of the activity of serum Gamma-glutamyl transferase (GGT). Those patients whose health did not improve were obese and/or were diabetics with another additional cause of fatty liver.[18]

Abstinence for alcoholic hepatitis

In mild-to-moderate ASH, alcohol abstinence also results in the reversibility of inflammatory and degenerative alterations.[6] The seven-year survival in patients with AH was found to be 80% compared to 50% when alcohol consumption was continued.[5] In severe cases with AH alcohol abstinence is a prerequisite for survival.

Abstinence for alcoholic liver cirrhosis

Abstinence also improves survival in cirrhotic patients. Five-year survival in patients with alcoholic cirrhosis who stopped drinking was 50–75% as compared to 40% in patients who continued drinking. This advantage is also true for patients with decompensated cirrhosis of the liver.[19] In a study of 283 patients with compensated alcoholic cirrhosis of the liver, five-year survival was found to be 89% under abstinence as compared to 68%. An improvement was especially seen in patients with jaundice, but not in patients with variceal bleeding. This shows that abstinence improves liver function, but not portal hypertension.

Borowski and coworkers studied the survival of 54 male cirrhotics with ascites over a time interval of 32 months. Forty-three percent stayed abstinent for 14 months, while 28% continued to drink heavily. Twelve out of 15 heavy drinkers died within 7.2 months, while all patients, except one, who stayed abstinent survived.[20] This result was statistically significant ($P < 0.001$). Similar data came from England. These studies show clearly that continuous drinking has a poor prognosis and decreases survival. Finally, Schenker and coworkers also studied the natural course of ALD. These authors reported that the five-year mortality in alcoholic cirrhosis Child A was 10% with abstinence which increased to 30% when alcohol drinking was continued. The corresponding results for Child C cirrhosis were 40 and 70%, respectively.[21]

How to achieve abstinence

Following alcohol detoxification, psychosocial interventions for alcohol use disorders (AUDs) have been implemented. This may include brief interventions including motivational interviewing as well as cognitive behavior therapy (CBT). In addition, family and couple therapy is sometimes employed in the treatment of AUD (for the review of psychosocial intervention, see Ref. 22).

Psychosocial intervention can be combined by anticraving medication.[23] Acamprosate acts by normalizing the protracted dysregulation of the N-methyl-D-Aspartate (NMDA)-mediated glutamatergic neurotransmission. Many

European studies showed positive effects. However, a large clinical trial did not find any effect of acamprosate alone or in combination with naltrexone and/or CBT compared to placebo.[24]

Naltrexone, an opioid antagonist which is thought to reduce alcohol craving by blocking the μ-opioid receptor, seems to be effective in reducing relapse and diminishing the percentage of drinking days when combined with several interventions (for review, see Ref. 25). Topiramate reduces the reinforcing effects of alcohol by facilitating the gamma-aminobutyric acid (GABA) function and inhibiting glutaminergic pathways in the corticomesolimbic system. Baclofen is a GABA-B receptor agonist and may also be effective in AUD. Nalmefene, an opioid receptor modulator, has been recently introduced into the treatment of alcohol dependency with some success to reduce the alcohol intake associated with improvement of ALD.[26–28]

Therapy of AH

At present, the therapy of severe AH consists of abstinence, the treatment of the complications of the liver disease, hyperalimentation, and the administration of corticosteroids. The additional administration of NAC may also be helpful.[5–7] A variety of other drugs have been investigated in clinical trial without significant success, including the tumor necrosis factor-α (TNF-α) antibody infliximab, and finally also the non-selective phosphodiesterase inhibitor pentoxifylline.[29] Liver transplantation for AH is presently an issue of intensive worldwide discussion.[30,31] Established therapy of ALD has been summarized.[5–7,17,32]

General measures

As discussed previously, complete abstinence is the therapeutic backbone in patients with AH, but even in those who manage to stop drinking, AH may persist and progress toward liver failure. Patients developing severe withdrawal symptoms or delirium tremens can be treated with both short-acting benzodiazepines and chlormethiazole (CMZ), but the risk of worsening encephalopathy should be kept in mind. Apart from the specific treatments of AH that have been outlined in the following, the treatment of AH does not differ from that for decompensated liver disease due to non-alcoholic causes.

Current guidelines issue evidence-based recommendations for the treatment of ascites and associated spontaneous bacterial peritonitis with paracentesis, and of HRS with the administration of vasoconstrictors such as terlipressin or norepinephrine in combination with albumin.[5–7] Portosystemic encephalopathy can be treated with lactulose and gut-cleaning antibiotics, and possibly rifaximin, although its safety and efficacy in patients with AH have not been investigated. Due to the high prevalence of infections in patients with AH, therapeutic and prophylactic antibiotics, ideally third generation cephalosporins, should be used.

Hyperalimentation

Many patients with significant ALD reveal a certain degree of protein calorie malnutrition and deficiencies of numerous micronutrients,[33] and malnutrition is present in nearly all patients with severe AH. Interestingly, the nutritional status was part of the initial Child–Pugh–Turcotte score, but was omitted for practicability reasons, and malnutrition constitutes an independent risk factor for reduced survival.[33] Thus, counterbalancing nutritional deficiencies may theoretically improve the prognosis of patients with AH.

Several trials have been made to study the efficacy of oral or total enteral nutritional (TEN) support in patients with AH. Particularly interesting is the study by Cabré and associates because it emphasizes the potential of sufficient nutritional support.[33] Herein, investigators compared four weeks of TEN via a nasoduodenal tube providing 2,000 kcal/day versus prednisolone at 40 mg/day in combination with a diet containing 2,000 kcal/day in 71 patients with severe AH defined by the discriminant factor, DF > 32. While the mortality during treatment between groups was similar in both groups, it was significantly higher with steroids during follow-up, mostly due to infections. Based on the evidence derived from this and other studies, TEN by oral nutritional supplements in patients with AH is recommended by the European Society for Parenteral and Enteral Nutrition (ESPEN) since it improves nutritional status and survival in severely malnourished patients with AH.[34]

Corticosteroids

The use of corticosteroids is the most widely studied intervention in patients with AH. A recent meta-analysis included 15 trials with a total of 721 randomized patients.[35] Overall results were inconsistent, only 3 trails reported a significant improvement in mortality, whereas the remaining 12 trials did not. However, the reanalysis of individual patient data from the five most recent placebo-controlled studies with an adequate number of patients and appropriate quality demonstrated that 28-day survival was significantly higher in corticosteroid-treated patients than in non-corticosteroid-treated patients (80% vs. 66%). These trials only included patients with severe AH as defined by DF ≥ 32 or encephalopathy, and the survival benefit derived from corticosteroids was predominantly observed in patients classified as responders or partial responders by the Lille model confirming the predictive role of this composite score.[36]

Optimal dosage and type of corticosteroid have not been systematically assessed, but prednisolone at 40 milligrams per day for 28 days and then stopped or tapered down over two weeks is suggested. The full course of corticosteroids, however, should only be administered in patients who show an adequate response to corticosteroids, whereas patients with a Lille score above 0.45 after seven days of corticosteroids are unlikely to respond and more likely to develop corticosteroid-associated adverse effects.[6,7,36] The interruption of corticosteroids is particularly recommended in those identified as non-responders as per a Lille score of >0.56.[35]

N-Acetylcysteine

NAC is well established in the treatment of fulminant hepatic failure due to paracetamol overdose, and it increases transplant-free survival in early-stage non-paracetamol acute liver failure. Two recent trials have tested the efficacy of NAC also in patients with severe AH based on the concept that the consumption of large amounts of alcohol causes oxidative stress and depletion of glutathione. Moreno and coworkers randomized 52 patients into either a group receiving adequate enteral nutrition plus intravenous NAC at 100 mg/kg body weight, or enteral nutrition with an intravenous placebo solution for two weeks.[37] Survival, surrogate parameters of liver dysfunction, and rates of infection at months 1 and 6 were not different between groups, but the study was underpowered due to a small sample size.

The second study randomly assigned patients with severe AH as defined by a DF ≥ 32, and a liver biopsy consistent with AH to receive either prednisolone at 40 mg/day plus NAC at 50–150 mg/kg body weight (n = 85) or prednisolone alone (n = 89).[38] Both groups received an oral hospital diet with 1,800–2,000 kcal/day. Mortality at 6 months was selected as the primary end point, but not significantly decreased in the prednisolone/NAC group compared to the prednisolone-only group at months 3 and 6. However, mortality was significantly lower at 1 month (8% vs. 24%, $P = 0.006$), mainly due to a lower frequency of the HRS and of infections in the prednisolone/NAC group.

Liver transplantation

In many countries, patients with decompensated ALD are only listed for liver transplantation, provided they can substantiate a six-month period of abstinence. This, however, cannot be applied to patients with AH as the majority of such patients will die prior to the achievement of this goal. In most countries, AH is still regarded as a contraindication for liver transplantation, for reasons which are only in part of medical nature.[31,39] Retrospective histological analyses of liver explants for criteria of AH showed that AH patients and patients with ALD but without ASH have comparable outcomes. Another reason for denying liver transplantation for patients with AH is that medical therapies, such as corticosteroids and nutritional support, are available and effective to only a set of patients. The remaining fraction of non-responders to this kind of medical therapy, however, reveals a six-month mortality of up to 75%, and they preponderantly die without additional therapeutic options.

A French multicenter study showed that liver transplantation could significantly improve the outcome of such non-responders to prior corticosteroid therapy.[30] Mathurin and colleagues selected 26 patients with severe AH with a median Lille score of 0.88, indicating a high risk of short-term death who were non-responsive to corticosteroid therapy.[30] The cumulative six-month survival rate was higher among patients who received early transplantation than among those who did not (77% vs. 23%, $P < 0.001$). This figure is comparable to those for other indications, and was sustained through two years of follow-up. Patients were carefully selected based on the following criteria: (1) first decompensation episode; (2) non-response to medical therapy; (3) supportive family background; (4) exclusion of psychiatric illnesses; (5) commitment to lifelong abstinence; and (6) complete consensus among team members to select the patient for transplantation. It should be emphasized that only three patients returned to occasional or harmful drinking. Meanwhile, similar excellent results for liver transplantation in AH have been achieved in the United States,[40] which has further challenged the six-month rule.

Therapy of alcoholic cirrhosis of the liver

Since there is at present no effective antifibrogenic therapeutic approach besides abstinence, alcoholic cirrhosis of the liver needs to be treated by treating or preventing their complications, as pointed out under the section "General measures." Future directions for basic and clinical research on alcoholic liver fibrosis have been focused on recently.

New Therapeutic Approaches in ALD

While treatment for AUD comprises total abstinence using psychotherapeutic and pharmacological treatment modalities, these results show that many individuals are not able or willing to achieve abstinence, resulting in an undertreated medical condition. This is reflected in the latest guidelines from the European Medicines Agency (EMA, 2010), the US National Institute on Alcohol Abuse and Alcoholism (NIAAA, 2007), the Canadian Centre for Addiction and Mental Health (CAMH, 2012), and the British National Institute for Health and Clinical Excellence (NICE, 2011). Nalmefene (Selincro®, H Lundbeck A/S) is an opioid system modulator, with antagonist activity at the μ- and δ-opioid receptors, and partial agonist activity at the κ-opioid receptor. It diminishes the reinforcing effects of alcohol, helping the patient to reduce drinking. Nalmefene was approved in February 2013 by the EMA for the reduction of alcohol consumption in adult patients with alcohol dependence who have a high drinking risk level, without physical withdrawal symptoms and who do not require immediate detoxification.

Three randomized, multicenter, double-blind, placebo-controlled, parallel-group phase III studies were designed to assess the efficacy and safety of nalmefene in reducing alcohol consumption.[26–28] This phase III program enrolled about 2,000 patients with alcohol dependence. Two studies comprised a 24-week treatment period followed by a 4-week run-out phase (ESENSE 1 & 2), while the third one (SENSE) was a 52-week study. While the ESENSE 1 & 2 studies aimed to evaluate the effect of nalmefene on alcohol consumption at study end,[26,27] the SENSE study aimed to evaluate the safety and tolerability of nalmefene at study end, as well as the effect of nalmefene on alcohol consumption at 6 months.[28] Differences to placebo at 6 months in heavy drinking days (HDDs) were of –2.3, –1.7, and –0.9 HDDs per month in the ESENSE 1 ($P < 0.05$), ESENSE 2 ($P < 0.05$), and SENSE studies, respectively. Differences to placebo at 6 months in terms of total alcohol consumption were of –11.0, –5.0, and –3.5 grams per day in the ESENSE 1, ESENSE 2, and SENSE studies, respectively. Notably, these results were consistent with liver function test outcomes for the same sample of patients with high Drinking risk levels (DRLs), as GGT and alanine aminotransferase levels at 24 weeks were significantly reduced versus placebo in almost all outcomes (adjusted geometric means, $P < 0.05$ for GGT/Alanine amino transferase (ALT) in ESENSE 1, $P < 0.05$ for ALT in ESENSE 2, $P = 0.244$ for GGT in ESENSE 2). Safety results from a pooled analysis of all three phase III studies showed that the most frequent (>10% of patients) adverse events in the nalmefene arm (n = 1,144) were nausea, dizziness, insomnia, and headache.

In conclusion, there remains a large treatment gap for alcohol dependence, but the reduced risks associated with reduced alcohol consumption supported by nalmefene in combination with psychosocial support are meaningful. Patients with a high or very high drinking risk level at baseline and randomization showed a greater benefit from nalmefene treatment, which was generally well tolerated. An ongoing study (Study No.: 15871A, DELIVER, EudraCT: 2014-000413-31) aims at further validating potentially hepatoprotective effects of nalmefene due to the reduction in alcohol consumption.

Endotoxins and cytokines as therapeutic targets: Anti-inflammatory and anti-fibrotic strategies

ASH is characterized by a typical histomorphological appearance. In addition to fat accumulation and MDBs, a dense neutrophilic infiltrate and pronounced activation of Kupffer cells are visible. The marked inflammation is commonly ascribed to endotoxins shifted from the gut to the liver due to an alcohol-mediated disruption of the mucosal barrier function and changes in GI bacteria composition. Endotoxins stem predominantly from gram negative bacteria and bind to and activate Kupffer cells. These secrete chemokines and cytokines lead to hepatic inflammation via various mechanisms.[5–7] Several specific inflammatory targets, for example, interleukin 1 (IL-1), interleukin-8 (IL-8), interleukin-22 (IL-22), osteopontin (OPN), Lipopolysaccharide (LPS), and gut microbiota are currently under investigation for the treatment of AH.

One approach would be the prevention of Kupffer cell activation by lowering endotoxin uptake or increasing endotoxin elimination from the serum. In rat experiments using the Tsukamoto–French model, the administration of antibiotics decreasing bacterial endotoxins has alleviated ASH. Besides the administration of non-absorbable antibiotics, several studies have shown that the modulation of gut microbiota seems to be a promising strategy to reduce alcohol-induced liver injury. For example, in mice, Lactobacillus rhamnosus GG culture supernatant increases the intestinal occludin expression and protects them from ALD.[41] Furthermore, the anti-LPS substance Travelan produced by vaccination of cows to 13 common *Escherichia coli* (*E. coli*) strains, a hyperimmune IgG directed against LPS in colostrums and resistant to digestion in the GI tract, is presently used in AH.

Mookerjee and coworkers investigated whether the full activation of neutrophils by endotoxins renders them unable to respond to further bacterial challenge.[42] The authors found the defective neutrophil function in most cases of ASH associated with a greater risk of infection, organ failure, and mortality. This defective neutrophilic function was transmissible through the patient's plasma to normal neutrophils, and the patient's neutrophilic function could be restored by normal plasma. The removal of endotoxins from the patient's plasma by using LPS-neutralizing antihuman, anti-CD14, antibody, or by a polymyxin B column decreased the resting burst of neutrophils and increased the phagocytic function.[42] Thereby, an early decision could be made whether the patients need endotoxin removal (poor phagocytic function) or steroid therapy with a lower risk for infections.

In another approach, Horie introduced granulocytes/monocytes apheresis for severe AH and found improved prognosis in patients with white blood counts >10(4)/μL.[43] Since some cytokines and chemokines are associated with severity and survival of ALD, they could function as a therapeutic target. In ASH, IL-1 levels are approximately 10 times higher compared to normal livers. It was shown that resveratrol decreases IL-1 in mice with an improvement of liver injury.[44] Blockade of IL-1 also improves systemic inflammation. Therefore, suitable IL-1 antagonists could provide an option in severe ASH. Another cytokine associated with short-term survival is IL-6 and Il-8.[45]

Interleukin-22 (IL-22) produced by Th17 and natural killer cells controls bacterial infection, homeostasis, and tissue repair, upregulates several antioxidant, anti-apoptotic, and antimicrobial genes, has antifibrotic effects, and improves experimental ALD in mice. IL-22 also ameliorates kidney injury. It is currently under investigation in preclinical and clinical studies for AH.[46]

Hepatic expressions of CXC chemokines (IL-8, CXCL5, CXCL6, CXCL7, Gro-α, Gro-β, and Gro-γ are members of the ELR+ CXC family, whereby the ELR motif appears to be important in ligand/receptor interactions on neutrophils) predict portal hypertension and survival in patients with AH.[45] Both IL-8 and ENA-78 significantly predict survival probability. CCL20, one of the most upregulated chemokines in AH, has been identified as an important mediator linking inflammation, injury, and fibrosis in AH. The GRO-α as well as DUOX-2 gene expression correlates with neutrophilic infiltration and with the severity of AH, so do MMP-2 and TIMP-1. TGF-β and Procollagen 4a(1) correlate with portal infiltration.[45,47]

The intrahepatic gene expression profile of human ASH revealed the elevated expression of OPN.[48] OPN modulates hepatic inflammation by CD44 and integrin binding motifs (SLAYGLR), and the subsequent recruitment of neutrophils and mononuclear cells. The neutrophilic infiltrate is associated with a high hepatic OPN expression, and the administration of neutralizing antibodies against OPN improved inflammatory features and liver injury. OPN-mediated neutrophilic infiltration evolves through ligand binding of an N-terminal integrin binding motif of OPN to its receptor a9β1 and a4β1 integrin on neutrophils. In theory, alcohol elicits OPN secretion from bile duct epithelial cells and hepatocytes exposing the cryptic SLAYGLR sequence, followed by integrin binding, subsequent neutrophil adhesion and migration, and neutrophil-mediated liver damage. OPN is induced by LPS and stimulates inflammatory actions in hepatic stellate cells.[48] OPN knockout mice are protected against ALD.[48] Thus, an elimination of OPN by an adequate antibody could prevent this mechanism.

Ethanol enhances cytokine production in monocytes by increasing histone acetylation of pro-inflammatory genes.[49] Histone deacetylation may silence these genes. Thus, a stimulation of deacetylation by a compound like theophylline could be of interest, particularly as it is widely used to treat bronchopulmonary obstruction.[49] The cannabinoid CB2 receptor (CB2) displays potent anti-inflammatory properties, while the cannabinoid CB1 receptor (CB1) mediates fibrogenesis.[50] While alcohol administration to rodents increased CB1 receptor activity, possibly due to acetaldehyde resulting in increased fibrogenesis, the concomitant administration of CB2 agonist improved ALD. Thus, CB2 agonists could be potential therapeutic agents for the therapy of ALD.[51]

Counteracting oxidative stress and cytochrome P4502E1 induction

Besides the action of cytokines, oxidative stress and the production of reactive oxygen species (ROS) and lipid peroxides are of major importance in ALD. A variety of factors may contribute to the generation of ROS following alcohol ingestion. However, animal experiments have convincingly demonstrated the important role of CYP2E1 in the production of ROS and ALD (for review, see Refs. 52 and 53).

Chronic alcohol consumption leads to a 10–20-fold induction of CYP2E1, which metabolizes ethanol to acetaldehyde.[5,53] In chronic alcoholics, almost 30% of ethanol degradation is mediated by CYP2E1. In humans, the extent of CYP2E1 induction varies between individuals. CYP2E1 induction can be observed following the consumption of 40 gram alcohol/day, corresponding to 400 milliliter of 12.5 vol% wine, after one week.[54] CYP2E1 induction disappears in most patients after days of abstinence; however, some patients sustain elevated CYP2E1 activity for longer periods. It has been shown in animal experiments that CYP2E1 induction is associated with fat accumulation, inflammation, fibrosis, and cancer (for review, see Ref. 52).

The role of CYP2E1 induction and cell injury has been studied in detail. For example, oxidized DNA products have been found to be lower in CYP2E1 knockout mice compared to wild-type mice, while this was more pronounced in transgenic mice overexpressing CYP2E1. Hepatic CYP2E1 also correlates with the generation of carcinogenic exocyclic etheno-DNA adducts via lipid peroxidation products such as 4-hydroxynonenal.[55]

CYP2E1-derived ROS contributes to alcohol-induced fatty liver[56] by inhibiting fatty acid oxidation via impaired upregulation of PPARα. Moreover, hepatic free fatty acids (FFA) may also induce CYP2E1 and form ROS. Thus, fatty liver enhances the production of ROS with lipid peroxidation. Diets enriched with polyunsaturated fatty acids such as fish oil worsen liver injury following alcohol consumption as compared to unsaturated fatty acid enriched diets. In this context, PPARα protects from the development of ALD,[57] and the PPARα agonist Wy-14,643 reverses fibrosis and steatohepatitis in mice.[58]

CYP2E1 can be induced in animals by chronic alcohol feeding, and its inhibition by CMZ improves liver damage.[52] It has been concluded that this effect is mainly due to the inhibition of free radical formation. The inhibition of CYP2E1 by a specific inhibitor not only leads to a decrease in fat accumulation but also to a significant improvement in experimental ALD. CYP2E1 inhibition also leads to a significant decrease in DNA lesions in cell cultures, animal experiments, and humans.[55] The most selective inhibitor of CYP2E1 is CMZ which has been used in many experimental studies. In Germany, CMZ is a drug approved for humans for alcohol detoxification; however, it is only applicable for a short time interval because the drug itself has potency for causing dependence. We are presently investigating the effect of CMZ versus Diazepam in the treatment of alcohol detoxification with respect to the short-term course of ALD by measuring the serum enzyme profile, liver fat, and stiffness as well as CYP2E1 using a special micro chlorzoxazone assay (Figure 2).

Interestingly Lee and colleagues reported most recently that interleukin-32Y attenuated ethanol-induced liver injury by the inhibition of the CYP2E1 expression and inflammatory responses.[59]

Homocysteine, endoplasmic reticulum stress, and apoptosis: The use of betaine and antiapoptotic strategies

In ALD, severe alterations in the metabolism of homocysteine and methionine are observed resulting in an increase of hepatic homocysteine and a decrease of hepatic methionine. Various mechanisms including deficiencies

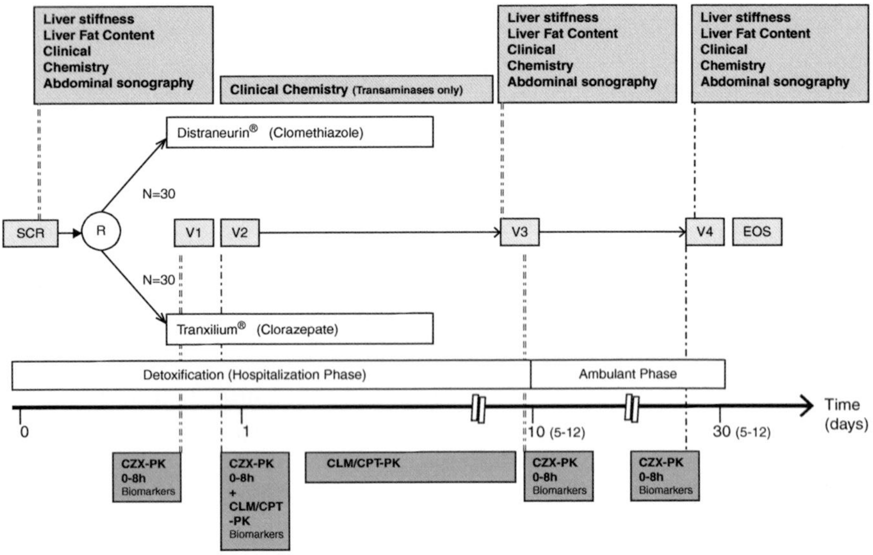

Figure 2. Protocol of our ongoing trial to test the effect of CMZ: a specific cytochrome P4502E1 inhibitor, on hepatic parameters in the alcoholic. Chronic alcoholics who are admitted to the hospital for alcohol detoxification are screened and are integrated into the study when AST was found to be elevated and cirrhosis was excluded by a liver stiffness less than 12 kPa measured by Fibroscan. Patients were randomized for chlormethiazole or clorazepate treatment. Before, during, and after treatments, a chlorzoxazone test was performed to measure total cytochrome P4502E1. In addition, clomethiazole blood levels were also measured during medication. Various parameters such as liver stiffness, hepatic fat content, and laboratory values were recorded.
Abbreviations: SCR: screening, CZX-PK: chlorzoxazone pharmacokinetic, CLM: clormethiazole, CPT: clorazepate, V: visit.

of folate, vitamin B12, and vitamin B6 as well as acetaldehyde-mediated inhibition of enzymes in the metabolism of methionine and S-adenosylmethionine (SAMe) contribute to these changes.[60] A profound reduction of SAMe is responsible for a severely impaired methylation capacity, resulting in altered methylation of DNA and phospholipids.[60] On the other hand, elevated hepatic homocysteine results in endoplasmic reticulum (ER) stress. Homocysteinylation of ER proteins leads to a malfolding-induced ER stress response, resulting in the activation of transcription factors which upregulate proapoptotic genes via the ER transcription factors

SREBPs, ATF6, ATF4, and ER kinases (IRE1a, PERK).[61] As a result of ER stress, TRAF 2 translocation occurs, leading to the release of caspase 12 and consecutive apoptosis.[61] Indeed, apoptosis in ASH is correlated with disease severity.[62] Although it has been shown that TNF-α contributes to necro-inflammation and apoptosis in ASH, it does not contribute to hyperhomocysteinemia and ER stress in intragastric alcohol fed mice.[63]

An inhibition of ER stress may reduce apoptosis. For example, the administration of betaine to alcohol-fed rats prevented fatty liver.[61,64] Although the activity of betaine-homocysteine methyltransferase (BHMT) is upregulated in rodents, this may not be fully sufficient to decrease homocysteine and to increase methionine. An additional administration of betaine may be necessary to increase methionine and finally SAMe. Indeed, betaine decreases hyperhomocysteinemia, ER stress, and liver injury in alcohol-fed mice.[61]

Alcohol and LPS may enhance hepatic apoptosis synergistically through different mechanisms. Deaciuc *et al.*[65] demonstrated that the caspase inhibitor IDN1965 not only inhibited caspases and apoptosis, but also reversed the effect of LPS on plasma ALT levels in alcohol-fed animals and prevented LPS-induced necrosis.[65] However, it was also reported that caspase activation is associated with a spontaneous recovery from acute liver failure, and it was emphasized that caspase-independent cell death might be more relevant in severe forms of liver failure.

Hepatic cell regeneration: Induction of proliferation of hepatic progenitor cells, mesenchymal stem cell transplantation, and bone marrow transplantation granulocyte colony stimulating factor

It has been shown that hepatic cell proliferation plays an important role in the prognosis of AH.[66] Liver cell regeneration is decreased in AH. To stimulate liver cell regeneration, insulin and glucagon were used in a clinical trial with disappointing results and poor tolerability due to hypoglycemia.

The granulocyte colony stimulating factor (G-CSF) has been used to induce the proliferation of hepatic progenitors in ASH. In a small study in patients with severe ASH, G-CSF was administered for five days.[67] CD34+ cells and hepatocyte growth factor (HGF) increased significantly in the group receiving G-CSF. Changes in Ki67+/cytokeratin7+ cells are correlated with changes in CD34+ cells, and it was concluded from these preliminary data that G-CSF mobilizes CD34+ cells, increases HGF, and drives hepatic progenitor cells to proliferate within seven days following administration. This, together with an inhibition of apoptosis, could be an interesting approach in future therapies of ASH. Another randomized pilot study with G-CSF in severe AH has been published demonstrating an increased short term survival.[68]

Liver progenitor cells in AH: Stem cell transplantation therapy

ALD is generally accompanied by a ductular reaction that is characterized by the periportal accumulation of atypical bile duct cells closely paralleling the severity of liver disease. Ductular cells and myofibroblasts extend into the parenchyma, revealing proliferative activity often associated with markers of immature cells. It has been shown that several of the major cell types that participate in the ductular reaction,[70] namely pluripotent hepatic progenitors, immature cholangiocytes, and liver myofibroblasts, produce and respond to Hedgehog (Hh) ligands.[69] The Hh pathway signals to cells to assure proper embryogenesis. However, Hh regulates stem cells involved in the maintenance and regeneration of organ tissues in adults, and has been implicated in the development of some cancers.

Upregulated Hh signaling and increased numbers of Hh-responsive cells were found in mice that were chronically fed alcohol.[71] Both progenitors and stromal cells populations harbored Hh-positive cells, while more ductular-type progenitors were noted after alcohol. In addition, Hh-responsive cells were also increased in patients with AH, especially in severely ill patients with a Maddrey index of more than 32. The lobular accumulation of Gli2/CK7 double positive ductular cells in patients with AH is correlated with high short-term mortality risk. If these preliminary new results could be confirmed in a more extended protocol, an intervention leading to an appropriate Hh pathway activation may be a prerequisite for eventually recovery from severe ALD. However, it is important to note that liver progenitor cell (LPC) markers correlate positively with the severity and short-term mortality of AH. Obviously, an expansion of LPCs is inefficient to yield mature hepatocytes. Thus, strategies to promote the differentiation of LPCs into mature hepatocytes should be focused on.

In a recent review by Levine *et al.*,[72] molecular mechanisms of stem cell therapy have been discussed in detail. The therapeutic mechanisms of multipotent mesenchymal stem cells are based on their potential to differentiate into hepatocytes, on their immunomodulatory properties, their potential to promote residual hepatocyte regeneration, and their capacity to inhibit hepatic stellate cells. In summary, it seems that mesenchymal stem cell transplantation is a promising therapeutic strategy to manage AH onset and progression.

Bone marrow transplantation

Few data exist for autologous bone marrow transplantation (BMT) in patients with alcoholic liver cirrhosis. Saito *et al.*[73] reported BMT in five patients with ALD. The authors found an improvement of liver function and hepatic fibrosis.[73] In another study of 12 patients with alcoholic liver cirrhosis, the administration of autologous BM-derived mesenchymal stem cells induced the histological and quantitative improvement of hepatic fibrosis.[74]

Summary and Conclusion

ALD is the most common liver disease in Europe with high mortality, a high burden of disease, associated with enormous health costs. Preventive measures have not resulted in much success. Present therapy is limited to alcohol abstinence and liver transplantation at end-stage liver disease. AH is a serious disease with extremely high mortality, but without convincing therapy. Therefore, new therapeutic approaches are urgently needed. Figure 3 reflects a simplified summary of the major principles in the pathogenesis of ALD with possible therapeutic.

Although the knowledge of the mechanisms in ALD has grown significantly, especially within the last decade, we are far from exploiting this for novel therapies. However, the latest research focusing on endotoxins and cytokines as therapeutic targets for inflammation and antifibrosis and on oxidative stress as well as apoptosis are promising. New strategies stimulating hepatocellular regeneration and using stem cell therapy and BMT may find their way into clinical trials. The European Association for the Study of the Liver (EASL) has, therefore, supported a European Initiative of Hepatologist

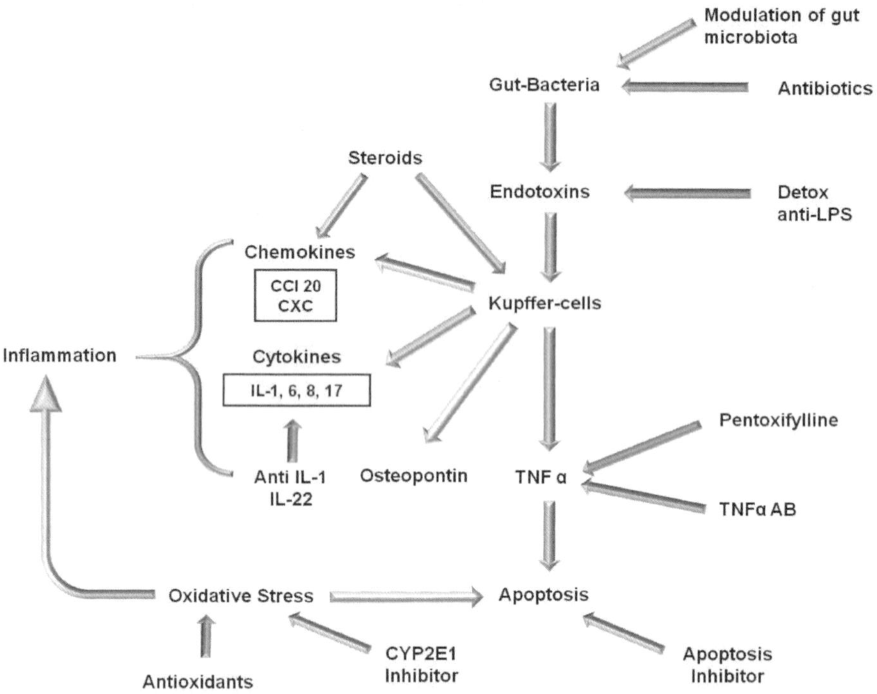

Figure 3. Simplified mechanisms of the toxic action of ethanol on the liver. Endotoxins from the gut are bound to Kupffer cells which secrete a number of chemokines and cytokines leading to inflammatory responses. In addition, apoptosis occurs due to secretion of TNF-α and oxidative stress. Various experimental and clinical approaches have been tried to interact with the cascade of this process or to counteract the action of some cytokines, chemokines, apoptosis, or oxidative stress (for more details, see text).

(SALVE) to develop strategies in the risk management of ALD and in new therapeutic approaches especially for AH.

Acknowledgments

Original studies included in this review have been supported by the Dietmar Hopp Foundation, St. Leon Roth, Germany. The author thanks Mrs Heike Grönebaum for typing the manuscript.

References

1. WHO (2015) Global status Report.
2. OECD Report (2015) Tackling Harmful Alcohol Use.
3. J Rehm, KD Shield (2013) Global alcohol-attributable deaths from cancer, liver cirrhosis, and injury in 2010. *Alcohol Res* **35**: 174–183.
4. R Williams (2015) Liver disease in the UK: Startling findings and urgent need for action. *J Hepatol* **63**: 297–299.
5. HK Seitz, S Mueller (2010) Alcoholic liver diseases. In: H Dancygier (ed.), *Clinical Hepatology: Principles and Practice of Hepatobiliary Diseases*, pp. 1111–1151. Springer, New York.
6. European Association for the Study of the Liver (2012) EASL clinical practical guidelines: Management of alcoholic liver disease. *J Hepatol* **57:** 399–420.
7. F Stickel, HK Seitz (2013) Update on the management of alcoholic steatohepatitis. *J Gastrointestin Liver Dis* **22**: 189–197.
8. F Stickel, S Buch, K Lau, H Meyer zu Schwabedissen, T Berg, M Ridinger, M Rietschel, C Schafmayer, F Braun, H Hinrichsen, R Gunther, A Arlt, M Seeger, S Muller, HK Seitz, M Soyka, M Lerch, F Lammert, C Sarrazin, R Kubitz, D Haussinger, C Hellerbrand, D Broring, S Schreiber, F Kiefer, R Spanagel, K Mann, C Datz, M Krawczak, N Wodarz, H Volzke, J Hampe (2011) Genetic variation in the PNPLA3 gene is associated with alcoholic liver injury in caucasians. *Hepatology* **53**: 86–95.
9. S Buch, F Stickel, E Trepo, M Way, A Herrmann, HD Nischalke, M Brosch, J Rosendahl, T Berg, M Ridinger, M Rietschel, A McQuillin, J Frank, F Kiefer, S Schreiber, W Lieb, M Soyka, N Semmo, E Aigner, C Datz, R Schmelz, S Brückner, S Zeissig, A-M Stephan, N Wodarz, J Devière, N Clumeck, C Sarrazin, F Lammert, T Gustot, P Deltenre, H Völzke, MM Lerch, J Mayerle, F Eyer, C Schafmayer, S Cichon, MM Nöthen, M Nothnagel, D Ellinghaus, K Huse, A Franke, S Zopf, C Hellerbrand, C Moreno, D Franchimont, MY Morgan, J Hampe (2015) A genome-wide association study confirms PNPLA3 and identifies TM6SF2 and MBOAT7 as risk loci for alcohol-related cirrhosis. *Nat Genet* **47**: 1443–1448.
10. JB Whitfield, K Rahman, PS Haber, CP Day, S Masson, AK Daly, HJ Cordell, S Mueller, HK Seitz, S Liangpunsakul, C Westerhold, T Liang, L Lumeng, T Foroud, B Nalpas, P Mathurin, F Stickel, M Soyka, GJ Botwin, TR Morgan, D Seth, for the GenomALC Consortium (2015) Brief report: Genetics of alcoholic cirrhosis-GenomALC multinational study. *Alcohol Clin Exp Res* **39**: 836–842.
11. JE Tirnitz-Parker, A Glanfield, JK Olynyk, GA Ramm (2013) Iron and hepatic carcinogenesis. *Crit Rev Oncog* **18**: 391–407.

12. S Mueller, G Millonig, HK Seitz (2009) Alcoholic liver disease and hepatitis C: A frequently underestimated combination. *World J Gastroenterol* **15**: 3462–3471.
13. CJ Chen, KY Liang, AS Chang, YC Chang, SN Lu, YF Liaw, WY Chang, MC Sheen, TM Lin (1991) Effects of hepatitis B virus, alcohol drinking, cigarette smoking and familial tendency on hepatocellular carcinoma. *Hepatology* **13**: 398–406.
14. HK Seitz, S Mueller, C Hellerbrand, S Liangpunsakul (2015) Effect of chronic alcohol consumption on the development and progression of non-alcoholic fatty liver disease (NAFLD). *Hepatobiliary Surg Nutr* **4**: 147–151.
15. HK Seitz, S Mueller (2012) Ethanol metabolism and its consequences. In: P Anzenbacher, U Zanger (eds.) *Metabolism of Drugs and Other Xenobiotics*, pp. 493–516. Wiley, Weinheim.
16. E Patsenker, M Stoll, G Millonig, A Agaimy, T Wissniowski, V Schneider, S Mueller, R Brenneisen, HK Seitz, M Ocker, F Stickel (2011) Cannabinoid receptor type I modulates alcohol-induced liver fibrosis. *Mol Med* **17**: 1285–1294.
17. J Ursic-Bedoya, S Faure, H Donnadieu-Rigole, GP Pageaux (2015) Liver transplantation for alcoholic liver disease: Lessons learned and unresolved issues. *World J Gastroenterol* **21**: 10994–11002.
18. B Simonis, FM Reimann, R Waldherr, HK Seitz (2007) Sonographic course of alcoholic fatty liver by interobserver and digital evaluation of liver echogenicity. *Zeitschr Gastroenterol* **45**: 689–696.
19. G D'Amico, A Morabito, L Pagliaro, E Marubini (1986) Survival and prognostic indicators in compensated and decompensated cirrhosis. *Dig Dis Sci* **31**: 468–475.
20. SA Borowsky, S Strome, E Lott (1981) Continued heavy drinking and survival in alcoholic cirrhotics. *Gastroenterology* **80**: 1405–1409.
21. S Schenker (1984) Alcoholic liver disease: Evaluation of natural history and prognostic factors. *Hepatology* **4**: 36S–43S.
22. WR Miller, PL Wilbourne, JA Hettema (2003) What works? A summary of treatment outcome research. In: RK Hester, WR Miller (eds.), *Handbook of Alcoholism Treatment Approaches: Effective Alternatives*, pp. 13–63. Allyn & Bacon, Needham Heights, MA.
23. JC Garbutt (2009) The state of pharmacotherapy for the treatment of alcohol dependence. *J Subst Abuse Treat* **36**: S15–23; quiz S24–25.
24. RF Anton, SS O'Malley, DA Ciraulo, RA Cisler, D Couper, DM Donovan, DR Gastfriend, JD Hosking, BA Johnson, JS LoCastro, R Longabaugh, BJ Mason, ME Mattson, WR Miller, HM Pettinati, CL Randall, R Swift, RD Weiss, LD Williams, A Zweben (2006) Combined pharmacotherapies and behavioral

interventions for alcohol dependence: The COMBINE study: A randomized controlled trial. *JAMA* **295**: 2003–217.

25. HG Roozen, R de Waart, DA van der Windt, W van den Brink, CA de Jong, AJ Kerkhof (2006) A systematic review of the effectiveness of naltrexone in the maintenance treatment of opioid and alcohol dependence. *Eur Neuropsychopharmacol* **16**: 311–323.
26. K Mann, A Bladstrom, L Torup, A Gual, W van den Brink (2012) Extending the treatment options in alcohol dependence: A randomized controlled study of as-needed nalmefene. *Biol Psychiatry* **73**: 706–713.
27. W van den Brink, HJ Aubin, A Bladstrom, L Torup, A Gual, K Mann (2013) Efficacy of as-needed nalmefene in alcohol-dependent patients with at least a high drinking risk level: Results from a subgroup analysis of two randomized controlled 6-month studies. *Alcohol Alcohol* **48**: 570–578.
28. A Gual, Y He, L Torup, W van den Brink, K Mann (2013) A randomised, double-blind, placebo-controlled, efficacy study of nalmefene, as-needed use, in patients with alcohol dependence. *Eur Neuropsychopharmacol* **23**: 1432–1442.
29. MR Thursz, P Richardson, M Allison, A Austin, M Bowers, CP Day, N Downs, D Gleeson, A MacGilchrist, A Grant, S Hood, S Masson, A McCune, J Mellor, J O'Grady, D Patch, I Ratcliffe, P Roderick, L Stanton, N Vergis, M Wright, S Ryder, EH Forrest, for the STOPAH Trial (2015) Prednisolone or pentoxifylline for alcoholic hepatitis. *New Engl J Med* **372**: 1619–1628.
30. P Mathurin, C Moreno, D Samuel, J Dumortier, J Salleron, F Durand, H Castel, A Duhamel, GP Pageaux, V Leroy, S Dharancy, A Louvet, E Boleslawski, V Lucidi, T Gustot, C Francoz, C Letoublon, D Castaing, J Belghiti, V Donckier, FR Pruvot, JC Duclos-Vallee (2011) Early liver transplantation for severe alcoholic hepatitis. *New Engl J Med* **365**: 1790–1800.
31. M Gelu-Simeon, JC Duclos-Vallee, D Samuel (2014) Liver transplantation for alcoholic hepatitis. Current situation and future. *Hepatol Int* **8** (Suppl 2): 481–485.
32. P Mathurin, R Bataller (2015) Trends in the management and burden of alcoholic liver disease. *J Hepatol* **62**: S38–S46.
33. F Stickel, B Hoehn, D Schuppan, HK Seitz (2003) Review article: Nutritional therapy in alcoholic liver disease. *Aliment Pharmacol Ther* **18**: 357–373.
34. M Plauth, E Cabre, O Riggio, M Assis-Camilo, M Pirlich, J Kondrup, P Ferenci, E Holm, S Vom Dahl, MJ Muller, W Nolte (2006) ESPEN guidelines on enteral nutrition: Liver disease. *Clin Nutr* **25**: 285–294.
35. A Rambaldi, HH Saconato, E Christensen, K Thorlund, J Wetterslev, C Gluud (2008) Systematic review: Glucocorticosteroids for alcoholic hepatitis — A

Cochrane Hepato-Biliary Group systematic review with meta-analyses and trial sequential analyses of randomized clinical trials. *Aliment Pharmacol Ther* **27**: 1167–1178.

36. P Mathurin, J O'Grady, RL Carithers, M Phillips, A Louvet, CL Mendenhall, MJ Ramond, S Naveau, WC Maddrey, TR Morgan (2011) Corticosteroids improve short-term survival in patients with severe alcoholic hepatitis: Meta-analysis of individual patient data. *Gut* **60**: 255–260.
37. C Moreno, P Langlet, A Hittelet, L Lasser, D Degre, S Evrard, I Colle, A Lemmers, J Deviere, O Le Moine (2010) Enteral nutrition with or without N-acetylcysteine in the treatment of severe acute alcoholic hepatitis: A randomized multicenter controlled trial. *J Hepatol* **53**: 1117–1122.
38. E Nguyen-Khac, T Thevenot, MA Piquet, S Benferhat, O Goria, D Chatelain, B Tramier, F Dewaele, S Ghrib, M Rudler, N Carbonell, H Tossou, A Bental, B Bernard-Chabert, JL Dupas (2011) Glucocorticoids plus N-acetylcysteine in severe alcoholic hepatitis. *New Engl J Med* **365**: 1781–1789.
39. J Neuberger (2007) Public and professional attitudes to transplanting alcoholic patients. *Liver Transpl* **13**: S65–S68.
40. GY Im, L Kim-Schluger, A Shenoy, E Schubert, A Goel, SL Friedman, S Florman, TD Schiano (2015) Early liver transplantation for severe alcoholic hepatitis in the United States — A single-center experience. *Am J Transplant* **16**: 841–849.
41. H Zhao, C Zhao, Y Dong, M Zhang, Y Wang, F Li, X Li, C McClain, S Yang, W Feng (2015) Inhibition of miR122a by Lactobacillus rhamnosus GG culture supernatant increases intestinal occludin expression and protects mice from alcoholic liver disease. *Toxicol Lett* **234**: 194–200.
42. RP Mookerjee, M Malaki, NA Davies, SJ Hodges, RN Dalton, C Turner, S Sen, R Williams, J Leiper, P Vallance, R Jalan (2007) Increasing dimethylarginine levels are associated with adverse clinical outcome in severe alcoholic hepatitis. *Hepatology* **45**: 62–71.
43. Y Horie (2012) Granulocytapheresis and plasma exchange for severe alcoholic hepatitis. *J Gastroenterol Hepatol* **27** (Suppl 2): 99–103.
44. L Bujanda, M Garcia-Barcina, V Gutierrez-de Juan, J Bidaurrazaga, MF de Luco, M Gutierrez-Stampa, M Larzabal, E Hijona, C Sarasqueta, M Echenique-Elizondo, JI Arenas (2006) Effect of resveratrol on alcohol-induced mortality and liver lesions in mice. *BMC Gastroenterol* **6**: 35.
45. M Dominguez, R Miquel, J Colmenero, M Moreno, JC Garcia-Pagan, J Bosch, V Arroyo, P Gines, J Caballeria, R Bataller (2009) Hepatic expression of CXC chemokines predicts portal hypertension and survival in patients with alcoholic hepatitis. *Gastroenterology* **136**: 1639–1650.

46. X Kong, D Feng, S Mathews, B Gao (2013) Hepatoprotective and anti-fibrotic functions of interleukin-22: Therapeutic potential for the treatment of alcoholic liver disease. *J Gastroenterol Hepatol* **28** (Suppl 1): 56–60.
47. J Colmenero, R Bataller, P Sancho-Bru, P Bellot, R Miquel, M Moreno, P Jares, J Bosch, V Arroyo, J Caballeria, P Gines (2007) Hepatic expression of candidate genes in patients with alcoholic hepatitis: Correlation with disease severity. *Gastroenterology* **132**: 687–697.
48. O Morales-Ibanez, M Dominguez, SH Ki, M Marcos, JF Chaves, E Nguyen-Khac, H Houchi, S Affo, P Sancho-Bru, J Altamirano, J Michelena, JC Garcia-Pagan, JG Abraldes, V Arroyo, J Caballeria, FJ Laso, B Gao, R Bataller (2013) Human and experimental evidence supporting a role for osteopontin in alcoholic hepatitis. *Hepatology* **58**: 1742–1756.
49. SF Kendrick, E Henderson, J Palmer, DE Jones, CP Day (2010) Theophylline improves steroid sensitivity in acute alcoholic hepatitis. *Hepatology* **52**: 126–131.
50. E Patsenker, M Stoll, G Millonig, A Agaimy, T Wissniowski, V Schneider, S Mueller, R Brenneisen, HK Seitz, M Ocker, F Stickel (2011) Cannabinoid receptor type I modulates alcohol-induced liver fibrosis. *Mol Med* **17**: 1285–1294.
51. A Louvet, F Teixeira-Clerc, MN Chobert, V Deveaux, C Pavoine, A Zimmer, F Pecker, A Mallat, S Lotersztajn (2011) Cannabinoid CB2 receptors protect against alcoholic liver disease by regulating Kupffer cell polarization in mice. *Hepatology* **54**: 1217–1226.
52. A Dey (2013) Cytochrome P450 2E1: Its clinical aspects and a brief perspective on the current research scenario. *Subcell Biochem* **67**: 1–104.
53. HK Seitz, F Stickel (2007) Molecular mechanisms of alcohol-mediated carcinogenesis. *Nat Rev Cancer* **7**: 599–612.
54. CM Oneta, CS Lieber, J Li, S Ruttimann, B Schmid, J Lattmann, AS Rosman, HK Seitz (2002) Dynamics of cytochrome P4502E1 activity in man: Induction by ethanol and disappearance during withdrawal phase. *J Hepatol* **36**: 47–52.
55. Y Wang, S Mueller, G Millonig, J Nair, H Bartsch, HK Seitz (2008) The role of cytochrome P4502e1 in DNA damage and ethanol-mediated hepatic carcinogenesis. *Gastroenterology* **134** (Suppl 1): A-18.
56. A Mahli, WE Thasler, E Patsenker, S Muller, F Stickel, M Muller, HK Seitz, AI Cederbaum, C Hellerbrand (2015) Identification of cytochrome CYP2E1 as critical mediator of synergistic effects of alcohol and cellular lipid accumulation in hepatocytes in vitro. *Oncotarget* **6**: 41464–41478.
57. T Nakajima, Y Kamijo, N Tanaka, E Sugiyama, E Tanaka, K Kiyosawa, Y Fukushima, JM Peters, FJ Gonzalez, T Aoyama (2004) Peroxisome proliferator-activated receptor alpha protects against alcohol-induced liver damage. *Hepatology* **40**: 972–980.

58. E Ip, G Farrell, P Hall, G Robertson, I Leclercq (2004) Administration of the potent PPARalpha agonist, Wy-14,643, reverses nutritional fibrosis and steatohepatitis in mice. *Hepatology* **39**: 1286–1296.
59. DH Lee, DH Kim, CJ Hwang, S Song, SB Han, Y Kim, HS Yoo, Y Jung, SH Kim, Y Yoon do, JT Hong (2015) Interleukin-32gamma attenuates ethanol-induced liver injury by the inhibition of cytochrome P450 2E1 expression and inflammatory responses. *Clin Sci (Lond)* **128**: 695–706.
60. F Stickel, C Herold, HK Seitz, D Schuppan (2006) Alcohol and methyl transfer: Implication for alcohol related hepatocarcinogenesis. In: S Ali, SL Friedman & DA Mann (eds.), *Liver Disease: Biochemical Mechanisms and New Therapeutic Insights*, Science Publ. Enfield, Jersey, Plymouth.
61. C Ji, N Kaplowitz (2003) Betaine decreases hyperhomocysteinemia, endoplasmic reticulum stress, and liver injury in alcohol-fed mice. *Gastroenterology* **124**: 1488–1499.
62. PS Ribeiro, H Cortez-Pinto, S Sola, RE Castro, RM Ramalho, A Baptista, MC Moura, ME Camilo, CM Rodrigues (2004) Hepatocyte apoptosis, expression of death receptors, and activation of NF-kappaB in the liver of nonalcoholic and alcoholic steatohepatitis patients. *Am J Gastroenterol* **99**: 1708–1717.
63. C Ji, Q Deng, N Kaplowitz (2004) Role of TNF-alpha in ethanol-induced hyperhomocysteinemia and murine alcoholic liver injury. *Hepatology* **40**: 442–451.
64. KK Kharbanda, ME Mailliard, CR Baldwin, HC Beckenhauer, MF Sorrell, DJ Tuma (2007) Betaine attenuates alcoholic steatosis by restoring phosphatidylcholine generation via the phosphatidylethanolamine methyltransferase pathway. *J Hepatol* **46**: 314–321.
65. IV Deaciuc, NB D'Souza, WJ de Villiers, R Burikhanov, TG Sarphie, DB Hill, CJ McClain (2001) Inhibition of caspases in vivo protects the rat liver against alcohol-induced sensitization to bacterial lipopolysaccharide. *Alcohol Clin Exp Res* **25**: 935–943.
66. N Lanthier, L Rubbia-Brandt, N Lin-Marq, S Clement, JL Frossard, N Goossens, A Hadengue, L Spahr (2015) Hepatic cell proliferation plays a pivotal role in the prognosis of alcoholic hepatitis. *J Hepatol* **63**: 609–621.
67. L Spahr, JF Lambert, L Rubbia-Brandt, Y Chalandon, JL Frossard, E Giostra, A Hadengue (2008) Granulocyte-colony stimulating factor induces proliferation of hepatic progenitors in alcoholic steatohepatitis: A randomized trial. *Hepatology* **48**: 221–229.
68. V Singh, AK Sharma, RL Narasimhan, A Bhalla, N Sharma, R Sharma (2014) Granulocyte colony-stimulating factor in severe alcoholic hepatitis: A randomized pilot study. *Am J Gastroenterol* **109**: 1417–1423.

69. JK Sicklick, YX Li, A Melhem, E Schmelzer, M Zdanowicz, J Huang, M Caballero, JH Fair, JW Ludlow, RE McClelland, LM Reid, AM Diehl (2006) Hedgehog signaling maintains resident hepatic progenitors throughout life. *Am J Physiol Gastrointest Liver Physiol* **290**: G859–G870.
70. A Omenetti, L Yang, YX Li, SJ McCall, Y Jung, JK Sicklick, J Huang, S Choi, A Suzuki, AM Diehl (2007) Hedgehog-mediated mesenchymal-epithelial interactions modulate hepatic response to bile duct ligation. *Lab Invest* **87**: 499–514.
71. Y Jung, KD Brown, RP Witek, A Omenetti, L Yang, M Vandongen, RJ Milton, IN Hines, RA Rippe, L Spahr, L Rubbia-Brandt, AM Diehl (2008) Accumulation of hedgehog-responsive progenitors parallels alcoholic liver disease severity in mice and humans. *Gastroenterology* **134**: 1532–1543.
72. P Levine, K McDaniel, H Francis, L Kennedy, G Alpini, F Meng (2014) Molecular mechanisms of stem cell therapy in alcoholic liver disease. *Dig Liver Dis* **46**: 391–397.
73. T Saito, K Okumoto, H Haga, Y Nishise, R Ishii, C Sato, H Watanabe, A Okada, M Ikeda, H Togashi, T Ishikawa, S Terai, I Sakaida, S Kawata (2011) Potential therapeutic application of intravenous autologous bone marrow infusion in patients with alcoholic liver cirrhosis. *Stem Cells Dev* **20**: 1503–1510.
74. YO Jang, YJ Kim, SK Baik, MY Kim, YW Eom, MY Cho, HJ Park, SY Park, BR Kim, JW Kim, HS Kim, SO Kwon, EH Choi, YM Kim (2014) Histological improvement following administration of autologous bone marrow-derived mesenchymal stem cells for alcoholic cirrhosis: a pilot study. *Liver Int* **34**: 33–41.

Section III
Carcinogenesis and Therapeutic Targets in the Gastrointestinal Tract

Chapter 6

Targets of Tumor Epigenetics and Its Microenvironment in Gastrointestinal Cancer

Ssu-Yin Yen, Hong-Meng Chuang, Mao-Hsuan Huang, Sheng-Feng Tsai, Tzyy-Wen Chiou, Hong-Lin Su, Li-Ing Ho, Shinn-Zong Lin, and Horng-Jyh Harn

Abstract

Gastrointestinal (GI) cancers, including gastric, liver, pancreatic, and colorectal cancers, are the major cause of death worldwide. One of the carcinogenic pathways associated with GI cancer is chronic inflammation. Also, the tumor microenvironment, including cells like fibroblasts and immune cells and other modulators, such as growth factors, cytokines, and proteins, can support the growth of cancer cells. The interaction between cancer cells and stromal cells is essential for tumor growth, progression, and metastasis. Moreover, tumor progression involves various genetic modifications and epigenetic alterations, leading to gain-of-function in oncogenes and loss of function in tumor suppressor genes. In gastric cancer, *Helicobacter pylori* infection is probably a predisposing factor. This may cause chronic inflammation. In addition, it has been reported that *H. pylori* infection enhances irregular DNA methylation in gastric cancer cells and silences tumor suppressor genes to promote gastric carcinogenesis. In this chapter, we shall introduce the mechanism of epigenetics, endoplasmic reticulum stress, cytokine regulation, and epithelial–mesenchymal transition in GI cancer. We believe that targeting the tumor microenvironment or modifying epigenetic changes may be the potential and effective therapeutic strategies in the treatment of GI cancer.

Introduction

Cancer is a difficult issue in the world, and it is also a leading cause of death. In 1863, the German pathologist Virchow was the first suggesting a link between inflammation and cancer. Many scientists demonstrated that inflammation is the initiation and progression of gastrointestinal (GI) cancer. Besides, several genetic and epigenetic alterations have been implicating a strong association between the inflammation mechanism and that might be responsible for cancer carcinogenesis.

The common mechanism involved in inflammation and its association with cancer is the NF-κB (nuclear factor-κ-light-chain-enhancer of activated B cells) pathway. Activation of NF-κB in the GI tract leads to the induction of pro-inflammatory cytokines and plays an important role in tumor development. NF-κB activation in tissues has been found in patients with some GI tract diseases. Targeting cytokines, chemokines, and inflammation responsive transcription factors represents a potential target and promising therapeutic strategy. The mechanisms of epigenetics, endoplasmic reticulum stress, cytokine regulation, and epithelial–mesenchymal transition (EMT) association with inflammation in GI cancer are described in detail below.

Histone Modifications and Inflammation in Gastrointestinal Cancer Epigenetics

Epigenetic change can be influenced by several factors including age, environment, lifestyle and also the disease state. The term epigenetics refers to heritable changes in gene expression (activation of oncogenes and/or inactivation of tumor suppressor genes) that does not involve changes to the underlying DNA sequence (i.e. a change in phenotype without a change in genotype). Currently, it is thought that DNA methylation, histone modification, and non-coding RNA-associated gene silencing are responsible for initiating and sustaining epigenetic change. Epigenetic change can produce more damaging effects that can result in diseases such as cancer. Epigenetic regulation may be involved in tumor progression, metastasis, invasiveness, and the response to chemotherapy. Nowadays, researchers are becoming more aware of the roles of epigenetics in a variety of human disorders, particularly cancer.

Epigenetics in cancer

Cancer is caused by the accumulation of gene aberrations during the multistep process of carcinogenesis. Abnormal patterns of epigenetic modifications are common in numerous human diseases. The epigenetic modifications involve cell differentiation, cell proliferation, and patient survival during malignant development. In 1983, DNA methylation was first used to investigate human cancer cases, since then, many other diseases have been linked to epigenetics.[1]

DNA methylation

DNA methylation is one type of epigenetic modification and is crucial for the following reasons: for maintaining genomic DNA in genome imprinting, for the stability of the chromosome, and in transcriptional silencing of repetitive genes. DNA methylation is mediated by a family of highly related DNA methyltransferase enzymes (DNMT1, DNMT3A, and DNMT3B) which transfers a methyl group from S-adenosyl-L-methionine to cytosines in CpG dinucleotides. Typically, the maintenance of DNA methylation patterns in somatic cells is attributed to DNMT1, whereas de novo DNA methylation during embryonic development is performed by DNMT3A and DNMT3B. However, DNMT1 can also contribute to de novo DNA methylation both *in vitro* and *in vivo*, and the maintenance of methylation in certain regions of the genome requires DNMT3A and DNMT3B.[2] In DNMT3a-null mice, each passage resulted in a lowered differentiation capacity of hematopoietic stem cells. DNMT3a was determined to be indispensable for the proper differentiation of these cells.[3] Some contributing factors have been identified in the aberrant methylation pattern in gastric epithelia, such as aging, diet, chronic inflammation, and microbial infection in gastric cancer.[4,5]

Histone modification

Epigenetic alterations frequently occur in cancer development and it plays a critical role in cancer pathogenesis. A high expression of histone deacetylase (HDAC) class I enzymes has been reported in different tumor types, including gastric cancer.[6] In addition, other studies have described a decrease in acetylated histones and overexpression of HDAC2 in gastric cancer patients. Panobinostat (LBH589) is a novel pan-deacetylase inhibitor that overcomes imatinib resistance in preclinical models of GI stromal tumors.[7,8] It belongs to the hydroxamate class of compounds and has potent inhibitory activity at low nanomolar concentrations. LBH589 has shown great promise as a monotherapy for cutaneous T-cell lymphoma and high efficacy in preclinical studies of GI stromal tumors.[9,10] LBH589 has also been proven to cause the regression of colon cancer in animal models, and in phase I trials. This agent has been shown to be well tolerated.[9]

Epigenetic events in inflammation

Inflammation is the physical response of an organism to harmful stimuli such as pathogens, damaged cells, or irritants. Macrophages play an important role in cancer response and allergy response. Recent research data indicated that chromatin modifications are mechanistically crucial when acquiring the macrophage phenotype.[11] NF-κB, forkhead box P3 (FOXP3), interferon regulatory factor (IRF), and signal transducer and activator of transcription (STAT) families are involved in epigenetic changes, including DNA methylation and covalent histone modifications. It has been shown to be of great importance in regulating inflammatory genes. Also, epigenetic mechanisms in T-cells and monocytes are controlled by several of these regulatory factors. *H. pylori* infection induces both acute and chronic gastritis, which leads to superficial mucosal inflammation in the gastric mucosa.[12] Although most infected individuals have no clinical manifestations, approximately 10–20% of patients develop peptic ulcers, and 1% of patients develop gastric cancer.

Regulation of microRNA Profiles by Cytokines and Chemokines in Gastrointestinal Cancer

microRNA in general

microRNA (miRNA) is a new class of regulatory molecule that was recently discovered. They are involved in the process of inflammation and cancer growth, and belong to the group of non-coding RNAs with short 18–24-bp RNA duplex that does not translate to proteins. They function as posttranscriptional regulators of target messenger RNAs (mRNAs), which promotes target mRNA degradation. Primary miRNAs contain 7-methylguanosine and are polyadenylated and transcripted by RNA polymerase II. Primary miRNAs are broken down by the enzyme Drosha, within the nucleus, into 60–80-bp stem-loop precursor miRNAs. The precursor miRNAs are then exported into the cytoplasm, and the RNase Dicer breaks them down further into short 18–24-bp mature miRNAs. The mature miRNAs then synthesize the RNA-induced silencing complex, which leads to the downregulation of specific genes where the binding of complementary sequences in the 3′ untranslated regions (3′-UTRs) of the target mRNAs occur.

microRNAs in gastrointestinal cancer

Several studies have reported that miRNAs are involved in GI cancer development and progression. For example, members of the miR-17-92 cluster, miR-19a and miR-19b, can be upregulated in multidrug resistance (MDR) cell lines, and they can also be modulated in MDR in gastric cancer cells by targeting phosphatase and tensin homolog (PTEN).[13] Furthermore, miRNA profiling has revealed that miR-153 is highly expressed in colorectal cancer.[14] In colorectal cancer patients who were followed for 50 months, 21 of 30 patients with high levels of miR-153 had greater disease progression when compared with others in the same group with low levels of miR-153.[15] The studies have shown that miR-153 upregulation can increase colorectal cancer invasiveness and resistance to oxaliplatin and cisplatin, both *in vitro* and *in vivo*.[14]

A recent study involving a unique 95 miRNAs expression profile in human pancreatic cancer tissues and cell lines identified eight miRNAs (miR-196a, miR-190, miR-186, miR-221, miR-222, miR-200b, miR-15b, and miR-95). Their expressions were significantly increased in most of the pancreatic cancer tissues and cell lines when compared with those in normal pancreatic tissues.[16] miR-21 is overexpressed in various human cancer types, including pancreatic and colon cancer types. Its expression is associated with an advanced clinical stage and limited patient survival.[17] miR-21 could downregulate its target programmed cell death 4 and stimulate colorectal cancer cell proliferation and invasion.[18] On the other hand, miR-155 could repress tumor protein 53-induced nuclear protein 1 expression and increase pancreatic tumor development.[19] Moreover, miR-155 could reprogram normal adjacent fibroblasts into cancer-associated fibroblasts (CAFs), which are the major constituent in the pancreatic cancer microenvironment.[20] miR-451 regulates macrophage migration inhibitory factor production and the proliferation of GI cancer cells,[21] while miR-223 promotes gastric cancer invasion and metastasis by targeting tumor suppressor EPB41L3.[22] The previously mentioned miRNAs serve as oncogenes. There are other groups of miRNAs which serve as tumor suppressor genes. miR-34 could interfere with pancreatic cancer stem cell (CSC) self-renewal by restoring the tumor-suppressing function of p53 in p53-deficient human pancreatic cancer cells.[23] miR-143 was markedly reduced in colon cancer cells, and ERK5 had been determined to be the target gene of such microRNA. The restoration of the miR-143 expression had resulted in a significant inhibition of human colon cancer growth.[24]

microRNA regulation by cytokines and chemokines

The miRNA expression can be regulated by a variety of mechanisms including transcription factor binding, epigenetic modifications, and genomic amplification or deletion. In addition, inflammatory stress also alters the miRNA expression. Experiments in which lipopolysaccharides have been used to stimulate mouse immune response show that inflammatory stress alters the miRNA expression. In malignant tissues, miR-21 is one of the most frequently upregulated miRNAs in solid tumors, including pancreatic and colon cancer tumors. Although miR-21 regulation is complicated, IL-6, a pro-inflammatory cytokine, was reported to drive the expression of miR-21 through a STAT3-dependent mechanism in colon cancer. Furthermore, miR-21 has been known to directly target and repress the IL12-p35 expression in mouse models.[25] In humans, the miR-21binding site in the 3′-UTR of IL12-p35 is conserved. These *in vitro* data suggest that the connections among IL6, IL12-p35, and miR-21 are probably relevant in the context of human colon cancer and that miR-21 may contribute to inflammation-induced carcinogenesis. In addition to miR-21, IL-6 has been determined to be able to regulate another miRNA, miR-370, in human malignant cholangiocytes. IL-6 alerts the DNA methyltransferase-1 and the HASJ4442 expression. The miR-370 expression is strictly dominated by DNA methylation.[26] Thus, IL-6 could induce tumor progression by modulating the expression of selected miRNAs, such as miR-21 and miR-370. miR-155 is another miRNA which is widely expressed in malignant tissues. Interferon-γ has been determined to be able to stimulate the expression of miR-155 in an inflammatory environment. miR-155 can target the suppressor of cytokine 1, leading to the induction of the *NOS2* gene.[27] In addition, the transforming growth factor-β (TGF-β) signaling pathway can also regulate miRNA biogenesis. TGF-β signaling promotes the nuclear localization of R-Smad proteins, which stimulates the Drosha-mediated production of pre-miR-21. miR-21 is rapidly induced by TGF-β, subsequently causing programmed cell death, protein-4 inhibition, and tumor progression.[28] These studies have identified the crucial pathway through which inflammation-associated cytokines and chemokines can epigenetically modulate the gene expression and directly contribute to tumor progression. In the future, targeting miRNAs and their related cytokines may become therapeutic targets for cancer patients.

Targeting Epithelial–Mesenchymal Transition Attenuates Gastrointestinal Tumor Invasion and Metastasis

What is epithelial–mesenchymal transition?

When cells change their properties and differentiate into a variety of cell types, some of the cells lose their cell polarity and cell–cell adhesion, especially if they transition from epithelial to mesenchymal cell type. This is called EMT.[29] EMT is essential for numerous developmental processes, tissue remodeling, and cell migration. However, cancer cells also undergo EMT to obtain additional abilities aside from their overgrowth properties. In normal states, epithelial cells express E-cadherin to enable the tight junctions to attach rigidly to a specific position for a specific function. In previous studies,

EMT was controlled by the expression of E-cadherin, which was downregulated by Snail1/2 and ZEB1/2 in this process, causing cells to lose their polarity[30] and cell–cell adhesion, as well as tumor mobility, invasive properties, and stemness character.

Regulation of epithelial–mesenchymal transition in cancer cells

Regulators of EMT in cancer cells include Notch, Wnt, and especially TGF-β, which is a particularly efficient inducer of EMT.[31] TGF-β signaling activates Smad or non-Smad pathways.[32] The phosphorylated Smad translocates into nuclei and forms the DNA-binding complex, thus activating EMT genes such as Snail and Twist.[33] Several studies have demonstrated that EMT promotes cancer cell invasion and metastasis. Bone morphogenetic proteins (BMPs) belong to the TGF-β super family, demonstrating the inhibitory effect of TGF-β-induced EMT pathways.[33] BMP7 activates Smad 1/5/8 to induce the expression of E-cadherin, which is considered a natural antagonist of TGF-β and can reverse EMT. In addition, the Wnt signaling pathway regulates the dynamic and reversible EMT and MET, and the progression of cancer is consistent with β-catenin/TCF transcriptional target genes. Likewise, the Notch signaling pathway regulates the expressions of miR-21 and miR-200, and also their targets ZEB1 and E-cadherin.[34] These regulators may be the candidates in targeting EMT for cancer therapies.

Tumor stroma and its epithelial–mesenchymal transition induction

In hepatic tumors, stroma crosstalk may induce EMT at the tumor edge and also control the microenvironment where reprogramming of different cytokines or chemokines takes place. These types of extracellular matrix remodeling involve collagen type I and III synthesis and also the expression of matrix metalloproteinases (MMPs).[35] The elevated MMP expression might help tumor cells to escape the cell–cell junction, promoting the ability of cancer cells to metastasize.[36]

Microenvironmental regulators of epithelial–mesenchymal transition

CAFs surrounding the tumor stroma are believed to support tumor carcinogenesis.[37] CAFs enhance tumor or peripheral cell growth by secreting growth factors such as vascular endothelial growth factor (VEGF), fibroblast growth factor, and TGF-β. Moreover, the hypoxic state is also associated with the Warburg effect, which benefits the metabolism of cancer cells. Consequently, the CAFs and the cancer and peripheral cells can migrate into an appropriate microenvironment which leads to tumor growth.

Epithelial–mesenchymal transition regulates inflammation in cancer

EMT and inflammation are commonly associated with the development of organ fibrosis and the progression of cancer.[38] Although EMT events have been well documented, the cause-and-effect relationship between EMT and inflammation is not well understood. To our knowledge, inflammation, oxidative stress, and hypoxia work together through different pathways, leading to the induction of EMT in the progression of organ fibrosis and cancer metastasis. Cyclooxygenase-2 (COX-2) inactivates Smad 2/3 pathways.[39] In addition, transcription factors such as Snail1 also seem to cause serial inflammatory reactions by upregulating the expression of IL-8. Moreover, inducing migration and inflammatory reactions in the microenvironment that has been altered by EMT is considered to be a worldwide disease model.[33]

Epithelial–mesenchymal transition confers a cancer stem cell phenotype

CSCs were identified according to their greater proliferation rate and higher resistance to chemotherapeutic drugs than non-CSCs. The expression of CSC markers such as CD133, OCT4, and Sox2 may be able to predict distant recurrence when the prognosis is poor. A recent study has shown the potential link between EMT and CSC-like phenotypes, with the EMT-associated properties of stemness, drug resistance, and metastasis. The developmentally dependent signaling pathways such as Wnt and Notch can also be used to maintain CSC properties.[40] The most direct evidence shows that EMT may force the emergence of stem-like cells by blocking E-cadherin or giving TGF-β treatment.[41] However, recent studies have suggested that EMT can directly contribute to both drug resistance and metastasis.[42,43] It is likely that EMT might have the potential to obtain CSC properties through some unknown mechanisms.

Targets of epithelial–mesenchymal transition as a therapeutic strategy

Potential targets of EMT are TGF-β receptors and Wnt signaling pathway. Recently, AP-12009 (Trabedersen) was used to target TGF-β, a TGF-β-specific antisense oligonucleotide, in a clinical trial for glioma and pancreatic cancer.[44] LGK974 and CWP232291 are small-molecule inhibitors of Wnt signaling that have demonstrated their tumor-repressive ability in a rodent model.[45] Another small molecular compound, butylidenephthalide (BP), was reported to inhibit Axl, an essential regulator of cancer metastasis and patient survival. The downstream genes of EMT, Twist, and Snail were also reduced and accompanied by tumor migration and invasion.

Modulating the key effectors within the tumor stroma is a prime area for drug development (Figure 1). EMT regulation has important clinical implications in oncological research of tumor microenvironment. However, EMT is very difficult to target because it has different upstream inducers and may be connected to many molecular functions. It has become clear that small molecular drugs or RNA interference studies can become a promising agent for solving medical needs that have not been met. Controlling EMT through current therapeutic strategies may synergistically affect other efficient

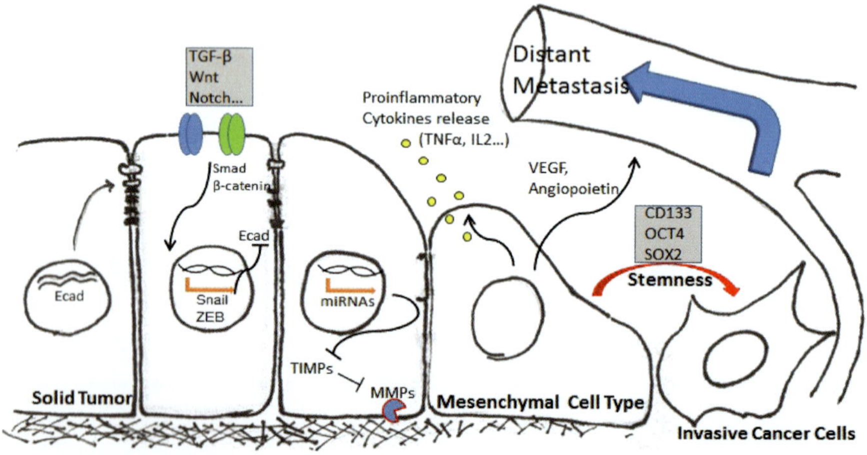

Figure 1. Strategy learned from other migrating cells. The step-by-step epithelial cell transformation into mesenchymal cells after the reduction of cell–cell junctions before digesting the cell–cell contact. EMT also releases pro-inflammatory cytokines and VEGF to enhance vascular growth and blood flow. Finally, the migrated cells become invasive and have stemness properties, and then they move into the blood vessels, and metastasize at a distant site.

cytotoxicity anti-tumor drugs. This could resolve the therapeutic failure and drug resistance in almost all cancer cells. If we cannot prevent these transformed cancer cells from growing, then we should stop their invasion.

Targeting Endoplasmic Reticulum Stress on the Tumor Unfolding Protein, Causing Apoptosis

Endoplasmic reticulum stress

The cell metabolism, protein synthesis, and energy production mechanisms inside tumors are unique. Tumor cells need to overcome many stress insults to accelerate cell proliferation.[46] Protein synthesis is the key factor in cancer cell proliferation and growth, and it also surpasses different cell cycle checkpoints.[47] The endoplasmic reticulum (ER) is a crucial organelle in controlling cell lipid synthesis as well as protein translation and protein folding. It also transports proteins to the Golgi apparatus for final modification or for making a vesicle for secretion. When the cell undergoes rapid proliferation and continued protein synthesis, the protein unfolding increases, and the unfolding protein accumulates in the ER lumen. This phenomenon is called "ER stress." Afterward, the ER lumen stress sensor activates the unfolding protein response (UPR) pathway. First, cells attempt to produce more chaperone proteins in order to increase the protein folding and to correct its efficiency. If the stress is still not corrected, then the cells proceed to the stage of apoptosis.[48]

Unfolding protein response pathway

After UPR activation, three ER stress sensors begin to function, namely (1) inositol-requiring enzyme 1 (IRE1),[49] (2) pancreatic ER kinase (PERK),[50] and (3) activating transcription factor 6 (ATF6). At normal states, the three ER stress sensors IRE1, PERK, and ATF6 are inactivated by binding with the chaperone GRP78. When ER stress occurs, GRP78 is disassociated from IRE1, ATF6, and PERK, and attempts to refold the unfolded or misfolded proteins. Meanwhile, the ER stress sensor PERK phosphorylation causes the α-subunit of eukaryotic initiation factor 2 (eIF2 alpha) to activate the downstream pathway, which can cease all cell protein synthesis. This prevents cell synthesis from accumulating more unfolding proteins in the ER lumen, which further damages the ER. PERK activation protects cell survival. However, if the unfolding response is not repaired, then the C/EBP homologous protein

(CHOP) is induced, and the transcription factor 4 (ATF4) begins to transcript; these are the two key factors in determining cell survival or cell apoptosis. IRE1 splices the transcription factor X box-binding protein 1 (XBP1). The XBP1 variants translocate to the nucleus to assist the ER chaperone in coding to mitigate the stress. In response to the ER stress, ATF6 leaves the ER lumen and moves to the Golgi apparatus where it can cleave ATF6 by using serine proteases S1P and S2P. The activated ATF6 also translocates to the nucleus to enhance GRP78 and GRP94 chaperone protein XBP1 transcription.[51]

Endoplasmic reticulum stress and gastrointestinal cancer

Cancer cells can adapt efficiently in different harsh conditions. This is entirely due to their extremely efficient chaperone, which prevents them from entering ER stress-associated apoptosis. The ER chaperone protein GRP78 is overexpressed in the following cancers: prostate,[52] liver,[53] stomach,[54] and colon.[55] The high level of GRP78 can prevent cancer cells from experiencing ER stress and other types of stress through different strategies. Furthermore, GRP78 can also suppress caspase-7 activation.[56] On the other hand, Chang used the siRNA knockdown GRP78 expression in colon cancer cell lines to increase 17-DMAG small-molecule toxicity.[57] Together, these two strategies for treating GI cancers are proposed as follows: (1) downregulate the GRP78 expression level and (2) activate the PERK-eIF2 alpha-CHOP axis apoptosis pathway. Moreover, the knockdown of the GRP78 expression can also increase the sensitivity of HCT-116 cells in chemotherapy drugs.[58] However, Xu has revealed that the Chinese natural compound oblongifolin C induced the CHOP expression in the HCT-116 cell line, leading to cell apoptosis.[59] In pancreatic cancers, avarol, the small molecule, can activate the PERK-eIF2alpha-CHOP axis and induce apoptosis,[60] and knockdown the GRP78 expression, which can also enhance the sensitivity of pancreatic cancer cells to anti-cancer agents.[61]

Endoplasmic reticulum stress signaling as a therapeutic target in clinical cancer research

UPR activation commonly occurs in the cancer environment. It can be applied as an effective target mechanism against cancer development.[62] Recently, an increasing number of targeting ER stress inhibitors have been identified, including the IRE1α inhibitors STF-083010, 3-ethoxy-5, and 6-dibromosalicylaldehyde, and the GRP78 inhibitors, verrucosidin and VER-155008. These molecules have been shown to be promising in *in vitro* studies.[63–65] However, the ER stress pathway in cancer is complicated, and by targeting only one of them may not be sufficient in generating cancer cell apoptosis. Thus, aiming to inhibit the produced chaperone cancer and simultaneously elevate the CHOP expression might be an effective approach in treating GI cancer in the future (Figure 2).

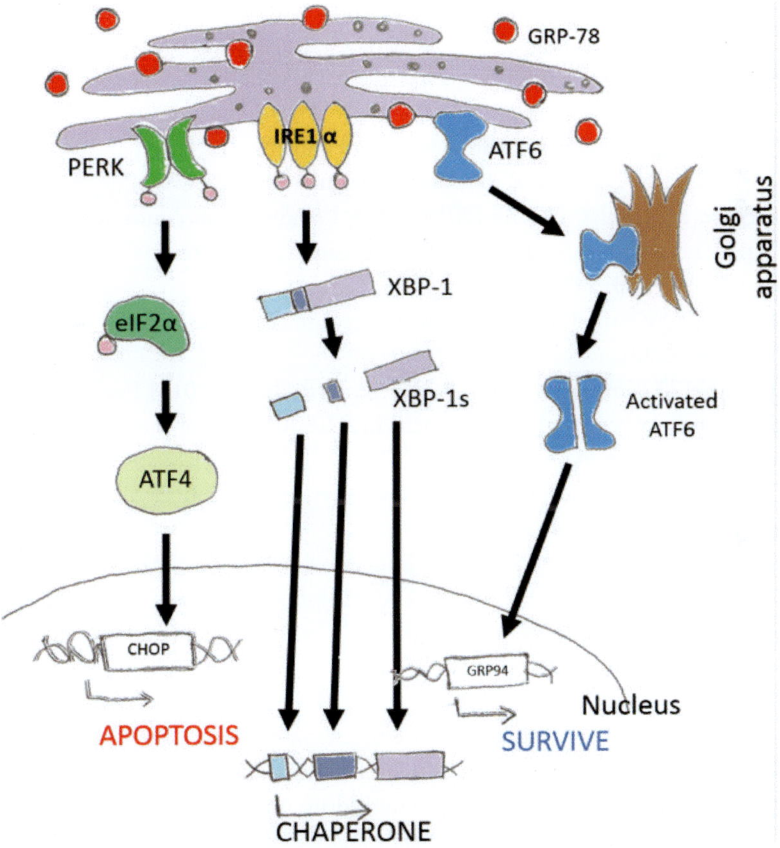

Figure 2. UPR response-signaling activation in a cell under ER stress. Cancer cells under rapid proliferation forced the tumor cells facing ER stress and activated UPR responses. Initially, GRP78 is released and PERK, IRE1α, and ATF6 become activated. IRE1α and ATF6 pathways increase cell chaperone protein translation and resolve ER stress. When the ER stress homeostasis is broken, PERK pathway will increase the CHOP expression, which is the key element in ER stress-mediated apoptosis.

References

1. B Weinhold (2006) Epigenetics: The science of change. *Environ Health Perspect* **114**: A160–167.
2. B Jin, Y Li, KD Robertson (2011) DNA methylation: Superior or subordinate in the epigenetic hierarchy? *Genes Cancer* **2**: 607–617.
3. S Shukla, SM Meeran (2014) Epigenetics of cancer stem cells: Pathways and therapeutics. *Biochim Biophys Acta* **1840**: 3494–3502.
4. Y Qu, S Dang, P Hou (2013) Gene methylation in gastric cancer. *Clin Chim Acta* **424**: 53–65.
5. D Bayarsaihan (2011) Epigenetic mechanisms in inflammation. *J Dent Res* **90**: 9–17.
6. S Ropero, M Esteller (2007) The role of histone deacetylases (HDACs) in human cancer. *Mol Oncol* **1**: 19–25.
7. S Bauer, RA Hilger, T Mühlenberg, F Grabellus, J Nagarajah, M Hoiczyk, A Reichardt, M Ahrens, P Reichardt, S Grunewald, ME Scheulen, A Pustowka, E Bock, M Schuler, D Pink (2014) Phase I study of panobinostat and imatinib in patients with treatment-refractory metastatic gastrointestinal stromal tumors. *Br J Cancer* **110**: 1155–1162.
8. J Zhang, Q Zhong (2014) Histone deacetylase inhibitors and cell death. *CMLS* **71**: 3885–3901.
9. M Anne, D Sammartino, MF Barginear, D Budman (2013) Profile of panobinostat and its potential for treatment in solid tumors: An update. *Onco Targets Ther* **6**: 1613–1624.
10. S Jain, J Zain, OO'connor (2012) Novel therapeutic agents for cutaneous T-cell lymphoma. *J Hematol Oncol* **5**: 24.
11. M Ishii, H Wen, CA Corsa, T Liu, AL Coelho, RM Allen, WF Carson, KA Cavassani, X Li, NW Lukacs, CM Hogaboam, Y Dou, SL Kunkel (2009) Epigenetic regulation of the alternatively activated macrophage phenotype. *Blood* **114**: 3244–3254.
12. L E Wroblewski, R M Peek, K T Wilson (2010) Helicobacter pylori and gastric cancer: Factors that modulate disease risk. *Clin Microbiol Rev* **23**: 713–739.
13. F Wang, T Li, B Zhang, H Li, Q Wu, L Yang, Y Nie, K Wu, Y Shi, D Fan (2013) MicroRNA-19a/b regulates multidrug resistance in human gastric cancer cells by targeting PTEN. *Biochem Biophys Res Commun* **434**: 688–694.
14. L Zhang, K Pickard, V Jenei, MD Bullock, A Bruce, R Mitter, G Kelly, C Paraskeva, J Strefford, J Primrose, GJ Thomas, G Packham, AH Mirnezami (2013) miR-153 supports colorectal cancer progression via pleiotropic effects

that enhance invasion and chemotherapeutic resistance. *Cancer Res* **73**: 6435–6447.

15. MD Bullock, K Pickard, R Mitter, AE Sayan, JN Primrose, C Ivan, GA Calin, GJ Thomas, GK Packham, AH Mirnezami (2015) Stratifying risk of recurrence in stage II colorectal cancer using deregulated stromal and epithelial microRNAs. *Oncotarget* **6**: 7262–7279.
16. Y Zhang, M Li, H Wang, WE Fisher, PH Lin, Q Yao, C Chen (2009) Profiling of 95 microRNAs in pancreatic cancer cell lines and surgical specimens by real-time PCR analysis. *World J Surg* **33**: 698–709.
17. M Dillhoff, J Liu, W Frankel, C Croce, M Bloomston (2008) MicroRNA-21 is overexpressed in pancreatic cancer and a potential predictor of survival. *J Gastrointest Surg* **12**: 2171–2176.
18. IA Asangani, SA Rasheed, DA Nikolova, JH Leupold, NH Colburn, S Post, H Allgayer (2008) MicroRNA-21 (miR-21) post-transcriptionally downregulates tumor suppressor Pdcd4 and stimulates invasion, intravasation and metastasis in colorectal cancer. *Oncogene* **27**: 2128–2136.
19. M Gironella, M Seux, MJ Xie, C Cano, R Tomasini, J Gommeaux, S Garcia, J Nowak, ML Yeung, KT Jeang, A Chaix, L Fazli, Y Motoo, Q Wang, P Rocchi, A Russo, M Gleave, JC Dagorn, JL Iovanna, A Carrier, MJ Pebusque, NJ Dusetti (2007) Tumor protein 53-induced nuclear protein 1 expression is repressed by miR-155, and its restoration inhibits pancreatic tumor development. *Proc Natl Acad Sci USA* **104**: 16170–16175.
20. W Pang, J Su, Y Wang, H Feng, X Dai, Y Yuan, X Chen, W Yao (2015) Pancreatic cancer-secreted miR-155 implicates in the conversion from normal fibroblasts to cancer-associated fibroblasts. *Cancer Sci* **106**: 1362–1369.
21. E Bandres, N Bitarte, F Arias, J Agorreta, P Fortes, X Agirre, R Zarate, JA Diaz-Gonzalez, N Ramirez, JJ Sola, P Jimenez, J Rodriguez, J Garcia-Foncillas (2009) microRNA-451 regulates macrophage migration inhibitory factor production and proliferation of gastrointestinal cancer cells. *Clin Cancer Res* **15**: 2281–2290.
22. X Li, Y Zhang, H Zhang, X Liu, T Gong, M Li, L Sun, G Ji, Y Shi, Z Han, S Han, Y Nie, X Chen, Q Zhao, J Ding, K Wu, F Daiming (2011) miRNA-223 promotes gastric cancer invasion and metastasis by targeting tumor suppressor EPB41L3. *Mol Cancer Res* **9**: 824–833.
23. Q Ji, X Hao, M Zhang, W Tang, M Yang, L Li, D Xiang, JT Desano, GT Bommer, D Fan, ER Fearon, TS Lawrence, L Xu (2009) MicroRNA miR-34 inhibits human pancreatic cancer tumor-initiating cells. *PloS One* **4**: e6816.

24. Y Akao, Y Nakagawa, T Naoe (2006) MicroRNAs 143 and 145 are possible common onco-microRNAs in human cancers. *Oncol Rep* **16**: 845–850.
25. TX Lu, A Munitz, ME Rothenberg (2009) MicroRNA-21 is up-regulated in allergic airway inflammation and regulates IL-12p35 expression. *J Immunol* **182**: 4994–5002.
26. F Meng, H Wehbe-Janek, R Henson, H Smith, T Patel (2008) Epigenetic regulation of microRNA-370 by interleukin-6 in malignant human cholangiocytes. *Oncogene* **27**: 378–386.
27. X Wang, Q Zhao, R Matta, X Meng, X Liu, CG Liu, LD Nelin, Y Liu (2009) Inducible nitric-oxide synthase expression is regulated by mitogen-activated protein kinase phosphatase-1. *J Biol Chem* **284**: 27123–27134.
28. A Hata, BN Davis (2009) Control of microRNA biogenesis by TGFβ signaling pathway—a novel role of Smads in the nucleus. *Cytokine Growth Factor Rev* **20**: 517–521.
29. S Lamouille, J Xu, R Derynck (2014) Molecular mechanisms of epithelial–mesenchymal transition. *Nat Rev Mol Cell Biol* **15**: 178–196.
30. G Moreno-Bueno, F Portillo, A Cano (2008) Transcriptional regulation of cell polarity in EMT and cancer. *Oncogene* **27**: 6958–6969.
31. CH Heldin, M Vanlandewijck, A Moustakas (2012) Regulation of EMT by TGFβ in cancer. *FEBS Lett.* **586**: 1959–1970.
32. M Yamashita, K Fatyol, C Jin, X Wang, Z Liu, YE Zhang (2008) TRAF6 mediates Smad-independent activation of JNK and p38 by TGF-beta. *Mol Cell* **31**: 918–924.
33. J M Lopez-Novoa, MA Nieto (2009) Inflammation and EMT: An alliance towards organ fibrosis and cancer progression. *EMBO Mol Med* **1**: 303–314.
34. B Bao, Z Wang, S Ali, D Kong, Y Li, A Ahmad, S Banerjee, AS Azmi, L Miele, FH Sarkar (2011) Notch-1 induces epithelial–mesenchymal transition consistent with cancer stem cell phenotype in pancreatic cancer cells. *Cancer Lett* **307**: 26–36.
35. M Roderfeld, R Weiskirchen, S Wagner, ML Berres, C Henkel, J Grotzinger, AM Gressner, S Matern, E Roeb (2006) Inhibition of hepatic fibrogenesis by matrix metalloproteinase-9 mutants in mice. *FASEB J* **20**: 444–454.
36. H Li, X Fan, J Houghton (2007) Tumor microenvironment: The role of the tumor stroma in cancer. *J Cell Biochem* **101**: 805–815.
37. D Hanahan, LM Coussens (2012) Accessories to the crime: Functions of cells recruited to the tumor microenvironment. *Cancer Cell* **21**: 309–322.
38. R Kalluri, RA Weinberg (2009) The basics of epithelial–mesenchymal transition. *J Clin Invest* **119**: 1420–1428.

39. JR Neil, KM Johnson, RA Nemenoff, WP Schiemann (2008) Cox-2 inactivates Smad signaling and enhances EMT stimulated by TGF-beta through a PGE2-dependent mechanisms. *Carcinogenesis* **29**: 2227–2235.
40. I Malanchi, H Peinado, D Kassen, T Hussenet, D Metzger, P Chambon, M Huber, D Hohl, A Cano, W Birchmeier, J Huelsken (2008) Cutaneous cancer stem cell maintenance is dependent on beta-catenin signalling. *Nature* **452**: 650–653.
41. SA Mani, W Guo, MJ Liao, EN Eaton, A Ayyanan, AY Zhou, M Brooks, F Reinhard, CC Zhang, M Shipitsin, LL Campbell, K Polyak, C Brisken, J Yang, RA Weinberg (2008) The epithelial–mesenchymal transition generates cells with properties of stem cells. *Cell* **133**: 704–715.
42. FH Sarkar, Y Li, Z Wang, D Kong (2009) Pancreatic cancer stem cells and EMT in drug resistance and metastasis. *Minerva Chir* **64**: 489–500.
43. F Nurwidya, F Takahashi, A Murakami, K Takahashi (2012) Epithelial–mesenchymal transition in drug resistance and metastasis of lung cancer. *Cancer Res Treat* **44**: 151–156.
44. L Vallieres (2009) Trabedersen, a TGFbeta2-specific antisense oligonucleotide for the treatment of malignant gliomas and other tumors overexpressing TGFbeta2. *IDrugs* **12**: 445–453.
45. J Liu, S Pan, MH Hsieh, N Ng, F Sun, T Wang, S Kasibhatla, AG Schuller, AG Li, D Cheng, J Li, C Tompkins, A Pferdekamper, A Steffy, J Cheng, C Kowal, V Phung, G Guo, Y Wang, MP Graham, S Flynn, JC Brenner, C Li, MC Villarroel, PG Schultz, X Wu, P Mcnamara, WR Sellers, L Petruzzelli, AL Boral, HM Seidel, ME Mclaughlin, J Che, TE Carey, G Vanasse, JL Harris (2013) Targeting Wnt-driven cancer through the inhibition of Porcupine by LGK974. *Proc Natl Acad Sci USA* **110**: 20224–20229.
46. LM Phan, S-C J Yeung, M-H Lee (2014) Cancer metabolic reprogramming: Importance, main features, and potentials for precise targeted anti-cancer therapies. *Cancer Biol Med* **11**: 1–19.
47. S White-Gilbertson, DT Kurtz, C Voelkel-Johnson (2009) The role of protein synthesis in cell cycling and cancer. *Mol Oncol* **3**: 402–408.
48. J Faitova, D Krekac, R Hrstka, B Vojtesek (2006) Endoplasmic reticulum stress and apoptosis. *Cell Mol Biol Lett* **11**: 488–505.
49. JS Cox, CE Shamu, P Walter (1993) Transcriptional induction of genes encoding endoplasmic reticulum resident proteins requires a transmembrane protein kinase. *Cell* **73**: 1197–1206.
50. HP Harding, Y Zhang, A Bertolotti, H Zeng, D Ron (2000) Perk is essential for translational regulation and cell survival during the unfolded protein response. *Mol Cell* **5**: 897–904.

51. M Li, P Baumeister, B Roy, T Phan, D Foti, S Luo, AS Lee (2000) ATF6 as a transcription activator of the endoplasmic reticulum stress element: Thapsigargin stress-induced changes and synergistic interactions with NF-Y and YY1. *Mol Cell Biol* **20**: 5096–5106.
52. N Li, A Zoubeidi, E Beraldi, ME Gleave (2013) GRP78 regulates clusterin stability, retrotranslocation and mitochondrial localization under ER stress in prostate cancer. *Oncogene* **32**: 1933–1942.
53. G Zhu, AS Lee (2015) Role of the unfolded protein response, GRP78 and GRP94 in organ homeostasis. *J Cell Physiol* **230**: 1413–1420.
54. X Wang, Y Li, G Xu, M Liu, L Xue, L Liu, S Hu, Y Zhang, Y Nie, S Liang (2015) Mechanism study of peptide GMBP1 and its receptor GRP78 in modulating gastric cancer MDR by iTRAQ-based proteomic analysis. *BMC Cancer* **15**: 1.
55. Y-J Chang, C-Y Huang, C-S Hung, W-Y Chen, P-L Wei (2015) GRP78 mediates the therapeutic efficacy of curcumin on colon cancer. *Tumor Biol* **36**: 633–641.
56. RK Reddy, C Mao, P Baumeister, RC Austin, RJ Kaufman, AS Lee (2003) Endoplasmic reticulum chaperone protein GRP78 protects cells from apoptosis induced by topoisomerase inhibitors role of ATP binding site in suppression of caspase-7 activation. *J Biol Chem* **278**: 20915–20924.
57. Y-J Chang, C-Y Huang, C-S Hung, H-H Liu, P-L Wei (2015) Glucose-regulated protein 78 mediates the therapeutic efficacy of 17-DMAG in colon cancer cells. *Tumor Biol* **36**: 4367–4376.
58. Y Wang, KK Auyeung, X Zhang, JK Ko (2014) Astragalus saponins modulates colon cancer development by regulating calpain-mediated glucose-regulated protein expression. *BMC Complement Altern Med* **14**: 1.
59. W Xu, M Cheng, Y Lao, X Wang, J Wu, L Zhou, Y Zhang, H Xu, N Xu (2015) DNA damage and ER stress contribute to oblongifolin C-induced cell killing in Bax/Bak-deficient cells. *Biochem Biophys Res Commun* **457**: 300–306.
60. T Namba, R Kodama (2015) Avarol induces apoptosis in pancreatic ductal adenocarcinoma cells by activating PERK–eIF2α–CHOP signaling. *Mar Drugs* **13**: 2376.
61. X Jiang, T Kanda, S Nakamoto, Y Haga, R Sasaki, M Nakamura, S Wu, R Mikata, O Yokosuka (2014) Knockdown of glucose-regulated protein 78 enhances poly (ADP-ribose) polymerase cleavage in human pancreatic cancer cells exposed to endoplasmic reticulum stress. *Oncol Rep* **32**: 2343–2348.
62. RK Yadav, S-W Chae, H-R Kim, HJ Chae (2014) Endoplasmic reticulum stress and cancer. *J Cancer Prevent* **19**: 75–88.

63. W Chien, L-W Ding, Q-Y Sun, LA Torres-Fernandez, SZ Tan, J Xiao, SL Lim, M Garg, KL Lee, S Kitajima (2014) Selective inhibition of unfolded protein response induces apoptosis in pancreatic cancer cells. *Oncotarget* **5**: 4881–4894.
64. AT Macias, DS Williamson, N Allen, J Borgognoni, A Clay, Z Daniels, P Dokurno, MJ Drysdale, GL Francis, CJ Graham (2011) Adenosine-derived inhibitors of 78 kDa glucose regulated protein (Grp78) ATPase: Insights into isoform selectivity. *J Med Chem* **54**: 4034–4041.
65. S Thomas, N Sharma, R Gonzalez, P-W Pao, FM Hofman, TC Chen, SG Louie, MC Pirrung, AH Schönthal (2013) Repositioning of verrucosidin, a purported inhibitor of chaperone protein GRP78, as an inhibitor of mitochondrial electron transport chain complex I. *PLoS One* **8**: e65695.

Chapter 7

Esophageal Cancer: From Bench to Bedside

Gang Ma and Zhihua Liu

Abstract

Esophageal cancer is a heavy health burden worldwide. The research community is continuously striving for understanding the initiation and progression of this malignance. Meanwhile, the clinical society is endeavoring to improve the 5-year survival rate and life quality of patients. In this chapter, we briefly discuss the esophageal development and homeostasis of mature esophagus, which can be a constructive starting point to elaborate how the epithelial cells in esophagus become cancerous. Afterward, we present genetic and environmental risk factors of two main types of esophageal cancer, namely the squamous cell carcinoma and adenocarcinoma. Importantly, several "omics" studies provide a full view of esophageal cancer, which will undoubtedly aid the research and clinical practice in this field. As metastases of surrounding lymph nodes and distant organs are usually present in the first-diagnosed cases with cancer, we shall focus on in discussing the genes and microenvironmental factors modulating the invasion-metastasis cascade of squamous cell carcinoma. Moreover, recent research advances of esophageal cancer stem cells are also discussed. All these offer options for diagnosis and/or treatment of metastatic esophageal cancer. Lastly, we introduce the current medication strategies, evaluate their strengths and weaknesses, and further propose some novel approaches in treatment (e.g. immunotherapy) at the preclinical stage of therapy.

Introduction

The function of the esophagus is relatively simple. The word ESOPHAGUS is derived from two Greek ancestors: *oisein*, meaning to carry, and *phagein*, meaning to eat. Thus, it well depicts the primary function of the esophagus: transporting liquids and foods from the pharynx to the stomach without other evident functions such as digestion and metabolism.[1] To this end, the esophagus consists of mucosa (a stratified squamous epithelium), submucosa (connective tissue), and smooth muscle layer.[2] Mucosa prevents damages caused by the swallowed liquids and foods, and peristaltic contractions of smooth muscle sustain the correctly unidirectional delivery of foods through the lumen of the esophagus.[2] As esophageal cancer remains a major health problem worldwide, in this chapter we discuss the homeostasis of esophageal epithelium, our current understanding of carcinogenesis and the invasion-metastasis cascade of esophageal cancer, and the potential translation from laboratory research to clinical treatment in metastatic esophageal cancer.

Regulation of Esophageal Development and Homeostasis

The esophagus is a simple organ. However, its embryonic development and homeostasis maintenance are nevertheless sophisticated. Understanding the mechanisms implicated in these two important biological processes is essential to know how esophageal malignancy arises and progresses.

Esophageal development and its regulation

Morphogenesis of the esophagus proceeds as a part of the foregut development. One vital event for the esophageal development is that the respiratory appendage (including one tracheal bud and two lung buds) separates from the foregut. This so-called tracheal–esophageal separation procedure starts at E9.5 for mice and at E26 for humans.[1] To date, studies have demonstrated that three transcription factors (Sox2, NKX2-1, and p63) and four signaling pathways (Wnt, hedgehog, bone morphogenetic protein [BMP], and fibroblast growth factor [FGF]) are involved in modulating the development of esophagus.[1] Here, we give a brief account on these key regulators.

The two transcription factors, Sox2 and NKX2-1, interact reciprocally to guarantee the proper execution of the tracheal–esophageal separation. Sox2 is expressed in endodermal cells that are destined to form the esophagus. It can be detected in epithelial cells of the adult esophagus.[1] Mutation of Sox2 leads to tracheoesophageal fistula (aberrant fusion between tracheal lumen and esophageal lumen) and esophageal atresia (abnormal disappearance of proximal esophagus) (Table 1), demonstrating that Sox2 is critical for the development of esophagus in humans.[3] On the other hand, NKX2-1 dictates endodermal cells to form the respiratory primordium and its expression is positive in adult alveolar epithelial cells.[1] Loss of this protein leads to the defects in separation of the trachea from the foregut, in proper branching organogenesis, and in differentiation of the pulmonary endoderm[1] (Table 1).

A third transcription factor required for the differentiation of the esophageal epithelium is p63; in particular, it is expressed in the basal layer of squamous epithelial cells to sustain proper proliferation.[1] In p63-mutated mice, goblet cells and cilia, two characteristics of the matured tracheal tract, are observed in the esophageal epithelium[4] (Table 1). In addition, the aberrant esophageal epithelium consists of pseudostratified columnar epithelial cells (as seen in normal airway tract) instead of cuboidal epithelial cells (as

Table 1. Mutations in genes of murine esophageal development.[1]

Gene mutation	Development phenotype
$Sox2^{EGFP/COND}$	Tracheoesophageal fistula and esophageal atresia
$NKX2\text{-}1^{-/-}$	Abnormal development of lung buds
$p63^{-/-}$	Aberrant esophagus with respiratory characteristics
$SHH^{-/-}$	Defects in tracheoesophageal separation
$Gli2^{-/-}$	Reduced esophageal lumen and underdeveloped mesenchyme
$Gli2^{-/-}/Gli3^{+/-}$	No trachea and lung appendages
$Foxf1^{-/-}$	Tracheoesophageal fistula and reduced esophageal lumen
$Bmp4^{-/-}$	One tube linking the pharynx, the stomach and the hypoplastic lungs
$Noggin^{-/-}$	Tracheoesophageal fistula and esophageal atresia
$Noggin^{-/-}$ $Bmp4^{+/-}$	No tracheoesophageal fistula and esophageal atresia

observed in normal esophagus).[4] These results underscore the critical regulatory roles of p63 in differentiation of the esophageal epithelium.

Besides these three transcription factors, the four morphogenetic signaling pathways, namely the hedgehog, BMP, FBF, and Wnt, regulate the tracheal–esophageal separation as well.[1] We make a concise discussion on hedgehog and BMP signaling pathways based on findings from murine esophagus.

In mammals, there are three secreted hedgehog proteins, the desert hedgehog (DHH), Indian hedgehog (IHH), and sonic hedgehog (SHH), among which SHH-induced signaling pathway plays a central role in the development of the esophagus, corroborated with the observed tracheoesophageal fistula in mice without SHH[1] (Table 1). Since the Gli family of transcription factors mediate the effects of SHH signaling pathway, it is not surprising to find that defects resulted from the deletion of Gli2 or/and Gli3 resemble those in $SHH^{-/-}$ mice[5] (Table 1). Similar aberrations between Sox2 deletion and SHH/Gli mutations imply the potential interaction between the Sox2 and SHH signaling pathways in the esophageal development. Although mechanistic details have not been clarified yet, Foxf1 was identified to be involved in the Sox2/SHH signaling axis.[6] Specifically, the forced expression of SHH increases the expression of Foxf1 in the mesenchyme of the foregut, suggesting that Foxf1 is probably a downstream effector of the SHH signaling pathway.[6] Moreover, $Foxf1^{+/-}$ mice fail to undergo accurate tracheal–esophageal separation and branching organogenesis,[6] demonstrating that the absence of Foxf1 would undermine the function of mesenchymal cells supporting the development of the esophageal epithelium.

Bmp4, one BMP, is expressed in mesenchyme that will develop into trachea. The tracheal–esophageal separation fails due to the conditional deletion of Bmp4 and this deficiency is the characteristic of a single tube linking the pharynx, the stomach, and the hypoplastic lungs.[7] Notably, the esophageal endodermal marker Pax9, instead of the tracheal mesenchymal marker Col2a and the tracheal endodermal marker NKX2-1, is detected in this tube, demonstrating that Bmp4 is vital in the development of trachea.[7] Noggin is an antagonist of the BMP signaling pathway. $Noggin^{-/-}$ mice manifest an opposite phenotype relative to $Bmp4^{-/-}$ counterparts: one tube with tracheal differentiation connecting the respiratory tract with the stomach.[8] However, $Noggin^{-/-}Bmp4^{+/-}$ could sustain the development of the esophagus in mice.[8]

Mechanistically, the BMP signaling pathway inhibits the expression of Sox2 in the tracheal endoderm.[9]

Collectively, these results demonstrate that SHH in the endoderm induces the expression of Foxf1 and further stimulates the expression of Bmp4 in the mesenchyme. Bmp4 then prevents the development of the esophagus by repressing Sox2 in the endoderm. Simultaneously, Noggin is expressed to liberate the expression of Sox2 in the endoderm to guarantee the proper esophageal development.[1]

Maintenance of homeostasis of esophageal epithelium

Carcinogenesis is a process of impairing homeostasis of intact tissues and molecular interactions. Accordingly, understanding the homeostasis of the esophageal epithelium and its regulation is crucial for deciphering the mechanisms underlying the malignant transformation of esophageal epithelial cells. To date, the key transcription factors and signaling pathways in the development of the esophagus have been identified to be essential for maintaining the homeostasis of the adult esophageal epithelium.

As described above, Sox2 marks the prospective esophageal epithelium during the development. In the matured esophageal epithelium of mice, Sox2 is expressed in all cells located in the basal layer.[1] The increased Sox2 expression leads to the expanded population of epithelia progenitor cells,[10] whereas the removal of Sox2-positive cells results in the complete loss of the basal layer in transgenic mice.[11] p63 is another transcription factor in favor of the proliferation of esophageal epithelial cells, which is corroborated by an *in vitro* organotypic study, demonstrating that the absence of p63 suppresses the self-renewal of epithelial cells.[12] In esophageal squamous cell carcinoma (ESCC) cell lines, the overexpression of p63 promotes proliferation and invasion through modulating the expression of several genes such as c-myc and β-catenin.[13] However, the lack of *in vivo* experiments hinders a deeper insight into the roles of p63 in the initiation and progression of ESCC.

Recent studies about ESCC at the genomic scale have revealed striking alternations in several signaling pathways, among which the hedgehog, Notch, and FGF signaling pathways also play critical roles in esophageal development and homeostasis. We briefly discuss the hedgehog signaling pathway in the following paragraph.

Table 2. Comparisons between adult human and mouse esophagus.

Properties	Human esophagus	Mouse esophagus
Morphology	Fewer cell layers without folding along papillae	More cell layers folded along papillae
Proliferating cells	Only the basal cells	Basal cells and suprabasal cells
Keratinization	Yes	No
Turnover of cells	Relatively inactive	Very active
Submucosal glands	No	Yes

The hedgehog signaling pathway of the esophageal development functions in a paracrine mode. However, the repressive smoothed receptor (Smo) and the downstream transcription factor Gli1 are expressed in the epithelial cells of adult esophagus simultaneously. Thus, this signaling pathway functions in an autocrine manner.[1] The enhanced hedgehog signaling pathway in two transgenic mouse models — one with the conditioned deletion in protein patched homolog1 (PTCH1) and the other with the conditioned upregulation of Gli1 — promotes the proliferation of epithelial cells.[14] The pro-proliferation function of the pathway is further corroborated by a few lines of evidence that inactive mutations in PTCH and the elevated expression of Gli1 are detected in ESCC specimens when compared with the adjacent normal counterparts.[15,16] Taking together the hedgehog signaling pathway sustains the proliferation of both prospective/adult epithelial cells and transforms epithelial cells in the esophagus.

Of note, most findings, especially *in vivo* evidence, are based on rodent models. Since the difference between human and mouse esophagi (Table 2), we should be cautious when applying these conclusions obtained from rodents to human applications.

Esophageal Carcinoma

Epidemiology of esophageal cancer

Worldwide, esophageal cancer ranks the sixth fatal cancer among males and the ninth among females according to the estimates in 2012.[17] In the United States, new cases of esophageal cancer and new deaths caused by this malignance are estimated to be 16,910 and 15,690 in 2016, respectively.[18] In China, 477,900 new cases of esophageal cancer and 375,000 new deaths are expected in 2015.[19] This is a reflection of geographic difference in the incidence of esophageal cancer. Esophageal cancer has two main subtypes: squamous cell carcinoma (ESCC) and adenocarcinoma (EAC). ESCC consists of 90% of cases of esophageal carcinoma worldwide and most of these victims live in the "esophageal cancer belt," stretching from Northern Iran through the Central Asia to North-Central China.[20] In the United States and some countries of Europe (such as England and France), the incidence of ESCC has been continuingly declining, while the incidence of EAC is increasing rapidly. Notably, males are more likely to suffer from esophageal cancer compared to females.[18] In the United States, the expected new cases and deaths in males are four times more than those of females.[18] Likewise, the prospective new cases and deaths in males double relative to female counterparts in China.[19] This sex distribution probably stems from different lifestyle between males and females.

Environmental risk factors contributing to esophageal cancer differ between ESCC and EAC. The risk factors for ESCC have not been fully understood yet. Smoking, alcohol consumption, and detrimental dietary habit make potential victims more vulnerable to esophageal cancer.[20] Sitas and colleagues reported a line of serological evidence showing a significant association between ESCC and human papillomavirus (HPV) 6 and 16, which demonstrates that HPV infection probably contributes to a subset of ESCC.[21] But this is still an open issue. Esophageal achalasia — one motility disorder — is characterized by a failure of smooth muscle surrounding the esophagus to relax and resultant inability to transport food. A retrospective cohort study shows that patients with esophageal achalasia are more likely to suffer from ESCC when compared with their counterparts without the same disorder.[22] Although the external risk factors are not fully understood, increased intake of fresh fruit and vegetables, constrained alcohol consumption, and quitting smoking would be in favor of lowering the incidence of ESCC.[20]

With respect to EAC, chronic gastroesophageal reflux disease (GERD), obesity (especially abdominal adiposity), and smoking are the three primary risk factors.[20] GERD is a process by which gastric acid enters into the esophagus from the stomach. Chronic GERD damages mucosa and elicits Barrett's esophagus under some circumstances. Barrett's esophagus has been identified as the precursor lesion of EAC. The risk of EAC increases by seven times in patients with daily GERD and by five times in patients with weekly GERD, when compared with the patients with less GERD symptoms.[23] Abdominal obesity, which is more prevalent in males than in females, probably promotes GERD by increasing intragastric pressure and gastroesophageal gradient.[24] Of note, approximately 40% of EAC patients have no GERD symptoms.[20] Interestingly, the infection of *Helicobacter pylori* in stomachs is associated with the decreased risk of EAC. One possible explanation is that this infection could reduce gastric acid secretion.[20] Smoking increases the risk of EAC by two times relatively to non-smoking.[18] However, alcohol consumption does not significantly contribute to the initiation of EAC as in ESCC.[18] Together, the management of body weight, abandon of tobacco usage, and treatment of GERD are valid strategies in preventing EAC.

Carcinogenesis is a vicious consequence of interactions between environmental risk factors and genetic backgrounds. To date, several studies at the genomic scale have revealed some molecular mechanisms. Genome wide association studies (GWAS) based on Chinese ESCC patients revealed seven susceptibility loci located on 5q11, 6p21, 10q23, 12q24, and 21q22.[25] The same group later identified that one single nucleotide polymorphism (SNP; rs1050631) in SLC39A6 is associated with the survival of ESCC patients.[26] Functional analyses demonstrate that the silence of SLC39A6 inhibits the proliferation and invasion of ESCC cells.[26] A recent joint analysis of three independent GWAS data of ESCC in China uncovered rs7447927, rs1642764, and rs35597309 as new susceptibility loci.[27] Three independent whole-genome and/or whole-exome sequencing assays show more details about ESCC. The group led by QM Zhan reported eight mutated genes (RB1, TP53, PIK3CA, CDKN2A, NOTCH1, ADAM29, NFE2L2, and FAM135B) and strikingly altered signaling pathways in ESCC.[28] They also found the pathological analog between ESCC and head and neck carcinoma.[28] Lin and colleagues identified more new mutated genes, such as FAT1, FAT2, KMT2D, and ZNF750.[29] A third exome sequencing assay verified the mutations reported by the two previous studies, and it, more importantly, underscored the critical roles of dysregulated epigenetic regulation in ESCC, which is corroborated by the fact that mutations of EP300 indicates poor survival in ESCC patients.[30] Similar molecular mutations were also detected in an independent cohort of ESCC patients from Japan.[31] Reanalysis of whole-genome sequencing data revealed a complex picture of somatic structural variations (SVs) of chromosome in ESCC. A high level of focal amplification caused by chromothripsis was detected in the genomic locus of FGFR1 and LETM2, which accounts for the elevated expression of these two genes.[32] Moreover, SVs lead to 173 in-frame fusion genes and 231 out-frame fusion genes, among which the EIF3E-RAD51B fusion transcript, for example, probably disrupts the functions of EIF3E and RAB51B simultaneously and thereby promotes the initiation and progression of ESCC.[32]

Besides, GWAS on Barrett's esophagus and EAC showed three significant susceptibility loci: rs10419226 in Crtc1, rs11789015 in Barx1, and rs2687201 in Foxp1.[33] Analyses of paired Barrett's esophagus and EAC showed a progression of malignancy using whole-exome sequencing. This sequential process begins with emerging mutations of TP53 in the early stage of Barrett's esophagus. Then, genome doubles corresponding to the absence of normal TP53 and oncogenes amplify accordingly without the loss of suppressor genes.[34] Further investigation in the spatial and temporal progression from Barrett's esophagus to EAC showed that the high frequency of mutation is present and distinct combinations of mutations mark variant clones in Barrett's esophagus.[35] In addition, mutations differ dramatically between EAC and adjacent Barrett's esophagus,[35] which is consistent with the idea that tumor is heterogeneous and molecular markers are needed to identify different subsets.

Metastasis of esophageal cancer

Invasion and metastasis account for more than 90% of cancer-caused deaths. It has become clear that invasion and metastasis occur in the early stage of cancer progression, instead of always as a late event. Additionally, an efficient strategy of early detection is lacking and this results in a locally advanced or metastasis in newly diagnosed patients. Treatments targeting primary lesions have been advancing gradually in recent decades, but a few disseminated malignant cells always survive from current treatments and flourish in distant organs. In this section, we discuss recent findings on ESCC invasion and metastasis.

Proteins regulating metastasis of ESCC

Dozens of genes implicated in the invasion and metastasis of esophageal cancer have been identified. Guan's group identified some genes involving in regulating the metastasis of ESCC, among which Uroplakin 1A (UPK1A), SOX6, and Ras-like small GTPase DIRAS1 inhibit, whereas adenosine deaminases acting on RNA (ADAR) promote migration and invasion *in vitro* or metastasis *in vivo*.[36–39] An elevated expression of the eukaryotic translation initiation factor 5A2 (eIF5A2) was recently found to be significantly associated with lymph node metastasis and poor prognosis of ESCC.[40] Mechanistically, the eIF5A2 expression increases in response to hypoxia, which is a common property among a wide range of solid tumors. In immunocompromised mice, elevated eIF5A2 dramatically promotes the genesis of more microvessels in xenograft tumors through partially stimulating the expression of HIF1α and VEGF.[40]

S100 protein family consists of 21 members and some of them play critical roles in proliferation, invasion-metastasis cascade, differentiation, and inflammation in cancer. We found that one SNP (461G>A) in S100A14 associates significantly with the decreased expression of S100A14 in ESCC and this SNP endows with a higher susceptibility to ESCC in smokers.[41] Further analysis revealed that 461G>A is located in the p53 binding site, suggesting that S10014 is probably a tumor suppressor gene dependent on p53.[42] Unexpectedly, S100A14 promotes rather than inhibiting the progression of ESCC. S100A14, like other siblings of this family, can be secreted into the extracellular space. We then found that this extracellular S100A14 directly binds to the receptor of advanced glycation end products (RAGE) and activates the NF-κB and ERK1/2 MAPK signaling pathways simultaneously to stimulate proliferation.[43] Besides, the forced expression of S100A14 enhances the expression of MMP2 to promote the invasion of ESCC cell lines.[42] Interestingly, the stimulative effect on the MMP2 expression requires p53 and this seemingly contradictory result stems from the influence of S100A14 on the transcription and stability of p53 protein.[42] Results from investigations into S100A14 exemplify how the protein–protein interaction complicates the regulations in motility in ESCC cells.

As the lymph node is a primary site of ESCC metastasis, several independent studies uncover that a few genes, such as PTTG, RASSF8, and GBP1, contribute to lymphangiogenesis or lymph nodes metastasis.[44–46]

An elevated expression of transducin (β)-like 1 X-linked receptor 1 (TBL1XR1) was detected in ESCC specimens, and it binds to the promoter of VEGF-C to stimulate its expression. Furthermore, the overexpression of TBL1XR1 promotes lymphangiogenesis and metastasis in a murine model.[47]

Non-coding RNAs and metastasis of ESCC

MicroRNAs (miRNAs) and long non-coding RNAs (lncRNAs) are two categories of non-coding RNA, extensively studied in cancer biology. As for the invasion and metastasis of ESCC, we previously described that miR-10b promotes the motility of ESCC cells *in vitro* by reducing the expression of Klf4.[48] Our latest study identified a new repressive microRNA — miR-92b — in the invasion-metastasis cascade of ESCC by silencing the expression of integrin αV.[49] Based on three murine models, we found that miR-92b undermines the local invasion into the adjacent smooth muscle layer, attenuates the pulmonary arrest, and reduces the final formation of overt metastases in lungs.[49] These results showed the inhibitory effect of miR-92b on an individual step of the invasion-metastasis cascade, providing more information about the functions of this microRNA.

In addition to microRNAs, lncRNAs also participate in regulating the motility of ESCC cells. The silence of MALAT1 in ESCC cells inhibits migration and invasion *in vitro*.[50] A second study started from the *in silico* analysis of the differentially expressed lncRNAs between 119 ESCC tissues and their adjacent normal counterparts. Then, the comparison of these differentially expressed lncRNAs among ESCC, head and neck carcinoma, and melanoma found that around 400 lncRNAs are implicated in metastasis. Among these candidates, the researchers, testing the role of a new identified lncRNA *Epist*, showed that the overexpression of this lncRNA significantly inhibited the migration and invasion of ESCC cells *in vitro*.[51] Nevertheless, further studies are needed to understand more mechanistic details about the inhibitory function of *Epist*.

Microenvironmental regulation of metastasis in ESCC

Tumor cells never live in an isolated environment. The importance of tumor-associated stromal cells and cytokines supporting progression of

ESCC has been realized recently. Cancer-associated fibroblasts (CAFs), for example, indicates the poor prognosis of ESCC patients. FGFR2-positive fibroblasts contribute greatly to the microenvironment, facilitating the migration and invasion of ESCC.[52] Considering the dysregulated FGF signaling pathway and its correlation with unfavorable outcome, there is probably a reciprocal stimulation between ESCC cells and CAFs; however, this theory still needs to be tested further. Moreover, CAFs in ESCC can secret Wnt2 to promote motility by inducing epithelial–mesenchymal transition (EMT) in malignant cells.[53]

Myeloid-derived suppressor cells (MDSCs) are one group of immune regulation cells, which are usually recruited to the microenvironment of solid tumors. In the peripheral blood of ESCC patients, MDSCs increase dramatically relative to that of healthy donors. This elevated level correlates positively with lymph node metastasis and the increased level of IL6.[54] This result was confirmed in a murine ESCC model induced by adding 4-nitroquinoline 1-oxide (4-NQO) into the drinking water for these domesticated mice.[54] Moreover, in one mouse model with the conditioned deletion of p120-catenin, the global gene expression in MDSCs obtained from the spontaneous ESCC showed that MDSCs with a higher expression of CD38 exert a stronger inhibitory effect on activating T cells than their counterparts with a lower expression of it. Moreover, the CD38 expression in MDSCs is induced by cytokines, such as IL6, CXCL16, and IGFBP3, secreted by ESCC cells.[55] Together, this finding corroborates again the reciprocal promotion between tumor-associated stromal cells and tumor cells. As our understanding of MDSCs in ESCC advances, the search for treatment strategy based on MDSCs is also on the way. In an experimental therapy against ESCC, the removal of IL6 using 1α-25-dihydroxyvitamin D3 (calcitriol) reduces the number of recruited MDSCs, and further retards the progression of ESCC.[56]

Although details of the invasion-metastasis cascade of ESCC have been uncovered continuously, findings in this field are somewhat fragmentary. This probably stems from different research interests of independent groups, resulting in the absence of a general and acceptable profile of the ESCC invasion-metastasis cascade. In breast cancer, for example, the EMT/MET model has been established and a hierarchy of regulation network linking metastasis, stem-like traits, and chemoradiotherapy resistance has also been under intensive investigation. Transcription factors, such as Snail and Twist, which are essential development modulators, have also been identified to promote the EMT program in malignant cells. In contrast, several critical transcription factors in esophageal development have been well described, but pieces of evidence about their potential contributions to the invasion-metastasis cascade of ESCC are few, which hinders further development of medication against metastasis of ESCC accordingly.

Esophageal cancer stem cells

In this section, we introduce what we have known about esophageal cancer stem cells (CSCs) or esophageal tumor-initiation cells (TICs) instead of detailing every aspect of CSC. To learn more about CSC, we recommend excellent reviews published recently.[57, 58]

Unlike hematologic cancer, the identification of CSC population in solid cancers is a more burdensome task largely because specific CSC markers are not completely certain. As for TIC of ESCC, the widely accepted markers are CD90, CD44, and aldehyde dehydrogenases (ALDHs). CD90-positive population isolated from the KYSE140 and KYSE520 cell lines, respectively, possesses a stronger capacity of spheroid formation *in vitro* and tumor growth *in vivo*. Moreover, CD90 stimulates the expression of the Ets-1/MMPs pathway and subsequent invasion and metastasis.[59] Interestingly, when examining the expression of the other two TIC markers — CD44 and CD271 — in CD90-positive population, the researchers found a low frequency of the overlapping expression of the three proteins, suggesting that various subsets of TIC exist in ESCC.[59] ALDHs are a group of enzymes to catalyze the oxidation process from aldehydes to carboxylic acids. Human genome encodes 19 ALDHs that fall into three classes. In breast cancer, colon cancer, head and neck cancer, melanoma, and pancreatic cancer, ALDH alone or with other markers identifies the CSC population.[60] In ESCC, Yang and colleagues found that high ALDH1A1 indicates the poor outcome of patients and marks a population of cells with the enhanced capacity of tumor initiation and metastasis.[60] The observed phenomena meet the functional criteria defined for TIC. However, further investigations are required to test the expression of previously reported TIC markers (CD90, CD44, or CD271) within the ALDH1A1-positive cells. This will facilitate us to determine whether ALDH1A1 is a relatively unique marker of a subset of TIC distinguished from the others (e.g. CD90-positive counterparts) or the elevated ALDH1A1 expression is just a shared property of TIC population in ESCC.

Several signaling pathways are also dysregulated to promote the stemness of ESCC. One report in 2013 described that the activated JAK2/STAT3 signaling pathway increases the proportion of CD44-positive population with stronger tumorigenesis capacity *in vitro* and *in vivo*.[61] Another pro-stemness signaling pathway in ESCC is the Wnt/β-catenin pathway, which increases CD90-positive population and enhances sphere formation and *in vivo* proliferation.[62] With respect to EAC, yes-associated protein (YAP), the key transcription factor of the Hippo signaling pathway, directly binds to the promoter of Sox9 to increase the expression of this gene. Sox9 then endows the malignant cells with cancer stem-like properties, which is represented by the elevated $ALDH^+CD44^+$ or $ALDH^+$ population.[63] The Notch signaling pathway also contributes to the stemness of EAC. The inhibition of this pathway using γ-secretase inhibitors suppresses the tumor growth *in vivo* and the expression of several CSC-related genes, such as ALDH and Lgr5.[64] There is a significant genetic difference between ESCC and EAC. Therefore, the identified regulations in TIC of each subtype are probably specific.

Before moving on to the next subject, we feel obliged to underscore the significance of investigations into esophageal CSC despite a little gloomy progress made in this field. Identification and characterization of CSC or TIC population facilitate the development of targeted therapy against these drivers of tumorigenesis and escapers of chemoradiotherapy. Since the striking difference exists between CSC and normal cells, the prospective therapy, in principle, is expected to exert far lower adverse effects compared with current medication.

Therapeutics in Metastatic Esophageal Cancer

As described previously, metastasis is the number one challenge in the management of cancers, including ESCC and EAC. In this section, we would introduce the current approach to address this conundrum and then discuss future development based on laboratory research.

Since the first anticancer compound was introduced into clinical practice in the late 1930s, the number of therapeutic compounds and their derivatives has amounted to 206, among which most aim at the machinery of the uncontrolled proliferation of malignant cells.[65] Currently, the treatment option for advanced esophageal cancer largely depends on chemotherapy. As for ESCC, the most widely adopted treatment is the combined administration of cisplatin and fluorouracil.[66] A phase II study testing the combination of oxaliplatin, fluorouracil, and leucovorin demonstrated a modest effect in metastatic ESCC.[66] A similar strategy is applied to treat metastatic EAC. The combined administration of two drugs, cisplatin and fluorouracil or oxaliplatin and capecitabine, has been adopted in clinical practice and significantly prolonged the overall survival rate. Although the simultaneous administration of three drugs (cisplatin, docetaxel, and fluorouracil) could further improve overall survival, the cytotoxicity of this solution cannot be neglected.[66] Another problem with chemotherapy in esophageal cancer is that patients usually suffer from comorbidities such as obesity, emphysema, and heart disease, and these symptoms would restrict the availability of some chemotherapy strategies under circumstances.[66] These weaknesses of the traditional chemotherapy call for the development of novel medication with high specificity and low toxicity.

In the late 1990s, targeted therapy emerged based on decades of investigations in cancer biology.[65] To date, imatinib and trastuzumab are two well-known symbols of success in targeted therapy. Imatinib is developed to target BCR-ABL1 fusion protein in chronic myeloid leukemia (CML). BCR-ABL1 chimeric tyrosine kinase stems from aberrant fusion between BCR located in chromosome 21 and ABL1 located in chromosome 9, and it is essential for the initiation and progression of CML.[65] Around 98% of CML patients are responsive to imatinib treatment. Although BCR-ABL1 kinase would acquire other mutations to neutralize the administration of imatinib, the second and the third generations of inhibitors, such as nilotinib and ponatinib, have been developed to address the relapse of CML patients.[65] Trastuzumab is the first humanized monoclonal antibody targeting HER2 (ERBB2), which is one of the four members of the ERBB protein family. HER2 could form heterodimers with EGFR (ERBB1) or ERBB3 to relay signals through RAS/MEK/ERK and PI3K/AKT/mTOR signaling pathways, which are usually aberrantly activated across a wide range of cancers.[65] Therefore, trastuzumab receives a great success in HER2-amplified breast cancer patients and the combined use of trastuzumab in adjuvant treatment significantly prolongs the overall survival by 37%.[65] In HER2-positive gastroesophageal junction adenocarcinomas, adding trastuzumab in chemotherapy is also accepted as a standard therapy strategy.[66] However, targeted therapy probably fails to assume the "Terminator" of all types of cancers because a tremendous amount of mutations exist in tumors.[67] Genetic diversity always makes sure that at least a few clones could survive in initial chemotherapy and radiotherapy. Furthermore, with the help of rapidly advancing technologies such as single-cell sequencing, people are aware that tumor cells are continuously evolving (acquirement of new genetic and epigenetic mutations) to adapt to constantly changing external microenvironment. That resistance of tumor cells is cultivated by continuing therapies (e.g. targeted therapy) well exemplifies the evolution of tumor cells. Specifically, 60% of melanoma patients carry a BRAF mutation V600E and thus are well responsive to one ATP-competitive BRAF inhibitor vemurafenib.[65] Unfortunately, at least 80% of these treated patients will relapse within a few months as several mutations simultaneously occur in key proteins of downstream signaling pathways such as MEK.[65] The combined administration of targeted inhibitors against BRAF and novel mutations could surmount this resistance for only a while and melanomas finally relapse again[65]. This circle is depressing; pioneering strategies are therefore needed to meet these challenges. Immunotherapy is now being considered as the most promising therapeutic strategy. The programmed cell death 1 (PD1) receptor is expressed in T cells and its ligand PD-L1 is expressed in malignant cells and infiltrating macrophages. Bind of PD-L1 to PD1 attenuates the antitumor function of T cells. In one multicenter phase I trial, the intravenous administration of anti-PD-L1 antibody significantly undermines the progression of several kinds of advanced cancers including melanoma, non-small-cell lung, and renal-cell cancer.[68] In esophageal cancer patients, PD-L1 indicates poor outcome as an independent prognostic factor,[69] suggesting that immunotherapy is probably an effective therapeutic alternative in the future treatment.

Before ending this chapter, we would like to propose a few considerations in developing effective treatments against metastasis of tumor cells. In principle, the promising treatment is better to be systematic. This means that both malignant cells themselves and surrounded microenvironmental factors are equally important therapeutical targets. On the one hand, the invasion-metastasis cascade of malignant cells consists of a serial of consecutive steps and cells would use a panel of different gene products to fulfill each process.

On the other hand, diverse tumor-tamed immune/stromal cells promote invasion and metastasis via complicated interactions with tumor cells.[70–71] Most present medications target individual specific proteins in malignant cells only. Therefore, broadening targeting spectrum in a single therapy and designing medications to disrupt the collusion between cancer cells and bad immune/stromal cells or to enhance antitumor effects of good immune cells are the future directions. Clinical trials and experimental therapeutic studies based on siRNAs, microRNAs, and lncRNAs exemplify a good start of aiming at multiple targets simultaneously.[72,73] Owing to the systematic property of metastasis, therapies, which can educate the internal microenvironment to be hostile to the disseminated tumor cells, are required to be developed and administered in the first-diagnosed patients. This strategy does not seek high specificity but focus on a broad spectrum. One emerging strategy is to harness extracellular vehicles (EVs) produced by cells. In one clinical trial, DC cells were collected from patients with metastatic melanoma. These DC cells were incubated with antigens of melanoma and then EVs secreted from the educated DC cells were harvested and introduced back into patients to stimulate immune response.[74] We believe that this idea can be applied in other antitumor immune cells as well.

In conclusion, the esophagus is a simple organ, but a comprehensive understanding of the mechanisms underlying its development requires further investigations, which will undoubtedly speed up the studies in carcinogenesis and progression of esophageal cancer. Metastasis is the leading lethal cause among most cancer patients, including victims suffered from esophageal cancer, whereas few effective treatment are available. However, the knowledge in metastasis of esophageal cancer is mounting, offering a promise in developing novel treatment strategies beyond current chemotherapy and target therapy.

References

1. SL Rosekrans, B Baan, V Muncan, GR van den Brink (2015) Esophageal development and epithelial homeostasis. *Am J Physiol Gastrointest Liver Physiol* **309**: G216–G228.
2. K Takubo, NA Shepherd (2013) In: NA Shepherd, BF Warren, GT Williams, JK Greenson, GY Lauwers, MR Novelli (eds.), *The Normal Oesophagus: Anatomy, Specimen Dissection and Histology Relevant to Pathological Practice*, pp. 3–10. Wiley-Blackwell, Oxford.

3. KA Williamson, AM Hever, J Rainger, RC Rogers, A Magee, Z Fiedler, WT Keng, FH Sharkey, N McGill, CJ Hill, A Schneider, M Messina, PD Turnpenny, JA Fantes, V van Heyningen, DR FitzPatrick (2006) Mutations in SOX2 cause anophthalmia-esophageal-genital (AEG) syndrome. *Hum Mol Genet* **15**: 1413–1422.
4. Y Daniely, G Liao, D Dixon, RI Linnoila, A Lori, SH Randell, M Oren, AM Jetten (2004) Critical role of p63 in the development of a normal esophageal and tracheobronchial epithelium. *Am J Physiol Cell Physiol* **287**: C171–C181.
5. J Motoyama, J Liu, R Mo, Q Ding, M Post, CC Hui (1998) Essential function of Gli2 and Gli3 in the formation of lung, trachea and oesophagus. *Nat Genet* **20**: 54–57.
6. M Mahlapuu, S Enerback, P Carlsson (2001) Haploinsufficiency of the forkhead gene Foxf1, a target for sonic hedgehog signaling, causes lung and foregut malformations. *Development* **128**: 2397–2406.
7. Y Li, J Gordon, NR Manley, Y Litingtung, C Chiang (2008) Bmp4 is required for tracheal formation: A novel mouse model for tracheal agenesis. *Dev Biol* **322**: 145–155.
8. J Que, M Choi, JW Ziel, J Klingensmith, BL Hogan (2006) Morphogenesis of the trachea and esophagus: Current players and new roles for noggin and Bmps. *Differentiation* **74**: 422–437.
9. ET Domyan, E Ferretti, K Throckmorton, Y Mishina, SK Nicolis, X Sun (2011) Signaling through BMP receptors promotes respiratory identity in the foregut via repression of Sox2. *Development* **138**: 971–981.
10. K Liu, M Jiang, Y Lu, H Chen, J Sun, S Wu, WY Ku, H Nakagawa, Y Kita, S Natsugoe, JH Peters, A Rustgi, MW Onaitis, A Kiernan, X Chen, J Que (2013) Sox2 cooperates with inflammation-mediated Stat3 activation in the malignant transformation of foregut basal progenitor cells. *Cell Stem Cell* **12**: 304–315.
11. K Arnold, A Sarkar, MA Yram, JM Polo, R Bronson, S Sengupta, M Seandel, N Geijsen, K Hochedlinger (2011) Sox2(+) adult stem and progenitor cells are important for tissue regeneration and survival of mice. *Cell Stem Cell* **9**: 317–329.
12. Y Jeong, H Rhee, S Martin, D Klass, Y Lin, XT Nguyen le, W Feng, M Diehn (2016) Identification and genetic manipulation of human and mouse oesophageal stem cells. *Gut* **65**: 1077–1086.
13. A Thepot, A Hautefeuille, MP Cros, B Abedi-Ardekani, A Petre, O Damour, V Krutovskikh, P Hainaut (2010) Intraepithelial p63-dependent expression of distinct components of cell adhesion complexes in normal esophageal mucosa and squamous cell carcinoma. *Int J Cancer* **127**: 2051–2062.

14. WA van Dop, SL Rosekrans, A Uhmann, V Jaks, GJ Offerhaus, MA van den Bergh Weerman, M Kasper, J Heijmans, JC Hardwick, HW Verspaget, DW Hommes, R Toftgard, H Hahn, GR van den Brink (2013) Hedgehog signalling stimulates precursor cell accumulation and impairs epithelial maturation in the murine oesophagus. *Gut* **62**: 348–357.
15. L Zhang, Y Zhou, C Cheng, H Cui, L Cheng, P Kong, J Wang, Y Li, W Chen, B Song, F Wang, Z Jia, L Li, Y Li, B Yang, J Liu, R Shi, Y Bi, Y Zhang, J Wang, Z Zhao, X Hu, J Yang, H Li, Z Gao, G Chen, X Huang, X Yang, S Wan, C Chen, B Li, Y Tan, L Chen, M He, S Xie, X Li, X Zhuang, M Wang, Z Xia, L Luo, J Ma, B Dong, J Zhao, Y Song, Y Ou, E Li, L Xu, J Wang, Y Xi, G Li, E Xu, J Liang, X Yang, J Guo, X Chen, Y Zhang, Q Li, L Liu, Y Li, X Zhang, H Yang, D Lin, X Cheng, Y Guo, J Wang, Q Zhan, Y Cui (2015) Genomic analyses reveal mutational signatures and frequently altered genes in esophageal squamous cell carcinoma. *Am J Hum Genet* **96**: 597–611.
16. N Hu, M Kadota, H Liu, CC Abnet, H Su, H Wu, ND Freedman, HH Yang, C Wang, C Yan, L Wang, S Gere, A Hutchinson, G Song, Y Wang, T Ding, YL Qiao, J Koshiol, SM Dawsey, C Giffen, AM Goldstein, PR Taylor, MP Lee (2016) Genomic landscape of somatic alterations in esophageal squamous cell carcinoma and gastric cancer. *Cancer Res* **76**: 1714–1723.
17. LA Torre, F Bray, RL Siegel, J Ferlay, J Lortet-Tieulent, A Jemal (2015) Global cancer statistics, 2012. *CA Cancer J Clin* **65**: 87–108.
18. RL Siegel, KD Miller, A Jemal (2016) Cancer statistics, 2016. *CA Cancer J Clin* **66**: 7–30.
19. W Chen, R Zheng, PD Baade, S Zhang, H Zeng, F Bray, A Jemal, XQ Yu, J He (2016) Cancer statistics in China, 2015. *CA Cancer J Clin* **66**: 115–132.
20. AK Rustgi, HB El-Serag (2014) Esophageal carcinoma. *N Engl J Med* **371**: 2499–509.
21. F Sitas, S Egger, MI Urban, PR Taylor, CC Abnet, P Boffetta, DL O'Connell, DC Whiteman, P Brennan, R Malekzadeh, M Pawlita, SM Dawsey, T Waterboer; InterSCOPE Collaboration (2012) InterSCOPE study: Associations between esophageal squamous cell carcinoma and human papillomavirus serological markers. *J Natl Cancer Inst* **104**: 147–158.
22. K Zendehdel, O Nyren, A Edberg, W Ye (2011) Risk of esophageal adenocarcinoma in achalasia patients, a retrospective cohort study in Sweden. *Am J Gastroenterol* **106**: 57–61.
23. JH Rubenstein, JB Taylor (2010) Meta-analysis: The association of oesophageal adenocarcinoma with symptoms of gastro-oesophageal reflux. *Aliment Pharmacol Ther* **32**: 1222–1227.
24. H El-Serag (2008) Role of obesity in GORD-related disorders. *Gut* **57**: 281–284.

25. C Wu, Z Hu, Z He, W Jia, F Wang, Y Zhou, Z Liu, Q Zhan, Y Liu, D Yu, K Zhai, J Chang, Y Qiao, G Jin, Z Liu, Y Shen, C Guo, J Fu, X Miao, W Tan, H Shen, Y Ke, Y Zeng, T Wu, D Lin (2011) Genome-wide association study identifies three new susceptibility loci for esophageal squamous-cell carcinoma in Chinese populations. *Nat Genet* **43**: 679–684.
26. C Wu, D Li, W Jia, Z Hu, Y Zhou, D Yu, T Tong, M Wang, D Lin, Y Qiao, Y Zhou, J Chang, K Zhai, M Wang, L Wei, W Tan, H Shen, Y Zeng, D Lin (2013) Genome-wide association study identifies common variants in SLC39A6 associated with length of survival in esophageal squamous-cell carcinoma. *Nat Genet* **45**: 632–638.
27. C Wu, Z Wang, X Song, XS Feng, CC Abnet, J He, N Hu, XB Zuo, W Tan, Q Zhan, Z Hu, Z He, W Jia, Y Zhou, K Yu, XO Shu, JM Yuan, W Zheng, XK Zhao, SG Gao, ZQ Yuan, FY Zhou, ZM Fan, JL Cui, HL Lin, XN Han, B Li, X Chen, SM Dawsey, L Liao, MP Lee, T Ding, YL Qiao, Z Liu, Y Liu, D Yu, J Chang, L Wei, YT Gao, WP Koh, YB Xiang, ZZ Tang, JH Fan, JJ Han, SL Zhou, P Zhang, DY Zhang, Y Yuan, Y Huang, C Liu, K Zhai, Y Qiao, G Jin, C Guo, J Fu, X Miao, C Lu, H Yang, C Wang, WA Wheeler, M Gail, M Yeager, J Yuenger, ET Guo, AL Li, W Zhang, XM Li, LD Sun, BG Ma, Y Li, S Tang, XQ Peng, J Liu, A Hutchinson, K Jacobs, C Giffen, L Burdette, JF Fraumeni, Jr., H Shen, Y Ke, Y Zeng, T Wu, P Kraft, CC Chung, MA Tucker, ZC Hou, YL Liu, YL Hu, Y Liu, L Wang, G Yuan, LS Chen, X Liu, T Ma, H Meng, L Sun, XM Li, XM Li, JW Ku, YF Zhou, LQ Yang, Z Wang, Y Li, Q Qige, WJ Yang, GY Lei, LQ Chen, EM Li, L Yuan, WB Yue, R Wang, LW Wang, XP Fan, FH Zhu, WX Zhao, YM Mao, M Zhang, GL Xing, JL Li, M Han, JL Ren, B Liu, SW Ren, QP Kong, F Li, I Sheyhidin, W Wei, YR Zhang, CW Feng, J Wang, YH Yang, HZ Hao, QD Bao, BC Liu, AQ Wu, D Xie, WC Yang, L Wang, XH Zhao, SQ Chen, JY Hong, XJ Zhang, ND Freedman, AM Goldstein, D Lin, PR Taylor, LD Wang, SJ Chanock (2014) Joint analysis of three genome-wide association studies of esophageal squamous cell carcinoma in Chinese populations. *Nat Genet* **46**: 1001–1006.
28. Y Song, L Li, Y Ou, Z Gao, E Li, X Li, W Zhang, J Wang, L Xu, Y Zhou, X Ma, L Liu, Z Zhao, X Huang, J Fan, L Dong, G Chen, L Ma, J Yang, L Chen, M He, M Li, X Zhuang, K Huang, K Qiu, G Yin, G Guo, Q Feng, P Chen, Z Wu, J Wu, L Ma, J Zhao, L Luo, M Fu, B Xu, B Chen, Y Li, T Tong, M Wang, Z Liu, D Lin, X Zhang, H Yang, J Wang, Q Zhan (2014) Identification of genomic alterations in oesophageal squamous cell cancer. *Nature* **509**: 91–95.
29. DC Lin, JJ Hao, Y Nagata, L Xu, L Shang, X Meng, Y Sato, Y Okuno, AM Varela, LW Ding, M Garg, LZ Liu, H Yang, D Yin, ZZ Shi, YY Jiang, WY Gu, T Gong, Y Zhang, X Xu, O Kalid, S Shacham, S Ogawa, MR Wang,

HP Koeffler (2014) Genomic and molecular characterization of esophageal squamous cell carcinoma. *Nat Genet* **46**: 467–473.

30. YB Gao, ZL Chen, JG Li, XD Hu, XJ Shi, ZM Sun, F Zhang, ZR Zhao, ZT Li, ZY Liu, YD Zhao, J Sun, CC Zhou, R Yao, SY Wang, P Wang, N Sun, BH Zhang, JS Dong, Y Yu, M Luo, XL Feng, SS Shi, F Zhou, FW Tan, B Qiu, N Li, K Shao, LJ Zhang, LJ Zhang, Q Xue, SG Gao, J He (2014) Genetic landscape of esophageal squamous cell carcinoma. *Nat Genet* **46**: 1097–1102.
31. G Sawada, A Niida, R Uchi, H Hirata, T Shimamura, Y Suzuki, Y Shiraishi, K Chiba, S Imoto, Y Takahashi, T Iwaya, T Sudo, T Hayashi, H Takai, Y Kawasaki, T Matsukawa, H Eguchi, K Sugimachi, F Tanaka, H Suzuki, K Yamamoto, H Ishii, M Shimizu, H Yamazaki, M Yamazaki, Y Tachimori, Y Kajiyama, S Natsugoe, H Fujita, K Mafune, Y Tanaka, DP Kelsell, CA Scott, S Tsuji, S Yachida, T Shibata, S Sugano, Y Doki, T Akiyama, H Aburatani, S Ogawa, S Miyano, M Mori, K Mimori (2016) Genomic landscape of esophageal squamous cell carcinoma in a Japanese population. *Gastroenterology* **150**: 1171–1182.
32. C Cheng, Y Zhou, H Li, T Xiong, S Li, Y Bi, P Kong, F Wang, H Cui, Y Li, X Fang, T Yan, Y Li, J Wang, B Yang, L Zhang, Z Jia, B Song, X Hu, J Yang, H Qiu, G Zhang, J Liu, E Xu, R Shi, Y Zhang, H Liu, C He, Z Zhao, Y Qian, R Rong, Z Han, Y Zhang, W Luo, J Wang, S Peng, X Yang, X Li, L Li, H Fang, X Liu, L Ma, Y Chen, S Guo, X Chen, Y Xi, G Li, J Liang, X Yang, J Guo, J Jia, Q Li, X Cheng, Q Zhan, Y Cui (2016) Whole-genome sequencing reveals diverse models of structural variations in esophageal squamous cell carcinoma. *Am J Hum Genet* **98**: 256–274.
33. DM Levine, WE Ek, R Zhang, X Liu, L Onstad, C Sather, P Lao-Sirieix, MD Gammon, DA Corley, NJ Shaheen, NC Bird, LJ Hardie, LJ Murray, BJ Reid, WH Chow, HA Risch, O Nyren, W Ye, G Liu, Y Romero, L Bernstein, AH Wu, AG Casson, SJ Chanock, P Harrington, I Caldas, I Debiram-Beecham, C Caldas, NK Hayward, PD Pharoah, RC Fitzgerald, S Macgregor, DC Whiteman, TL Vaughan (2013) A genome-wide association study identifies new susceptibility loci for esophageal adenocarcinoma and Barrett's esophagus. *Nat Genet* **45**: 1487–1493.
34. MD Stachler, A Taylor-Weiner, S Peng, A McKenna, AT Agoston, RD Odze, JM Davison, KS Nason, M Loda, I Leshchiner, C Stewart, P Stojanov, S Seepo, MS Lawrence, D Ferrer-Torres, J Lin, AC Chang, SB Gabriel, ES Lander, DG Beer, G Getz, SL Carter, AJ Bass (2015) Paired exome analysis of Barrett's esophagus and adenocarcinoma. *Nat Genet* **47**: 1047–1055.
35. CS Ross-Innes, J Becq, A Warren, RK Cheetham, H Northen, M O'Donovan, S Malhotra, M di Pietro, S Ivakhno, M He, JM Weaver, AG Lynch, Z Kingsbury, M Ross, S Humphray, D Bentley, RC Fitzgerald; Oesophageal Cancer Clinical

and Molecular Stratification (OCCAMS) Study Group; Oesophageal Cancer Clinical and Molecular Stratification OCCAMS Study Group (2015) Whole-genome sequencing provides new insights into the clonal architecture of Barrett's esophagus and esophageal adenocarcinoma. *Nat Genet* **47**: 1038–1046.
36. KL Kong, DL Kwong, L Fu, TH Chan, L Chen, H Liu, Y Li, YH Zhu, J Bi, YR Qin, SY Law, XY Guan (2010) Characterization of a candidate tumor suppressor gene uroplakin 1A in esophageal squamous cell carcinoma. *Cancer Res* **70**: 8832–8841.
37. YR Qin, H Tang, F Xie, H Liu, Y Zhu, J Ai, L Chen, Y Li, DL Kwong, L Fu, XY Guan (2011) Characterization of tumor-suppressive function of SOX6 in human esophageal squamous cell carcinoma. *Clin Cancer Res* **17**: 46–55.
38. YH Zhu, L Fu, L Chen, YR Qin, H Liu, F Xie, T Zeng, SS Dong, J Li, Y Li, Y Dai, D Xie, XY Guan (2013) Downregulation of the novel tumor suppressor DIRAS1 predicts poor prognosis in esophageal squamous cell carcinoma. *Cancer Res* **73**: 2298–2309.
39. YR Qin, JJ Qiao, TH Chan, YH Zhu, FF Li, H Liu, J Fei, Y Li, XY Guan, L Chen (2014) Adenosine-to-inosine RNA editing mediated by ADARs in esophageal squamous cell carcinoma. *Cancer Res* **74**: 840–851.
40. Y Li, L Fu, JB Li, Y Qin, TT Zeng, J Zhou, ZL Zeng, J Chen, TT Cao, X Ban, C Qian, Z Cai, D Xie, P Huang, XY Guan (2014) Increased expression of EIF5A2, via hypoxia or gene amplification, contributes to metastasis and angiogenesis of esophageal squamous cell carcinoma. *Gastroenterology* **146**: 1701–1713 e9.
41. H Chen, D Yu, A Luo, W Tan, C Zhang, D Zhao, M Yang, J Liu, D Lin, Z Liu (2009) Functional role of S100A14 genetic variants and their association with esophageal squamous cell carcinoma. *Cancer Res* **69**: 3451–3457.
42. H Chen, Y Yuan, C Zhang, A Luo, F Ding, J Ma, S Yang, Y Tian, T Tong, Q Zhan, Z Liu (2012) Involvement of S100A14 protein in cell invasion by affecting expression and function of matrix metalloproteinase (MMP)-2 via p53-dependent transcriptional regulation. *J Biol Chem* **287**: 17109–17019.
43. Q Jin, H Chen, A Luo, F Ding, Z Liu (2011) S100A14 stimulates cell proliferation and induces cell apoptosis at different concentrations via receptor for advanced glycation end products (RAGE). *PLoS One* **6**: e19375.
44. S Yan, C Zhou, X Lou, Z Xiao, H Zhu, Q Wang, Y Wang, N Lu, S He, Q Zhan, S Liu, N Xu (2009) PTTG overexpression promotes lymph node metastasis in human esophageal squamous cell carcinoma. *Cancer Res* **69**: 3283–3290.
45. L Zhang, JH Wang, RX Liang, ST Huang, J Xu, LJ Yuan, L Huang, Y Zhou, XJ Yu, SY Wu, RZ Luo, JP Yun, WH Jia, M Zheng (2015) RASSF8 downregulation promotes lymphangiogenesis and metastasis in esophageal squamous cell carcinoma. *Oncotarget* **6**: 34510–34524.

46. L Li, G Ma, C Jing, Z Liu (2015) Guanylate-binding protein 1 (GBP1) promotes lymph node metastasis in human esophageal squamous cell carcinoma. *Discov Med* **20**: 369–378.
47. L Liu, C Lin, W Liang, S Wu, A Liu, J Wu, X Zhang, P Ren, M Li, L Song (2015) TBL1XR1 promotes lymphangiogenesis and lymphatic metastasis in esophageal squamous cell carcinoma. *Gut* **64**: 26–36.
48. Y Tian, A Luo, Y Cai, Q Su, F Ding, H Chen, Z Liu (2010) MicroRNA-10b promotes migration and invasion through KLF4 in human esophageal cancer cell lines. *J Biol Chem* **285**: 7986–7994.
49. G Ma, C Jing, L Li, F Huang, F Ding, B Wang, D Lin, A Luo, Z Liu (2016) MicroRNA-92b represses invasion-metastasis cascade of esophageal squamous cell carcinoma. *Oncotarget* **7**: 20209–20222.
50. X Wang, M Li, Z Wang, S Han, X Tang, Y Ge, L Zhou, C Zhou, Q Yuan, M Yang (2015) Silencing of long noncoding RNA MALAT1 by miR-101 and miR-217 inhibits proliferation, migration, and invasion of esophageal squamous cell carcinoma cells. *J Biol Chem* **290**: 3925–3935.
51. G Wei, H Luo, Y Sun, J Li, L Tian, W Liu, L Liu, J Luo, J He, R Chen (2015) Transcriptome profiling of esophageal squamous cell carcinoma reveals a long noncoding RNA acting as a tumor suppressor. *Oncotarget* **6**: 17065–17080.
52. C Zhang, L Fu, J Fu, L Hu, H Yang, TH Rong, Y Li, H Liu, SB Fu, YX Zeng, XY Guan (2009) Fibroblast growth factor receptor 2-positive fibroblasts provide a suitable microenvironment for tumor development and progression in esophageal carcinoma. *Clin Cancer Res* **15**: 4017–4027.
53. L Fu, C Zhang, LY Zhang, SS Dong, LH Lu, J Chen, Y Dai, Y Li, KL Kong, DL Kwong, XY Guan (2011) Wnt2 secreted by tumour fibroblasts promotes tumour progression in oesophageal cancer by activation of the Wnt/beta-catenin signalling pathway. *Gut* **60**: 1635–1643.
54. MF Chen, FC Kuan, TC Yen, MS Lu, PY Lin, YH Chung, WC Chen, KD Lee (2014) IL-6-stimulated CD11b+ CD14+ HLA-DR- myeloid-derived suppressor cells, are associated with progression and poor prognosis in squamous cell carcinoma of the esophagus. *Oncotarget* **5**: 8716–8728.
55. TA Karakasheva, TJ Waldron, E Eruslanov, SB Kim, JS Lee, S O'Brien, PD Hicks, D Basu, S Singhal, F Malavasi, AK Rustgi (2015) CD38-expressing myeloid-derived suppressor cells promote tumor growth in a murine model of esophageal cancer. *Cancer Res* **75**: 4074–4085.
56. PT Chen, CC Hsieh, CT Wu, TC Yen, PY Lin, WC Chen, MF Chen (2015) 1alpha,25-dihydroxyvitamin D3 inhibits esophageal squamous cell carcinoma progression by reducing IL6 signaling. *Mol Cancer Ther* **14**: 1365–1375.

57. LV Nguyen, R Vanner, P Dirks, CJ Eaves (2012) Cancer stem cells: An evolving concept. *Nat Rev Cancer* **12**:133–143.
58. JE Visvader, GJ Lindeman (2012) Cancer stem cells: Current status and evolving complexities. *Cell Stem Cell* **10**: 717–728.
59. KH Tang, YD Dai, M Tong, YP Chan, PS Kwan, L Fu, YR Qin, SW Tsao, HL Lung, ML Lung, DK Tong, S Law, KW Chan, S Ma, XY Guan (2013) A CD90(+) tumor-initiating cell population with an aggressive signature and metastatic capacity in esophageal cancer. *Cancer Res* **73**: 2322–2332.
60. L Yang, Y Ren, X Yu, F Qian, BS Bian, HL Xiao, WG Wang, SL Xu, J Yang, W Cui, Q Liu, Z Wang, W Guo, G Xiong, K Yang, C Qian, X Zhang, P Zhang, YH Cui, XW Bian (2014) ALDH1A1 defines invasive cancer stem-like cells and predicts poor prognosis in patients with esophageal squamous cell carcinoma. *Mod Pathol* **27**: 775–783.
61. X Chen, Z Ying, X Lin, H Lin, J Wu, M Li, L Song (2013) Acylglycerol kinase augments JAK2/STAT3 signaling in esophageal squamous cells. *J Clin Invest* **123**: 2576–2589.
62. C Ge, S Wu, W Wang, Z Liu, J Zhang, Z Wang, R Li, Z Zhang, Z Li, S Dong, Y Wang, Y Xue, J Yang, Q Tan, Z Wang, X Song (2015) miR-942 promotes cancer stem cell-like traits in esophageal squamous cell carcinoma through activation of Wnt/beta-catenin signalling pathway. *Oncotarget* **6**: 10964–10977.
63. S Song, JA Ajani, S Honjo, DM Maru, Q Chen, AW Scott, TR Heallen, L Xiao, WL Hofstetter, B Weston, JH Lee, R Wadhwa, K Sudo, JR Stroehlein, JF Martin, MC Hung, RL Johnson (2014) Hippo coactivator YAP1 upregulates SOX9 and endows esophageal cancer cells with stem-like properties. *Cancer Res* **74**: 4170–4182.
64. Z Wang, TG Da Silva, K Jin, X Han, P Ranganathan, X Zhu, A Sanchez-Mejias, F Bai, B Li, DL Fei, K Weaver, RV Carpio, AE Moscowitz, VP Koshenkov, L Sanchez, L Sparling, XH Pei, D Franceschi, A Ribeiro, DJ Robbins, AS Livingstone, AJ Capobianco (2014) Notch signaling drives stemness and tumorigenicity of esophageal adenocarcinoma. *Cancer Res* **74**: 6364–6374.
65. MM Gottesman, O Lavi, MD Hall, JP Gillet (2016) Toward a better understanding of the complexity of cancer drug resistance. *Annu Rev Pharmacol Toxicol* **56**: 85–102.
66. MA Shah (2015) Update on metastatic gastric and esophageal cancers. *J Clin Oncol* **33**: 1760–1769.
67. S Ling, Z Hu, Z Yang, F Yang, Y Li, P Lin, K Chen, L Dong, L Cao, Y Tao, L Hao, Q Chen, Q Gong, D Wu, W Li, W Zhao, X Tian, C Hao, EA Hungate, DV Catenacci, RR Hudson, WH Li, X Lu, CI Wu (2015) Extremely high

genetic diversity in a single tumor points to prevalence of non-Darwinian cell evolution. *Proc Natl Acad Sci USA* **112**: E6496–E6505.

68. JR Brahmer, SS Tykodi, LQ Chow, WJ Hwu, SL Topalian, P Hwu, CG Drake, LH Camacho, J Kauh, K Odunsi, HC Pitot, O Hamid, S Bhatia, R Martins, K Eaton, S Chen, TM Salay, S Alaparthy, JF Grosso, AJ Korman, SM Parker, S Agrawal, SM Goldberg, DM Pardoll, A Gupta, JM Wigginton (2012) Safety and activity of anti-PD-L1 antibody in patients with advanced cancer. *N Engl J Med* **366**: 2455–2465.
69. Y Ohigashi, M Sho, Y Yamada, Y Tsurui, K Hamada, N Ikeda, T Mizuno, R Yoriki, H Kashizuka, K Yane, F Tsushima, N Otsuki, H Yagita, M Azuma, Y Nakajima (2005) Clinical significance of programmed death-1 ligand-1 and programmed death-1 ligand-2 expression in human esophageal cancer. *Clin Cancer Res* **11**: 2947–2953.
70. J Condeelis, JW Pollard (2006) Macrophages: Obligate partners for tumor cell migration, invasion, and metastasis. *Cell* **124**: 263–266.
71. SK Wculek, I Malanchi (2015) Neutrophils support lung colonization of metastasis-initiating breast cancer cells. *Nature* **528**: 413–417.
72. JE Zuckerman, ME Davis (2015) Clinical experiences with systemically administered siRNA-based therapeutics in cancer. *Nat Rev Drug Discov* **14**: 843–856.
73. H Ling, M Fabbri, GA Calin (2013) MicroRNAs and other non-coding RNAs as targets for anticancer drug development. *Nat Rev Drug Discov* **12**: 847–865.
74. B Gyorgy, ME Hung, XO Breakefield, JN Leonard (2015) Therapeutic applications of extracellular vesicles: Clinical promise and open questions. *Annu Rev Pharmacol Toxicol* **55**: 439–464.

Chapter 8

Angiogenesis and Lymphangiogenesis in Gastric MALT Lymphoma: Relation of VEGF and VASH2

Masahiko Nakamura, Anders Øverby, and Hidenori Matsui

Abstract

Using the gastric mucosa-associated lymphoid tissue (MALT) lymphoma model induced by *Helicobacter heilmannii* infection, the relation of the potent angiogenic molecule, vascular endothelial growth factor (VEGF) and vasohibin-2 (VASH2), a newly identified angiogenic protein, has been scrutinized. Massive angiogenesis and lymphangiogenesis have taken part in this tumor growth induced by the hypoxia and hypoxia-inducible factor-1α, angiogenic peptide, and its receptors on the microvessels. By the suppression of the VEGF pathway by axitinib, a multiple tyrosine kinase inhibitor, VASH 2 positive cells within the MALT lymphoma tissue have increased significantly, showing the reciprocal regulation between the angiogenic molecules during the tumor formation.

Introduction

A relationship between malignancy and blood vessels has been pointed out for more than a century.[1] The tumor microvessels have been shown to have a unique vascular pattern and permeability. Many reports have shown that a diffusible substance may be released from tumors which could stimulate the growth of the microvasculature.[2,3] In 1971, Folkman published a hypothesis that tumor growth is under angiogenesis dependency.[4] Using the cancer-transplant model, he described a model of tumor dormancy due to the blockade of angiogenesis and predicted a future discovery of angiogenesis inhibitors. In 1984, Shing *et al.* isolated and purified the first angiogenic endothelial cell mitogen,[5] which was later identified as basic fibroblast growth factor (bFGF). In 1989, Napoleone Ferrara purified a novel angiogenic protein from pituitary cells and named it vascular endothelial growth factor (VEGF).[6] Many pro-angiogenic molecules related to VEGF have later been discovered.

Among a variety of VEGF-inducible genes, *in vitro* functional assays for angiogenesis were performed on the undefined genes, and one gene having anti-angiogenic activity was identified. This gene was designated as vasohibin-1 (VASH1).[7] Further analyses revealed a gene homologous to VASH1 and designated as vasohibin-2 (VASH2), whose function was found to be opposite, that is, angiogenic.[8] The expression of VASH2 seems to be non-inducible, but constitutive, and it is not modulated by growth factors including VEGF and other cytokines.

The clinical challenge of VEGF-related antiangiogenic compounds is that they do not improve overall survival in patients with malignancy, as pointed out in the glioblastoma cases.[9] The interaction of VEGF and VASH2 in malignancy has not been fully clarified. In this chapter, the relation of VEGF and VASH2 is described in a *Helicobacter heilmannii*-induced gastric mucosa-associated lymphoid tissue (MALT) lymphoma model system.

Gastric MALT Lymphoma Induced by *Helicobacter heilmannii* Infection

We have established a mouse model of the gastric MALT lymphoma by the oral infection of *Helicobacter heilmannii* from a cynomolgus monkey.[10] *H. heilmannii* and related species, the so-called gastric non-*H. pylori* helicobacters (NHPH), have been known to be closely related to the formation of the gastric MALT lymphoma and other gastric diseases in human and domestic animals, such as cats, dogs, and pigs.[11,12] Infection in humans with these fastidious Gram negative spiral-shaped bacteria has been associated with diseases, including gastritis, ulcer, and gastric MALT lymphoma.

Hypoxia and Angiogenesis in Gastric MALT Lymphoma

Electron microscopic observation revealed that this MALT lymphoma has an irregular microvascular network composed of immature capillaries, venules, and lymphatics (Figure 1).[13] A markedly enhanced permeability is another

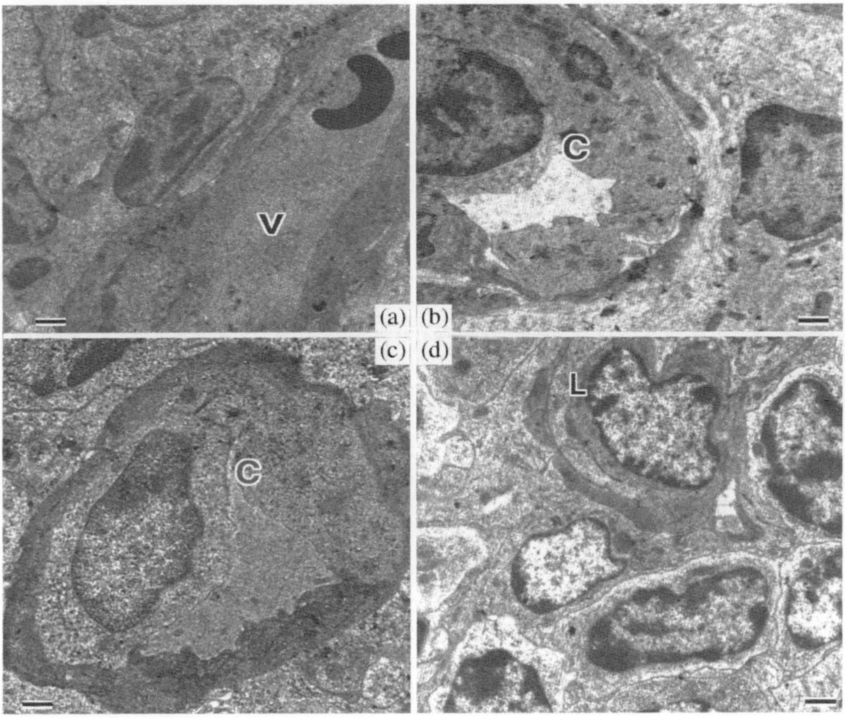

Figure 1. Angiogenesis in the gastric MALT lymphoma revealed by electron microscopy. (a), (b) Some of the pericytes of the venules (V) and capillary (C) are irregular and discontinuous and endothelial walls are very thick, which are the characteristics of immature microvessels. (c), (d) Some of the electron densities of the capillary endothelial cells are not homogeneous, which is also one of the characteristics of immature capillary. (d) The lumen of the some of the vessels (L) are occupied with amorphous substances, suggestive of lymphatic nature.

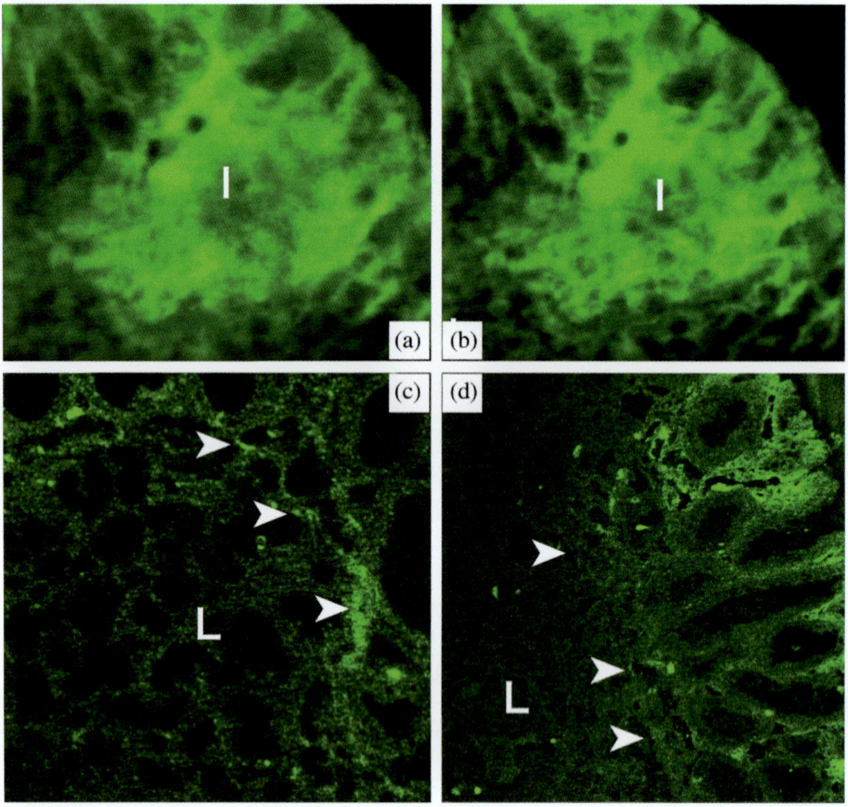

Figure 2. Increased vascular permeability, hypoxia and HIF-1α immunoreactivity in the gastric MALT lymphoma. (a), (b) By the infusion of FITC-dextran (MW50,000), the irregular microvascular network was visualized with the increased vascular permeability in the marginal area with the central ischemic zone (I) ×200. (c) Hypoxic area is shown by the hypoxyprobe administration and its immunohistochemistry. The marginal area (arrow heads) shows the positivity of the hypoxyprobe. L: the gastric MALT lymphoma ×400. (d) HIF-1alpha could be detected in the marginal area of the gastric MALT lymphoma (arrow heads) as well as the *lamina propria mucosae* between the overlying epithelial cells ×400.

pathological characteristic of this tumor as shown by FITC-dextran intravenous infusion (Figure 2). Angiogenesis within the tumor has been reported to start with the hypoxia induced by the outpacing of vasculature growth by tumor cell proliferation. The hypoxia activates an alpha/beta heterodimeric transcription factor, the hypoxia-inducible factor (HIF), followed by the expression of gene products, including VEGF-A and angiopoietin-2, which allows tumor cells to change the hypoxic situation by inducing the growth of the vascular network.[14,15] By the immunohistochemical analysis of the hypoxia using hypoxyprobe-1, and HIF1-α antibody, this MALT lymphoma clearly shows a hypoxic area and HIF1-α immunoreactivity with similar localization (Figure 2).[16]

Lymphangiogenesis of Gastric MALT Lymphoma

By immunohistochemistry using the markers of lymphatics, such as podoplanin, prox-1, and 5'-nucleotidase, marked lymphangiogenesis was detected in the gastric MALT lymphoma tissues (Figure 3), while in the control gastric mucosa lymphatics were detected only in the base of the mucosa and submucosal layers, suggesting the interaction of mediators stimulating the lymphangiogenesis in the MALT lymphoma formation. Some of the lymphatics in the MALT lymphoma were shown to be connected with the larger lymphatics in the surrounding tissues, suggesting that the origin could be derived from the surrounding area, possibly through the budding of the lymphatic endothelial cells.

VEGF and VEGF-R in Gastric MALT Lymphoma

As mentioned before, angiogenesis is very important in the proliferation of malignant tumors. The VEGF family exerts the most potent angiogenic activity in various kinds of cancers, and decreased overall survival has been reported for malignant tumors overexpressing VEGF.[17] At present, the VEGF family consists of VEGF-A, VEGF-B, VEGF-C, VEGF-D, VEGF-E, VEGF-F, and placenta growth factor (PlGF). The VEGF family is not only expressed in the endothelial cells, but also in the tumor cells. In our experimental model, VEGF-A and VEGF-C immunoreactivities, as well as their receptors, Flt-1, Flk-1, and Flt-4, were markedly enhanced (Figure 4).[18] Among these, VEGF-C has recently attracted attention as a mediator of lymphangiogenesis. High levels of the VEGF-C expression and signaling of VEGF-C/VEGFR3, that is, Flt-4, have recently been reported to correlate significantly with worse prognosis in a variety of malignancies,[19] which coincide with our present observation.

In addition, the administration of Flt-4 and Flt-1 antibodies significantly reduced the occupied surface area of the lymphoma in the fundic portion of

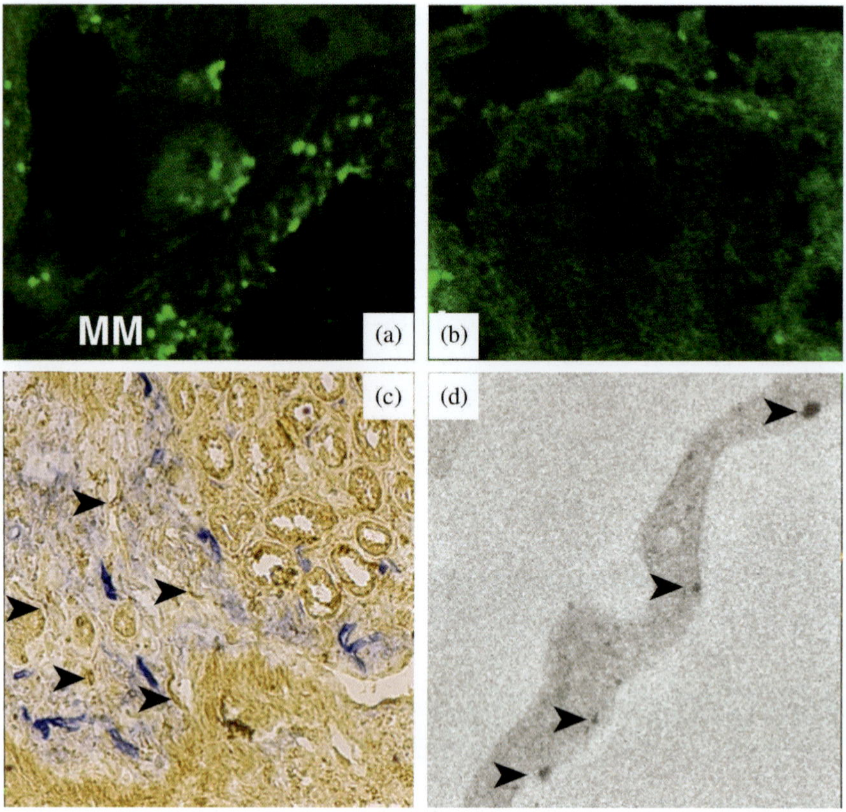

Figure 3. Lymphangiogenesis in the gastric MALT lymphoma. (a), (b) In the control stomach, lymphatics were only found in the base of the mucosa and submucosal layers by the prox-1 immunoreactivity. Many lymphatics were detected in the marginal area of the MALT lymphoma. MM: *muscularis mucosae*. (a): ×800, (b): ×400. (c) By the 5′-nucleotidase and alkaline phosphatase immunohistochemistry, many 5′-nucleotidase-positive brown lymphatics (arrow heads) were seen in the MALT lymphoma, while alkaline phosphatase-positive blue capillaries were distributed both in the MALT lymphoma and surrounding gastric mucosa ×400. (d) Many 5′-nucleotidase reaction products (arrowheads) were seen on the endothelium of the vessel, showing that this vessel belongs to the lymphatic ×20,000.

the mouse stomach as well as the average size of the tumor, and some of the apoptotic cells were shown to be lymphatic endothelial cells.[18] This clearly shows the role of a VEGF-related mechanism in the proliferation of gastric MALT lymphoma through regulation of angiogenesis and lymphangiogenesis.

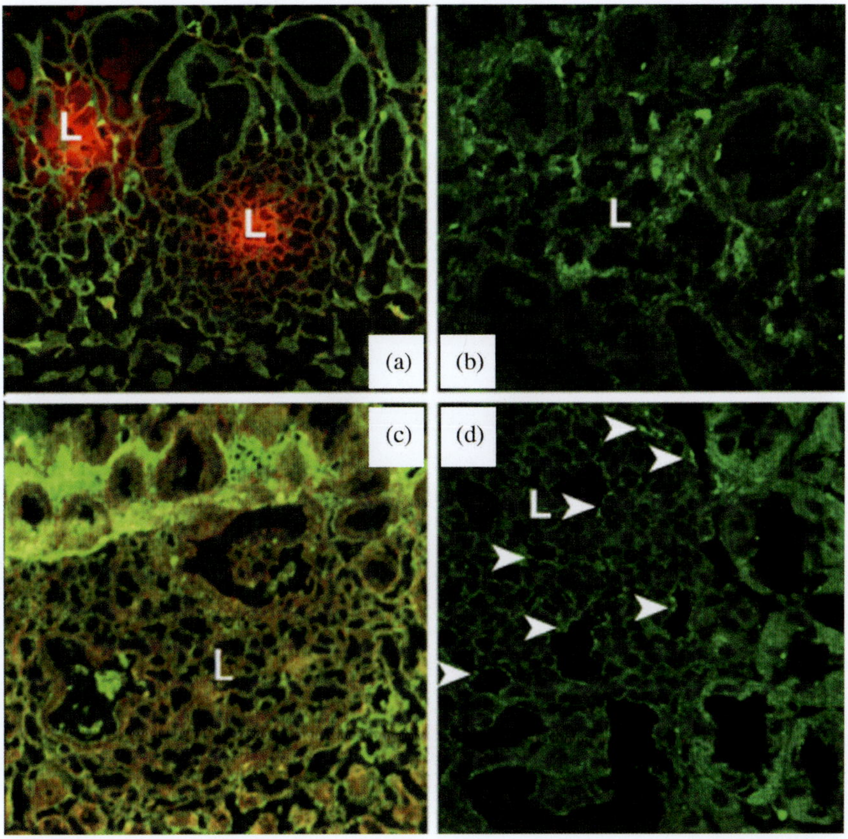

Figure 4. VEGF-A, -C and their receptors in the gastric MALT lymphoma. (a) Very marked immunoreactivity (red) against VEGF-A was exclusively localized in the MALT lymphoma. L: ×200. (b) Lymphangiogenesis-related VEGF-C immunoreactivity (green) was localized in the marginal zone of the MALT lymphoma. ×400. (c) Immunoreactivity of VEGF receptor-1, that is, Flt-1, was found in the MALT lymphoma and lamina propria above the tumor. L: ×400. (d) Immunoreactivity of VEGF receptor-3 (arrow heads), that is, Flt-4, which is related to lymphangiogenesis, was mostly seen in the marginal zone of the MALT lymphoma. L: ×400.

Significance of VASH2

As mentioned before, VASH2 is a newly identified angiogenic protein taking part in the regulation of neonatal growth and tumor formation. Similar to the localization of angiogenic protein, VASH2 has been reported to exist in the mononuclear cells other than endothelial cells in the postnatal period.[20]

To clarify the interaction of VASH2 and VEGF, the immunohistochemical study was performed using control gastric mucosa and the MALT lymphoma model. VEGF immunoreactivity was detected in capillaries and the parietal cells in the control gastric mucosa, while VASH2 immunoreactivity is more specific to the capillaries (Figure 5). In the MALT lymphoma, both VEGF and VASH2 immunoreactivities were detected in the lymphoma cells as well as microvessels, but few cells were doubly positive to VEGF-A and VASH2.

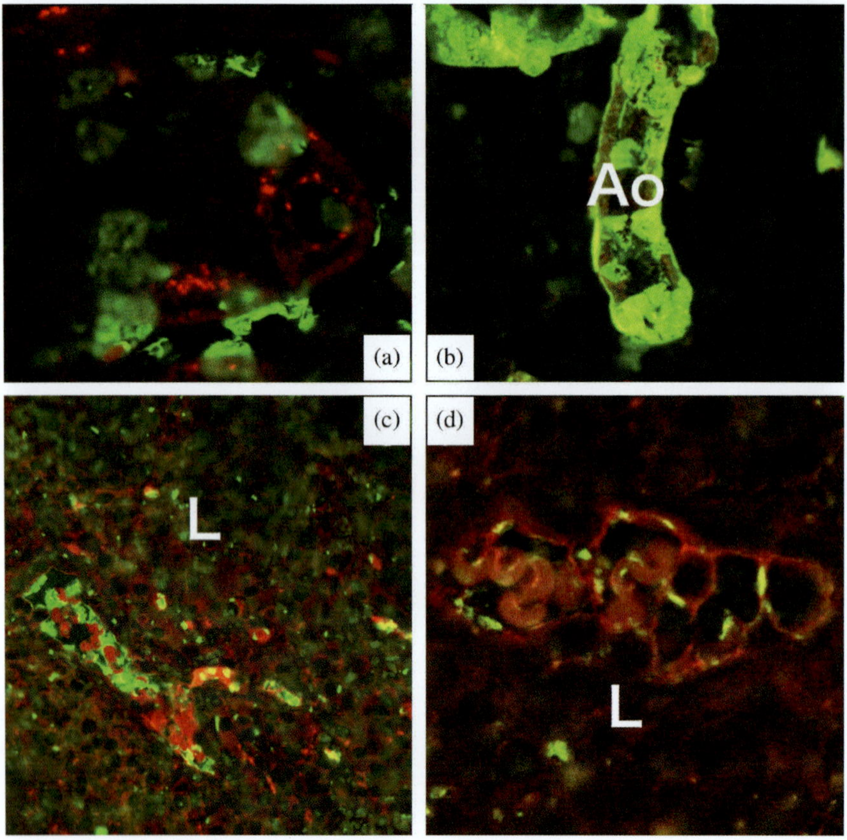

Figure 5. VASH2 and VEGFA immunoreactivities in the control gastric mucosa and the gastric MALT lymphoma. (a) VASH2 immunoreactivity (green) in the gastric mucosa was mostly seen in the interstitial cells in the lamina propria mucosae, while VEGF-A immunoreactivity (red) was detected in the capillaries as well as in the parietal cells ×800. (b) Both VASH2 (green) and VEFG-A (red) immunoreactivities were found in the arteriole (Ao) in the submucosal layer, while VEGF-A was mostly detected in the endothelial cells ×400. (c, d) Within the MALT lymphoma (L), both VASH2 and VEFG-A immunoreactivities were found, but the positive cells were not identical. c: ×400, d: ×800.

Effect of axitinib on VEGF and VASH2

Intraperitoneal administration of axitinib, a multiple tyrosine kinase inhibitor, induced the apoptosis of some of the MALT lymphoma cells, some of which were identified as the capillary endothelial cells (Figure 6). VEGF-A immunoreactivity was markedly reduced in these areas, while many cells were showing the immunoreactivity against VASH2.

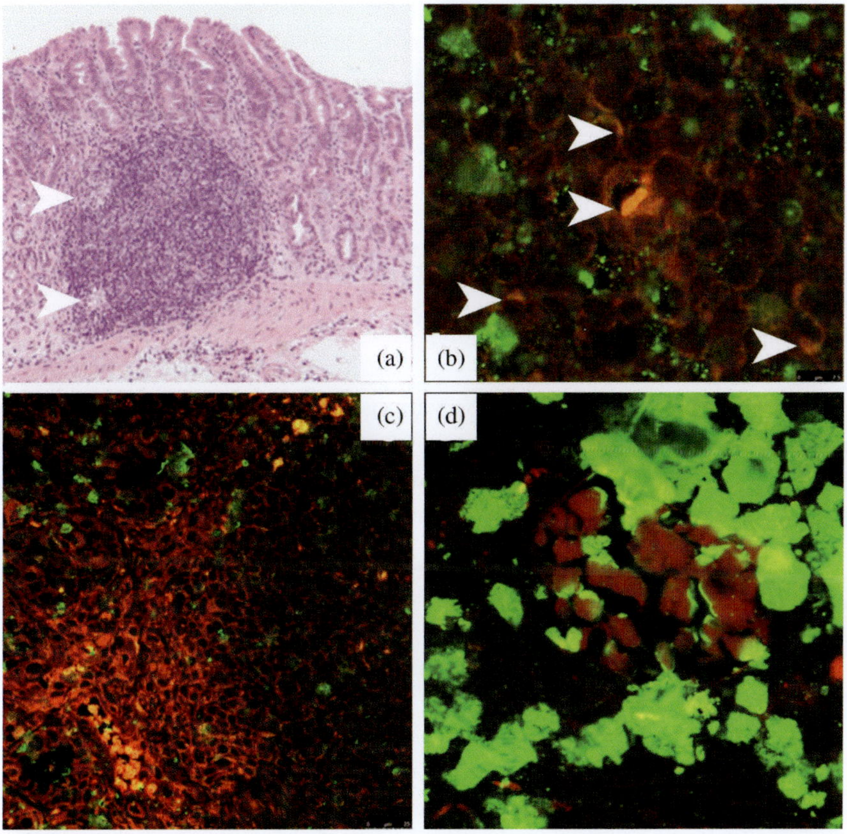

Figure 6. Effect of axitinib administration to the gastric MALT lymphoma. (a) By axitinib administration, some part of the MALT lymphoma became degenerated (arrow heads). HE staining ×200. (b) By the double immunostaining of CD31 (orange), that is, the marker of the endothelial cells and cleaved caspase 3 (green), some of the endothelia cells (arrow heads) became apoptotic by the axitinib administration ×800. (c, d) By the double immunostaining of VASH2 and VEGF-A, axitinib administration induced the decrease of VEGF positive cells (red), while the VASH2 positive cells (green) markedly increased within the MALT lymphoma. c: ×400, d: ×800.

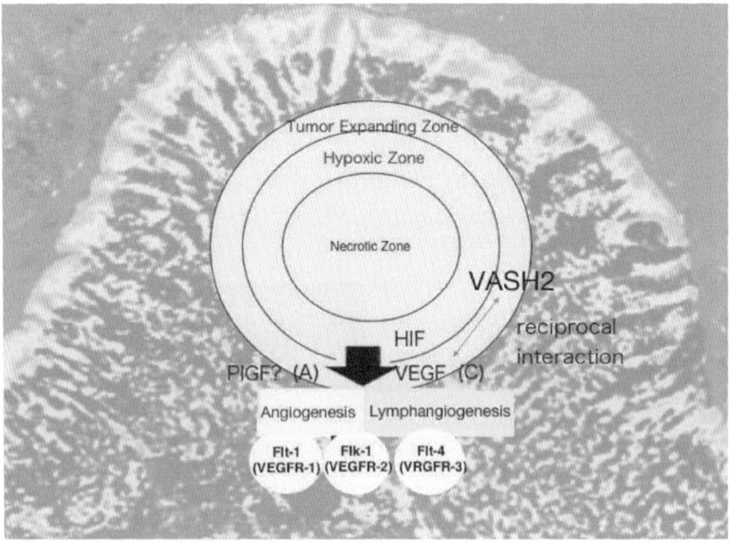

Figure 7. Reciprocal angiogenic regulation of the gastric MALT Lymphoma by VEGF family and VASH2.

In conclusion, from these observations, the reciprocal regulation could exist in the angiogenic mediators in tumor cells, a phenomenon which should be taken into account in the treatment of angiogenic tumors (Figure 7).

References

1. C Thiersch (1865) Der Epithelialkrebs namentlich der Haut mit Atlas. Leipzig. As cited in W Rogers, RF Edlich, DV Lewis, JB Aust. *Surg North Am* **47**: 1473.
2. AG Ide, NH Baker, SL Warren (1939) Vascularization of the Brown-Pearce rabbit epithelioma transplant as seen in the transparent ear chamber. *Am J Roentgenol* **42**: 891.
3. BW Zweifach (1977) Functional behavior of the microcirculation. Thomas Publisher Ltd., Springfield, IL, USA.
4. J Folkman (1971) Tumor angiogenesis: Therapeutic implications. *N Engl J Med* **285**: 1182–1186.
5. Y Shing, J Folkman, R Sullivan, C Butterfield, J Murray, M (1984) Heparin affinity: Purification of a tumor-derived capillary endothelial cell growth factor. *Science* **223**: 1296–1299.

6. N Ferrara, WJ Henzel (1989) Pituitary follicular cells secrete a novel heparin-binding growth factor specific for vascular endothelial cells. *Biochem Biophys Res Commun.* **161**: 851–858.
7. K Watanabe, Y Hasegawa, H Yamashita, K Shimizu, Y Ding, M Abe, H Ohta, K Imagawa, K Hojo, H Maki, H Sonoda, Y Sato (2004) Vasohibin as an endothelium-derived negative feedback regulator of angiogenesis. *J Clin Invest* **114**: 898–907.
8. T Shibuya, K Watanabe, H Yamashita, K Shimizu, H Miyashita, M Abe, T Moriya, H Ohta, H Sonoda, T Shimosegawa, K Tabayashi, Y Sato (2006) Isolation and characterization of vasohibin-2 as a homologue of VEGF-inducible endothelium-derived angiogenesis inhibitor vasohibin. *Arterioscler Thromb Vasc Biol* **26**: 1051–1057.
9. MR Gilbert, JJ Dignam, TS Armstrong, JS Wefel, DT Blumenthal, *et al.* (2014) A randomized trial of bevacizumab for newly diagnosed glioblastoma. *N Engl J Med* **370**: 699–708.
10. M Nakamura, SY Murayama, H Serizawa, *et al.* (2007) Candidatus Helicobacter heilmannii from cynomolgus monkey brought about gastric low grade MALT lymphoma in C57BL/6 mice. *Infect Immun* **75**: 1214–1222.
11. JL O'Rourke, JV Solnick, BA Neilan, K Seidel, R Hayter, LM Hansen, A Lee (2004) Description of "Candidatus Helicobacter heilmannii" based on DNA sequence analysis of 16S rRNA and urease genes. *Int J System Evolution Microbiol* **54**: 2203–2211.
12. F Haesebrouck, F Pasmans, B Flahou, A Smet, P Vandamme, R Ducatelle (2011) Non-*Helicobacter pylori Helicobacter* species in the human gastric mucosa: A proposal to introduce the terms *H. heilmannii Sensu Lato* and *Sensu Stricto*. *Helicobacter* **16**: 339–340.
13. K Nishikawa, M Nakamura, S Takahashi, *et al.* (2007) Increased apoptosis and angiogenesis in gastric low-grade mucosa-associated lymphoid tissue-type lymphoma by *Helicobacter heilmannii* infection in C57/BL6 mice. *FEMS Immunol Med Microbiol* **50**: 268–272.
14. R Gray, ME O'Donnell, P Maxwell, *et al.* (2012) Long-term follow-up of immunocytochemical analysis of vascular endothelial growth factor (VEGF), and its two receptors, VEGF-R1 (Flt-1) and VEGF-R2 (Flk-1/KDR), in oesophagogastric cancer. *Int J Biol Markers* **28**: 63–70.
15. P Carmeliet P, L Moons L, A Luttun A, *et al.* (2001) Synergism between vascular endothelial growth factor and placental growth factor contributes to angiogenesis and plasma extravasation in pathological conditions. *Nat Med* **7**: 575–583.

16. M Nakamura, H Matsui, SY Murayama, *et al.* (2007) Interaction of VEGF to gastric low grade MALT lymphoma by *Helicobacter heilmannii* infection in C57BL/6 mice. *Inflammopharmacology* **15**: 115–118.
17. Simonetti, G Lucarini, C Rubini *et al.* (2012) Microvessel density and VEGF, HIF-1α expression in primary oral melanoma: Correlation with prognosis. *Oral Dis* **19**: 620–627.
18. M Nakamura, S Takahashi, H Matsui H, *et al.* (2008) Microcirculatory alteration in low-grade mucosa-associated lymphoma by *Helicobacter heilmannii* infection: Its relation to vascular endothelial growth factor and cyclooxygenase-2. *J Gastroenterol Hepatol* **23** (**Suppl. 2**): S157–S160.
19. JC Chen, YW Chang, CC Hong, *et al.* (2012) The role of the VEGF-C/VEGFRs axis in tumor progression and therapy. *Int J Mol Sci* **14**: 88–107.
20. H Kimura, H Miyashita, Y Suzuki, M Kobayashi, K Watanabe, H Sonoda, H Ohta, T Fujiwara, T Shimosegawa, Y Sato (2010) Distinctive localization and opposed roles of vasohibin-1 and vasohibin-2 in the regulation of angiogenesis. *Blood* **113**: 4810–4818.

Chapter 9

NF-κB as a Potential Molecular Target for Therapy of Gastrointestinal Cancers

Nathan Palmer, Muthu K. Shanmugam, Gautam Sethi, and Philipp Kaldis

Abstract

Intensive research in the last two decades has identified NF-κB as a master transcription factor which has the potential to bridge the gap between inflammation and cancer development and may hold the key to the development of novel anti-cancer drugs. This review will focus on the effects of NF-κB dysregulation during the development and progression of gastrointestinal cancers such as those of colorectal, gastric, and liver cancers and the emerging therapeutic targets within the NF-κB pathway which may be exploited for their treatment.

Introduction

NF-κB is a ubiquitously expressed transcription factor which is able to rapidly activate a large and varied catalog of downstream effects. Under normal conditions, this transcription factor lies latent in the cytoplasm, ready to respond to an activating signal without the requirement for de novo synthesis; it is rendered functionally inactive due to constitutive and highly stringent negative regulation which sequesters it in the cytoplasm. Upon receipt of an upstream activating stimulus, however, this repression is relieved and NF-κB is able to translocate to the nucleus and activate the transcription of a large number of genes. NF-κB is able to transduce highly divergent activating signals due to its positioning downstream of multiple major cell signaling pathways and thus drives a diverse milieu of cellular effects which may have opposing functions depending on the origin of the activating signal. Although historically it was proposed by Rudolf Virchow as early as in 1863 that inflammation was associated with the presence of increased tumorigenesis, it was not until more recent times that large-scale epidemiological studies have been able to conclusively establish inflammation as a significant risk factor for cancer development. This phenomenon is now widely accepted and famously inflammation has been described as one of the initial six hallmarks of cancer development. Intensive research has subsequently identified NF-κB as a factor which has the potential to bridge the gap between inflammation and cancer development and may hold the key to the development of novel anti-cancer drugs. This review will focus on the effects of NF-κB dysregulation during the development and progression of cancers, especially those which arise within inflammatory microenvironments such as colorectal, gastric, and liver cancers and the emerging therapeutic targets within the NF-κB pathway which may be exploited for their treatment.

Structure and function of NF-κB

The naming of NF-κB as the nuclear factor-κ-light-chain-enhancer of activated B cells was prompted by the preliminary observation by David Baltimore in 1986 that a ubiquitously expressed protein NF-κB was able to bind a short immunoglobulin κ-light-chain-enhancer DNA sequence. Since its initial discovery, NF-κB has been heavily studied and identified as having roles in regulation of apoptosis and survival signaling, pro- and anti-inflammatory reactions, memory formation, cell adhesion maintenance, and many aspects of the immune response including viral infection response (reviewed by Gilmore[1]). Indeed, its central role in immune response control and the orchestration of cytokine and inflammatory signaling has led many to describe NF-κB as the prototypical pro-inflammatory signaling pathway. The

NF-κB signaling cascade interacts with several parallel pathways including the signaling cascades initiated by phosphatidylinositol 3-kinase (PI3K) and Akt.[2–4] Rather than a singular molecule, NF-κB is a broad term which refers to a collective family of ubiquitously expressed transcription factor subunits. Five NF-κB subunits are currently described in mammals. These subunits are also known as REL proteins due to the presence of an N-terminal REL homology domain which facilitates their DNA-binding activity, nuclear localization, dimerization with other REL homology domain containing proteins, and regulatory interaction with NF-κB inhibitory molecules such as the IκB class of proteins.[5]

The NF-κB/REL protein coding genes are highly conserved in eukaryotes and can be traced back to invertebrates including Drosophila and lower organisms such as sea sponges and the single-celled eukaryotes.[6–9] The REL proteins can be subdivided into two classes based on their transactivation properties and maturation state. These are the class II REL proteins, p65 (REL-A), REL-B, and c-REL and the class I REL proteins P105 and P100. Unlike the class II proteins that are synthesized as functionally active units, the class I REL proteins are synthesized as large immature precursors and must be processed by the ubiquitin-26S proteasome pathway. This is facilitated by the presence of degradable C-terminal ankyrin repeats. This post-translational modification yields the mature REL subunits p50 and p52, respectively, also commonly described in the literature as NF-κB1 and NF-κB2.

Although all combinations of both homodimers and heterodimers of the class I and class II REL proteins can be theoretically formed via the interaction of their REL homology domains, a heterodimer of p50 and REL-A (p65) is the predominantly formed and most well-studied complex.

Class I–Class II heterodimer protein complexes are able to translocate to the nucleus and activate gene transcription.[10] On the other hand, p50 and p52 homodimers have been shown to repress transcription at NF-κB DNA-binding sites.[11] NF-κB DNA binding sites are known as κB sites and have a highly degenerate 9–10 base pair consensus sequence of 5′GGGRNNYYCC3′. Although these sites are highly prevalent in eukaryotic genomes, their presence can be considered as a minimal requirement which depending on circumstance may require additional factors such as chromatin remodeling or post-translational modification for adequate NF-κB gene transcription.[12] Approximately around 150 genes have been shown to be directly regulated by NF-κB (an updated list is available at www.nf-kb.org). The actual number of possible NF-κB responsive genes is unknown as many genes which bind NF-κB strongly, conform weakly to the predicted κB binding site, and the relative importance of each nucleotide in this binding sequence seems to vary depending on the circumstance or factors such as the REL protein heterodimer concentration.[13]

NF-κB regulation

Many factors have been shown to be activators of NF-κB including, but not limited to, cytokines, antigens of bacterial and viral origin, free radicals and reactive oxidant species, and ultraviolet irradiation (reviewed by Pahl[14]). This broad spectrum of stimuli allows NF-κB to regulate a large number of vital processes, but it also means that the potential for NF-κB dysregulation is high and as a result tight regulation is needed to prevent activation in response to inappropriate signals. Under normal conditions, NF-κB activity is actively repressed by the IκB (inhibitor of κ B) family of molecules.[15] This family comprises of the catalytic subunits IκBα/β and also other IκB isoforms such as γ,ε[16] and the more recently characterized fourth IκB molecule, NF-κB2/p100, which is required in non-canonical NF-κB signaling.[17] The mechanism of this inhibition is primarily via the prevention of NF-κB nuclear translocation, although this is slightly different depending on the IκB family molecule interacting with the NF-κB dimer. IκBα, for example, contains a strong nuclear export signal, which lowers the concentration of NF-κB in the nucleus due to an increased rate of NF-κB export.[18] On the other hand, IκBβ is able to directly sequester NF-κB dimers in the cytoplasm through its interaction with their nuclear localization sequence, preventing nuclear-cytoplasmic shuttling entirely.[19] The IκB inhibition of NF-κB is constitutive and persists until an appropriate activating stimulus releases the IκB inhibition[20] Although IκB proteins are dispensable from an elegant depletion study which removed IκBα, IκBβ and IκBε protein from cells showed a basal level of p65 driven transcription in the absence of any activating stimulus. This suggests that these IκB proteins are required to prevent constitutive NF-κB signaling.[21]

All activating events of NF-κB converge upon the removal of IκB inhibition via phosphorylation of two conserved serine's (S32 and S36 in humans) within the destruction box domain on IκBα. This phosphorylation targets the IκB complex for ubiquitination and subsequent proteolytic degradation mediated by the 26S proteasome.[22] Alternate routes of negative regulation include the direct phosphorylation of the NF-κB subunit P65 by phosphatases such as WIP1 which inhibits the transactivation of NF-κB through the removal of an essential phosphorylation on serine 536.[23]

The primary driver phosphorylation events which stimulate the ubiquitination of IκB is a molecule known as IKK (inhibitor of κB kinase).[24] The IKK family contains five main catalytic subunits IKKα, IIKβ, IKKε, TANK-binding kinase 1 (TBK1) and also a further subunit, IKKγ also known as NF-κB essential modulator (NEMO) which contains no catalytic activity but is essential for NF-κB signaling.[25] The IKK molecules form complexes between family members and the most common of these is IKKα, IKKβ, and NEMO. These complexes are activated as a target of many diverse cell signaling pathways including MEK,[26] ERK,[27] Akt/PI3K,[28] and NF-κB-inducing kinase [TRAF/NIK].[29] These pathways culminate with the phosphorylation of Ser177 and Ser181 for IKKβ and Ser176 and Ser180 for IKKα in humans[30,31] within the activating T-loop structure.[32] Alternatively, IKK can undergo oligomerization-driven autophosphorylation. The IKK subunits are essential for normal development with IKKβ knockout causing embryonic lethality through massive apoptosis of embryonic hepatocytes and IKKα KO mice dying a few days perinatally displaying abnormalities in limb outgrowth and skin development due to a lack of NF-κB activation in these regions.[33–35] The knockout of the x-linked gene IKKγ (NEMO) causes male lethality development of an incontinentia pigmenti-like phenotype in heterozygous knockout females, causing skin lesions and apoptosis of keratinocytes.[36] This highlights the precise control and essential role of NF-κB needed both during embryonic and normal development.

Two main activation routes are available for the transduction of NF-κB signaling (Figure 1): the canonical and non-canonical pathways.[37] The canonical pathway results in the removal of the IκB inhibition of the p50–p65 dimer or less commonly the p50-c-REL dimer typically upon cytokine or pattern recognition receptor activation such as interleukin-1 receptor (IL-1R) or toll-like receptor 4.[10] Alternatively, the non-canonical pathway results in the IKKα-mediated phosphorylation by NF-κB-inducing kinase (NIK) and processing of p100-REL-B heterodimers leading to the production of

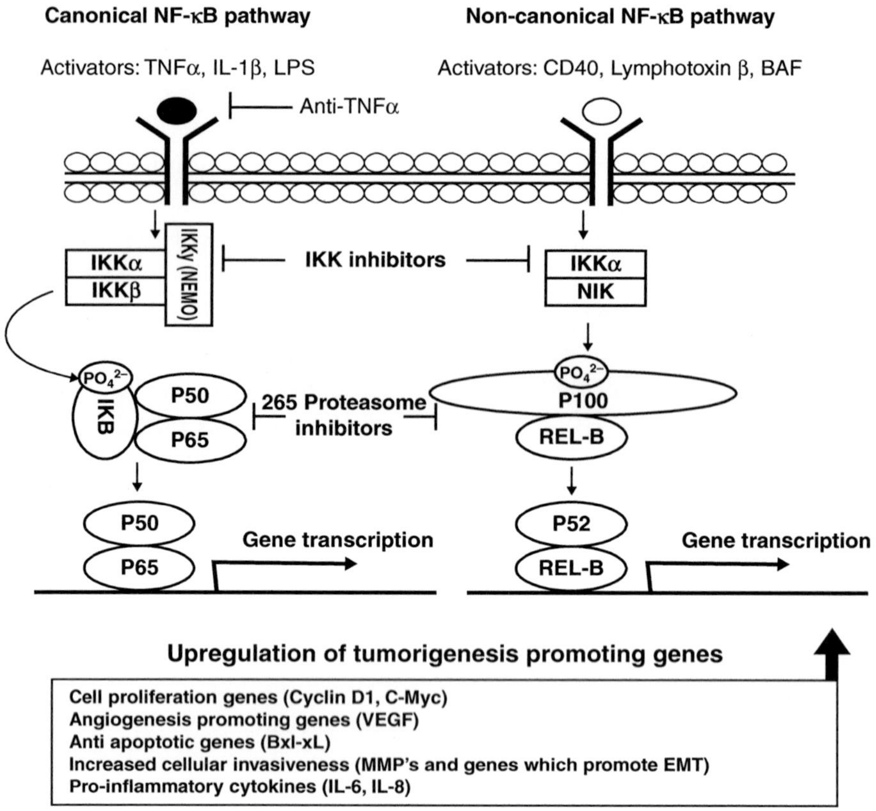

Figure 1. A schematic representation of the activation of the canonical and non-canonical NF-κB signaling pathways and their therapeutic targets.

p52-REL-B[38] upon stimulation primarily by tumor necrosis factor receptor cytokine ligands including lymphotoxin-*β*, CDC40, and BAFF.[39–41]

The role of NF-κB in cancer and its regulated genes in gastrointestinal (GI) tract cancer

The first indications that the NF-κB/REL family of proteins could be involved in oncogenesis were observations that their sequence was similar to a related molecule called V-REL. This protein was shown to be able to facilitate oncogenic transformation both *in vivo* and *in vitro* and has since been found to be oncogenic in transgenic mice which harbors mutations causing them to overexpress V-REL.[42] This inherent transforming ability is not seen in the REL/NF-κB family of proteins; however, transforming mutations result in hematopoietic malignancies rather than solid tumors.[43] An increase in C-REL protein expression, however, has been shown to transform primary chicken lymphoid cells *in vitro.*[44] This was proposed to be due to the overwhelming capacity of the IκB regulatory subunits to repress NF-κB nuclear translocation. This is supported by the fact that an increase in copy number of C-REL in humans has been shown in many cancers.[45] In addition to increased copy number the REL/NF-κB family of proteins is often indirectly upregulated via other means such as tumorigenic viruses,[43,46] inactivating mutations in the inhibitory IκB subunits IκBα, IκBβ, IκBε[46–48] which are seen in Hodgkin's lymphoma.[46] Mutations in activating molecules have also been shown to be oncogenic. Translocation of BCL-3, for example, which is a coactivator of p50 and p52 homodimers can also be seen in many lymphomas.[49] Confusingly, in some mouse models the opposite is true and some upstream activators such as IKKγ (NEMO) and IKKβ seem to have a role as tumor suppressor.[50,51]

The influence of inflammation on NF-κB dysregulation and cancer risk

The involvement of inflammation in tumor progression is now widely accepted and it is now recognized that infiltrating immune cells within the tumor microenvironment play a large role in secreting pro-inflammatory factors which drive tumorigenesis.[52] Anti-inflammatory therapies are now being sought as treatments or adjuvants to cancer therapy and evidence is building that anti-inflammatory pharmaceuticals may help to reduce lifetime cancer development risk[53] and may have beneficial effects in inhibiting tumor development.[54] The precise mechanisms whereby NF-κB becomes upregulated in cancers are unknown and the source of upregulation may be case specific. It has been proposed that inflammatory environments increase the risk of NF-κB dysregulation by feeding into the pre-existing NF-κB system as input stimuli and exaggerating its physiological functions. This is supported by the fact that a large number of cancers display elevated NF-κB activation independent of mutations in either IKK, IκB, or REL/NF-κB proteins or their upstream activators suggesting excessive physiological activation rather than a mutation in the existing NF-κB signaling pathways.[55,56] The typical downstream cellular functions upregulated by NF-κB encompass at least four of the six classical hallmarks of cancer.[57] These are the stimulation of cell growth, evasion of apoptosis, promotion of angiogenesis, and increased tissue invasiveness. NF-κB can drive cell growth by directly targeting cell cycle genes including cyclin D1. Cyclin D1 promotes G1/S phase transition through the hyperphosphorylation and inhibition of retinoblastoma protein, enhancing cell cycle proliferation[58] and also c-myc, an oncogenic signaling molecule, which also drives cell proliferation.[59] NF-κB can also augment proapoptotic factors including p53[60] and drive the expression of antiapoptotic proteins to facilitate the evasion of cancer cells from cell death.[61] NF-κB can also promote angiogenesis and the growth of blood vessels allowing vascularization of tumors through the expression of genes such as VEGF[62] and COX2.[63] Furthermore, NF-κB also employs multiple mechanisms which increase cell evasiveness such as the production of matrix metalloproteases[64] and upregulation of genes associated with epithelial–mesenchymal transition,[54] which can all promote the likelihood of extravasation into the bloodstream and metastasis. In addition to these cancer hallmarks, NF-κB drives the expression of a vast array of cytokines which are essential for its normal physiological role as a central mediator of the immune response allowing for its immune surveillance functions. These include 27 different cytokines and chemokines (reviewed by Pahl[14]). Interestingly, these also include the NF-κB activating molecules IL1-α[65] and TNF-α[66,67] allowing NF-κB to regulate its own expression. Usually, the cellular effects driven by these downstream effectors are purposeful and are propagated transiently until their purpose is served.

In chronic inflammation as is seen in many cancers, however, there is a persistence of inflammatory signaling prolonging the activation of NF-κB. This can either be due to environmental factors such as chronic infection by *Helicobacter pylori*, Hepatitis B and C, or Human papilloma virus or exposure to allergens such as smoke. In terms of GI tract cancers, genetic factors including predisposition to chronic inflammatory conditions such as ulcerative colitis or Crohn's disease[68] greatly increase the risk of cancer. Organs within the GI tract are typically at higher risk of inflammation-driven cancers

Table 1. A list of notable papers outlining the role of NF-κB signaling in the development of GI tact cancers (adapted from http://www.bu.edu/nf-kb/physiological-mediators/diseases/).

NF-κB associated cancers	Notable publications
Colon	105–107
Esophageal/gastric	108–111
Laryngeal	112,113
Stomach	114,115

(Table 1). This is due to the fact that the mucosal linings of the GI tract frequently come into contact with immune sensitizing external stimuli and must be prepared to mount an immune response to ingested pathogens or viruses. In addition, the mucosal layers of the GI tract are exposed to frictional shearing and must be constantly renewed to provide a constant protective layer increasing the need for maintained cell proliferation.

NF-κB signaling in cancers

To elucidate the role of NF-κB and its downstream gene targets in the development of solid tumors, cancer mouse models of the GI tract have been employed such as the colitis-associated cancer (CAC) mouse model. In this model, mice are administered with azoxymethane (AOM), which is a precarcinogen, which is metabolized by intestinal epithelial cells (IEC) to a genotoxic metabolite methylazoxymethanol; this leads to DNA damage and the development of large bowel adenomas.[69] Additional administration of second chemical dextran sulfate sodium (DSS) to AOM treated mice then leads to a progression of CAC. AOM treatment in mice with a conditional knockout of IKKβ in IEC cells, however, protects from the development of colonic adenoma. Subsequent analysis suggested that this was probably due to a loss of NF-κB-dependent upregulation of antiapoptotic factors such as Bcl-xL.[70] The additional effects that AOM treatment included are the stimulation of surrounding lamina propria macrophages to secrete pro-inflammatory cytokines such as IL-6 which are important in the development of CAC[71] and enhance adenoma growth.[72] In accordance with this observation, treatment of IL-6 knockout mice with AOM and DSS resulted in a reduced number and size of colonic adenomas as compared to wild-type mice receiving the same treatment suggesting that NF-κB stimulation of IL-6 or the downstream targets of IL-6 drive the development of CAC in this model. Indeed, IL-6 is a major downstream target which is activated by NF-κB[73] through binding of NF-κB to κB sequences occurring within the IL-6 gene promoter.[74,75] Many of the downstream effects of IL-6 signaling draw parallels with NF-κB activation including upregulation of genes involved in immune response cell survival and proliferation tissue homeostasis and regeneration.[76] This IL-6 signaling is mediated primarily through the activation of another transcription factor STAT3 which is also significantly upregulated in inflammatory cancers such as CAC.[77] It may be the case that NF-κB activation causes paracrine signaling through IL-6 to drive STAT3 activation in neighboring cells. p65 and p50 have previously been shown to physically interact with STAT3; although unclear, it has been suggested that this interaction may enhance NF-κB activation by removing IκB inhibition in the absence of IKK phosphorylation.[78] NF-κB in complex with STAT3 has also been shown to bind to unique DNA binding sites which NF-κB or STAT3 cannot bind in isolation.[79]

The combined action of NF-κB and STAT3 controls the expression of an array of inflammatory cytokine genes, which may lead to the perfect environment for premalignant cell transformation. The problem with targeting the NF-κB->IL-6->STAT3 axis is that ablation of IL-6 or STAT3 dramatically compromises normal IEC survival probably due to the interference of physiological STAT3 signaling. Other studies have shown that constitutive NF-κB upregulation in isolation is not sufficient to drive GI tract tumorigenesis. Additional signaling mechanism(s) such as activation of MAPK pathway has also been found to be involved in tumor initiation and progression.[80] Another mouse model was used to demonstrate that NF-κB activation was responsible for tumor growth under inflammatory conditions. In this model colonic adenoma cells were stimulated to generate lung metastases following LPS stimulation. LPS induced a strong NF-κB activation through the upregulation of circulating TNF-α levels causing heightened expression of antiapoptotic genes and tumor growth. When NF-κB was repressed by overexpressing IκB in the absence of an LPS stimulus, this prevented the upregulation of NF-κB driven antiapoptotic genes and subsequent tumor cell metastases. Interestingly repression of IκB combined with an LPS stimulus caused regression of metastases. This was proposed to be due to the LPS-driven upregulation of a type II TNF family transmembrane protein TRAIL which binds to death receptors such as DR4 and DR5 to promote apoptosis in the absence of the activation of NF-κB and its antiapoptotic effects. This elegant experiment highlights that cancer treatment often depends not just on preventing antiapoptotic signaling but also initiating apoptosis via other means.[81]

A further experiment utilized a mouse model in which Mdr2 knockout mice spontaneously developed hepatitis followed by hepatocellular carcinoma. This is characterized by sites of strong inflammation within the liver secreting TNF-α causing activation of NF-κB in a paracrine fashion. In this chapter, double-mutant mice which combine Mdr2 knockout with a secondary transgene, which encodes a hepatocyte-specific non-degradable super repressor IκBα, are also described. Using this model, it was shown that NF-κB inactivation at birth through the expression of the super repressor IκBa did not affect the onset of hepatitis or the initial Mdr2 driven transformation of hepatocytes. However, at later stages, it was clear that tumor burden of double-mutant mice with impaired NF-κB activation was far lower than either the Mdr2 single knockout mice or NF-κB-proficient, double-mutant mice, where the IκBα super repressor expression was inhibited.[82] This suggests that NF-κB inhibition was able to promote the apoptosis of transformed hepatocytes. Increased apoptosis was also seen as a result of upstream inhibition of NF-κB and other antiapoptotic proteins such as c-jun using anti-TNF-α antibody treatment highlighting the strong antiapoptotic signaling driven by the TNF-α–NF-κB axis.

Therapeutics targeting NF-κB in GI cancers

NF-κB is an extremely attractive target for novel anti-cancer therapeutics. Alongside the fact that NF-κB is upregulated in many GI tract cancers, upregulation of NF-κB is often associated with a resistance to existing cancer drugs.[83] The reduction of this apoptosis resistance may be key to improving outcomes using available drugs. One of the key therapeutic avenues, therefore, is to counteract the suppression of apoptosis driven by NF-κB. There are several options which could allow this, including reducing NF-κB activation within the inflammatory tumor microenvironment, targeting signaling pathways upstream of NF-κB, the direct targeting of NF-κB activating molecules such as IKK, or enhancement of physiological NF-κB inhibiting molecules such as the IκB family. Another possibility is to target the antiapoptotic transcriptional targets downstream of NF-κB.

Inflammation

In relation to controlling the inflammatory tumor microenvironment which often drives NF-κB activation in GI tract cancers, non-steroidal anti-inflammatory drugs (NSAIDs) may be of therapeutic value. This class of pharmacological regents targets the cyclooxygenase (COX) family of enzymes. Large-scale COX-2 specific clinical trials have recently shown great promise in reducing the incidence of colorectal cancers both in normal[84] and high-risk patients,[85] and also many others such as esophageal cancers.[86] Mechanistically, NF-κB is able to directly control the expression of the PGHS2 (COX-2) enzyme[87] and subsequently mediate the production of pro-inflammatory prostanoids including prostaglandin E_2 (PGE_2).[88] It has been shown that PGE_2 is upregulated in many colorectal cancers and can also work synergistically with TNF-α to strongly drive the activation of NF-κB providing a mechanism whereby NF-κB is able to continually drive COX-2 and PG production creating a positive feedback loop (Figure 2). A COX-2 inhibitor known as celecoxib and a similar compound rofecoxib, which has since been withdrawn, have already been used in clinics in patients with familial adenomatous polyposis for the reduction of polyp formation.[89] The COX-prostonoid pathway is very complex, however, and many other prostanoids including prostaglandin A1 (PGA1) have conversely been shown to reduce NF-κB through IKK inhibition and prevention of IKBα degradation.[90] It should also be taken into consideration that alongside all COX-2 inhibitors, there is a significant risk of GI bleeding, although the newer generation of drugs is being developed to reduce this side effect.

Upstream regulators, TNF-α, and Akt

In regard to the targeting of upstream NF-κB activation, both TNF-α and Akt are proposed as major influences contributing toward the activation of NF-κB. Anti-TNF-α cancer therapy is very attractive option due the fact that anti-TNF-α therapy has shown promise both in mice models[91] and early human clinical trials.[92] In this case, the lack of TNF-α signaling may lessen

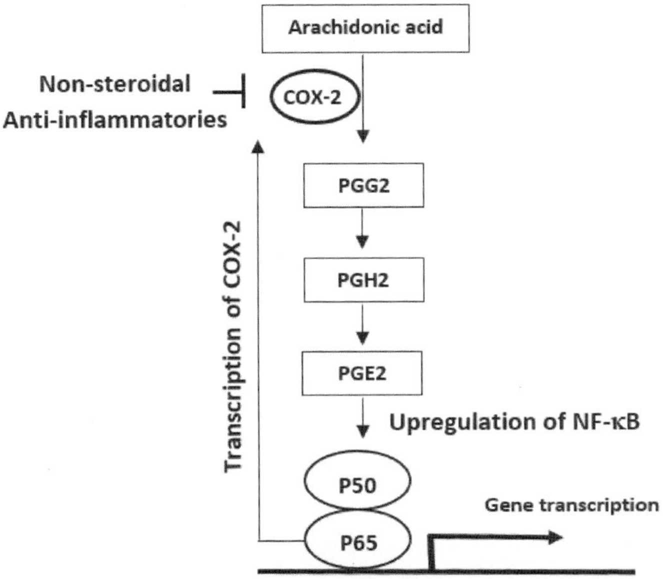

Figure 2. A simplified representation of the reduction in NF-κB activation following inhibition of COX-2 using non-steroidal anti-inflammatory drugs.

the activation of NF-κB reducing the overall expression of antiapoptotic genes, as under normal conditions IKK can be recruited to the TNFR-1 signaling complex and be activated to phosphorylate IκB causing its destruction.[93] Upstream Akt activation in cancer is also proposed to regulate NF-κB activation. Akt has been shown to phosphorylate Thr23 of IKKα in humans which is essential for the subsequent phosphorylation of both IκB and also p65 at Ser535 by IKKα/β leading to the subsequent activation of NF-κB. Constitutively, active Akt was also shown to transform cells and this was associated with a rise in NF-κB transcription which could be reduced by Akt inhibitors or was not seen using a kinase dead form of Akt.[94]

IKK/proteasome inhibitors

Another therapeutic target which is being explored is through the inhibition of the IKK complexes responsible for the normal activation of NF-κB through the ubiquitination of IκB inhibitory molecules. Several small pharmacological compounds have been described which report potent inhibition of NF-κB activation and the reduction of inflammation signaling.[95–99] Along similar lines, antisense oligonucleotides have also been shown to be efficacious in preventing the transcription of the IKK molecules effectively, decreasing the potential for NF-κB activation.[100] Alternatively, the inhibition of NF-κB can be preserved in the presence of active IKK through the prevention of proteolytic degradation of IKB's by the 26S proteasome. This has already been shown to be efficacious in the treatment of multiple myeloma cases which are often dependent on NF-κB activation.[101] This method has also been employed in cases of irritable bowel disease using drugs such as sulfasalazine and methotrexate to reduce proteasome-mediated IκB degradation and subsequently prevent NF-κB nuclear translocation, although this is currently used to treat acute symptoms rather than as a cancer therapy.[102,103] Although IKKγ (NEMO) is not functionally active, it plays an essential role in the activation of NF-κB, as such drugs have been designed to prevent its interaction with IKKα and IKKβ. One such drug known as the NEMO binding domain is a peptide inhibitor which acts to physically block the binding domain of IKKγ and thus its interaction with other IKK's.[104] Although preventing the activation of NF-κB is not directly cytotoxic to cancer cells, one would hope that these therapies may increase their susceptibility to other cytotoxic agents used in conjunction by lowering antiapoptotic resistance.

Conclusions

The role of NF-κB activation in cancers seems to fulfill a primary objective: to drive cell division and to prevent apoptosis. Rather than the result of a genetic mutation, NF-κB upregulation is often due to hijacking and enhancement of normal physiological signaling by aberrant inflammatory molecules originating from the tumor microenvironment. Unlike an oncogenic mutation which must be removed, or destroyed to treat the cancer, the dysregulation of NF-κB signaling has the potential to be righted by correcting the inflammation driving the NF-κB upregulation or by targeting NF-κB itself to be either unresponsive to the inflammatory stimuli or to prevent its transcriptional ability. As previously discussed, if excessive NF-κB signaling is allowed to continue, then the downstream targets of NF-κB may add fuel to the flames of inflammation and create a vicious cycle which may coactivate other cell signaling pathways. Future therapies may make it possible to counteract this overactivation of NF-κB using prophylactic anti-inflammatory treatments, although the full extent of this therapeutic value is still being explored. As light is shed on the full extent NF-κB regulated genes within the genome, it has become apparent that the potential effects of NF-κB activation are extremely far reaching and many of them play a role in normal cellular homeostasis. This makes the multitude of downstream effects of NF-κB extremely difficult to control, and instead the main focus for therapeutic agents should lie in breaking the chain of NF-κB activating signals before its effects can be propagated. However, in many cases the prevention of NF-κB activation alone is not sufficient to cause apoptosis of malignant cells within the tumor and additional pharmaceutical targets should include those pathways which integrate with NF-κB, such as Akt, TNF-α, and STAT3 to force the expression profile of the cancer cell toward apoptosis.

References

1. TD Gilmore (2006) Introduction to NF-κB: Players, pathways, perspectives. *Oncogene* **25**: 6680–6684.
2. LP Kane, VS Shapiro, D Stokoe, A Weiss (1999) Induction of NF-κB by the Akt/PKB kinase. *Curr Biol* **9**: 601–604.
3. N Sizemore, S Leung, GR Stark (1999) Activation of phosphatidylinositol 3-kinase in response to interleukin-1 leads to phosphorylation and activation of the NF-κB p65/RelA subunit. *Mol Cell Biol* **19**: 4798–4805.
4. JA Romashkova, SS Makarov (1999) NF-κB is a target of AKT in anti-apoptotic PDGF signalling. *Nature* **401**: 86–90.
5. AS Baldwin, Jr. (1996) The NF-κB and I κB proteins: New discoveries and insights. *Annu Rev Immunol* **14**: 649–683.
6. S Ghosh, MJ May, EB Kopp (1998) NF-κB and Rel proteins: Evolutionarily conserved mediators of immune responses. *Annu Rev Immunol* **16**: 225–260.
7. JC Sullivan, D Kalaitzidis, TD Gilmore, JR Finnerty (2007) Rel homology domain-containing transcription factors in the cnidarian Nematostella vectensis. *Dev Genes Evol* **217**: 63–72.
8. FS Wolenski, CA Bradham, JR Finnerty, TD Gilmore (2013) NF-κB is required for cnidocyte development in the sea anemone Nematostella vectensis. *Dev Biol* **373**: 205–215.

9. A Sebe-Pedros, A de Mendoza, BF Lang, BM Degnan, I Ruiz-Trillo (2011) Unexpected repertoire of metazoan transcription factors in the unicellular holozoan Capsaspora owczarzaki. *Mol Biol Evol* **28**: 1241–1254.
10. M Karin, Y Ben-Neriah (2000) Phosphorylation meets ubiquitination: The control of NF-[κ]B activity. *Annu Rev Immunol* **18**: 621–663.
11. H Guan, S Hou, RP Ricciardi (2005) DNA binding of repressor nuclear factor-κB p50/p50 depends on phosphorylation of Ser337 by the protein kinase A catalytic subunit. *J Biol Chem* **280**: 9957–9962.
12. G Natoli (2006) Tuning up inflammation: How DNA sequence and chromatin organization control the induction of inflammatory genes by NF-κB. *FEBS Lett* **580**: 2843–2849.
13. T Fujita, GP Nolan, S Ghosh, D Baltimore (1992) Independent modes of transcriptional activation by the p50 and p65 subunits of NF-κ B. *Genes Dev* **6**: 775–787.
14. HL Pahl (1999) Activators and target genes of Rel/NF-κB transcription factors. *Oncogene* **18**: 6853–6866.
15. Y Yamamoto, RB Gaynor (2004) IκB kinases: Key regulators of the NF-κB pathway. *Trends Biochem Sci* **29**: 72–79.
16. MS Hayden, S Ghosh (2008) Shared principles in NF-κB signaling. *Cell* **132**: 344–362.
17. S Basak, H Kim, JD Kearns, V Tergaonkar, E O'Dea, SL Werner, CA Benedict, CF Ware, G Ghosh, IM Verma, A Hoffmann (2007) A fourth IκB protein within the NF-κB signaling module. *Cell* **128**: 369–381.
18. TT Huang, N Kudo, M Yoshida, S Miyamoto (2000) A nuclear export signal in the N-terminal regulatory domain of IκBα controls cytoplasmic localization of inactive NF-κB/IκBα complexes. *Proc Natl Acad Sci USA* **97**: 1014–1019.
19. AA Beg, SM Ruben, RI Scheinman, S Haskill, CA Rosen, AS Baldwin, Jr. (1992) IκB interacts with the nuclear localization sequences of the subunits of NF-κB: A mechanism for cytoplasmic retention. *Genes Dev* **6**: 1899–1913.
20. H Hacker, M Karin (2006) Regulation and function of IKK and IKK-related kinases. *Sci STKE* **2006**: re13.
21. V Tergaonkar, RG Correa, M Ikawa, IM Verma (2005) Distinct roles of IκB proteins in regulating constitutive NF-κB activity. *Nat Cell Biol* 7: 921–923.
22. I Alkalay, A Yaron, A Hatzubai, A Orian, A Ciechanover, Y Ben-Neriah (1995) Stimulation-dependent I κ B α phosphorylation marks the NF-κ B inhibitor for degradation via the ubiquitin-proteasome pathway. *Proc Natl Acad Sci USA* **92**: 10599–10603.

23. J Chew, S Biswas, S Shreeram, M Humaidi, ET Wong, MK Dhillion, H Teo, A Hazra, CC Fang, E Lopez-Collazo, DV Bulavin, V Tergaonkar (2009) WIP1 phosphatase is a negative regulator of NF-κB signalling. *Nat Cell Biol* **11**: 659–666.
24. P Viatour, MP Merville, V Bours, A Chariot (2005) Phosphorylation of NF-κB and IκB proteins: Implications in cancer and inflammation. *Trends Biochem Sci* **30**: 43–52.
25. DM Rothwarf, E Zandi, G Natoli, M Karin (1998) IKK-gamma is an essential regulatory subunit of the IκB kinase complex. *Nature* **395**: 297–300.
26. MB Armstrong, X Bian, Y Liu, C Subramanian, AB Ratanaproeksa, F Shao, VC Yu, RP Kwok, AW Opipari, Jr., VP Castle (2006) Signaling from p53 to NF-κB determines the chemotherapy responsiveness of neuroblastoma. *Neoplasia* **8**: 967–977.
27. J Garaude, S Cherni, S Kaminski, E Delepine, C Chable-Bessia, M Benkirane, J Borges, A Pandiella, MA Iniguez, M Fresno, RA Hipskind, M Villalba (2006) ERK5 activates NF-κB in leukemic T cells and is essential for their growth *in vivo*. *J Immunol* **177**: 7607–7617.
28. A Agarwal, K Das, N Lerner, S Sathe, M Cicek, G Casey, N Sizemore (2005) The AKT/I κ B kinase pathway promotes angiogenic/metastatic gene expression in colorectal cancer by activating nuclear factor-κ B and β-catenin. *Oncogene* **24**: 1021–1031.
29. P Ramakrishnan, W Wang, D Wallach (2004) Receptor-specific signaling for both the alternative and the canonical NF-κB activation pathways by NF-κB-inducing kinase. *Immunity* **21**: 477–489.
30. F Mercurio, H Zhu, BW Murray, A Shevchenko, BL Bennett, J Li, DB Young, M Barbosa, M Mann, A Manning, A Rao (1997) IKK-1 and IKK-2: Cytokine-activated IκB kinases essential for NF-κB activation. *Science* **278**: 860–866.
31. M Delhase, M Hayakawa, Y Chen, M Karin (1999) Positive and negative regulation of IκB kinase activity through IKKβ subunit phosphorylation. *Science* **284**: 309–313.
32. C Scheidereit (2006) IκB kinase complexes: Gateways to NF-κB activation and transcription. *Oncogene* **25**: 6685–6705.
33. Y Hu, V Baud, M Delhase, P Zhang, T Deerinck, M Ellisman, R Johnson, M Karin (1999) Abnormal morphogenesis but intact IKK activation in mice lacking the IKKα subunit of IκB kinase. *Science* **284**: 316–320.
34. Q Li, Q Lu, JY Hwang, D Buscher, KF Lee, JC Izpisua-Belmonte, IM Verma (1999) IKK1-deficient mice exhibit abnormal development of skin and skeleton. *Genes Dev* **13**: 1322–1328.

35. K Takeda, O Takeuchi, T Tsujimura, S Itami, O Adachi, T Kawai, H Sanjo, K Yoshikawa, N Terada, S Akira (1999) Limb and skin abnormalities in mice lacking IKKα. *Science* **284**: 313–316.
36. M Schmidt-Supprian, W Bloch, G Courtois, K Addicks, A Israel, K Rajewsky, M Pasparakis (2000) NEMO/IKK gamma-deficient mice model incontinentia pigmenti. *Mol Cell* **5**: 981–992.
37. A Oeckinghaus, MS Hayden, S Ghosh (2011) Crosstalk in NF-κB signaling pathways. *Nat Immunol* **12**: 695–708.
38. G Xiao, EW Harhaj, SC Sun (2001) NF-κB-inducing kinase regulates the processing of NF-κB2 p100. *Mol Cell* **7**: 401–409.
39. SC Sun (2011) Non-canonical NF-κB signaling pathway. *Cell Res* **21**: 71–85.
40. B Razani, AD Reichardt, G Cheng (2011) Non-canonical NF-κB signaling activation and regulation: Principles and perspectives. *Immunol Rev* **244**: 44–54.
41. SC Sun (2012) The noncanonical NF-κB pathway. *Immunol Rev* **246**: 125–140.
42. D Carrasco, CA Rizzo, K Dorfman, R Bravo (1996) The v-rel oncogene promotes malignant T-cell leukemia/lymphoma in transgenic mice. *EMBO J* **15**: 3640–3650.
43. B Rayet, C Gelinas (1999) Aberrant rel/nfkb genes and activity in human cancer. *Oncogene* **18**: 6938–6947.
44. TD Gilmore, C Cormier, J Jean-Jacques, ME Gapuzan (2001) Malignant transformation of primary chicken spleen cells by human transcription factor c-Rel. *Oncogene* **20**: 7098–7103.
45. D Lu, JD Thompson, GK Gorski, NR Rice, MG Mayer, JJ Yunis (1991) Alterations at the rel locus in human lymphoma. *Oncogene* **6**: 1235–1241.
46. E Cabannes, G Khan, F Aillet, RF Jarrett, RT Hay (1999) Mutations in the IkBa gene in Hodgkin's disease suggest a tumour suppressor role for IκBα. *Oncogene* **18**: 3063–3070.
47. D Krappmann, F Emmerich, U Kordes, E Scharschmidt, B Dorken, C Scheidereit (1999) Molecular mechanisms of constitutive NF-κB/Rel activation in Hodgkin/Reed-Sternberg cells. *Oncogene* **18**: 943–953.
48. KM Wood, M Roff, RT Hay (1998) Defective IκBα in Hodgkin cell lines with constitutively active NF-κB. *Oncogene* **16**: 2131–2139.
49. M Nakagawa, H Sugiyama, H Ogawa, S Tone, H Morishita, H Ikeda, K Aozasa, M Taniwaki, T Abe, T Kishimoto (1995) Intermediate lymphocytic lymphoma with both t(14;19)(q32.3;q13.1) and t(3;22)(q27;q11.2). *Cancer Genet Cytogenet* **79**: 89–91.
50. T Luedde, N Beraza, V Kotsikoris, G van Loo, A Nenci, R De Vos, T Roskams, C Trautwein, M Pasparakis (2007) Deletion of NEMO/IKKgamma in liver parenchymal cells causes steatohepatitis and hepatocellular carcinoma. *Cancer Cell* **11**: 119–132.

51. U Keller, J Huber, JA Nilsson, M Fallahi, MA Hall, C Peschel, JL Cleveland (2010) Myc suppression of Nfkb2 accelerates lymphomagenesis. *BMC Cancer* **10**: 348.
52. LM Coussens, Z Werb (2002) Inflammation and cancer. *Nature* **420**: 860–867.
53. JA Baron, RS Sandler (2000) Nonsteroidal anti-inflammatory drugs and cancer prevention. *Annu Rev Med* **51**: 511–523.
54. A Mantovani, P Allavena, A Sica, F Balkwill (2008) Cancer-related inflammation. *Nature* **454**: 436–444.
55. M Karin (2009) NF-κB as a critical link between inflammation and cancer. *Cold Spring Harb Perspect Biol* **1**: a000141.
56. Y Ben-Neriah, M Karin (2011) Inflammation meets cancer, with NF-κB as the matchmaker. *Nat Immunol* **12**: 715–723.
57. D Hanahan, RA Weinberg (2000) The hallmarks of cancer. *Cell* **100**: 57–70.
58. M Hinz, D Krappmann, A Eichten, A Heder, C Scheidereit, M Strauss (1999) NF-κB function in growth control: Regulation of cyclin D1 expression and G0/G1-to-S-phase transition. *Mol Cell Biol* **19**: 2690–2698.
59. FA La Rosa, JW Pierce, GE Sonenshein (1994) Differential regulation of the c-myc oncogene promoter by the NF-κ B rel family of transcription factors. *Mol Cell Biol* **14**: 1039–1044.
60. V Tergaonkar, M Pando, O Vafa, G Wahl, I Verma (2002) p53 stabilization is decreased upon NFκB activation: A role for NFκB in acquisition of resistance to chemotherapy. *Cancer Cell* **1**: 493–503.
61. DJ Van Antwerp, SJ Martin, T Kafri, DR Green, IM Verma (1996) Suppression of TNF-α-induced apoptosis by NF-κB. *Science* **274**: 787–789.
62. A Shibata, T Nagaya, T Imai, H Funahashi, A Nakao, H Seo (2002) Inhibition of NF-κB activity decreases the VEGF mRNA expression in MDA-MB-231 breast cancer cells. *Breast Cancer Res Treat* **73**: 237–243.
63. S Wang, Z Liu, L Wang, X Zhang (2009) NF-κB signaling pathway, inflammation and colorectal cancer. *Cell Mol Immunol* **6**: 327–334.
64. S Huang, CA Pettaway, H Uehara, CD Bucana, IJ Fidler (2001) Blockade of NF-κB activity in human prostate cancer cells is associated with suppression of angiogenesis, invasion, and metastasis. *Oncogene* **20**: 4188–4197.
65. N Mori, D Prager (1996) Transactivation of the interleukin-1α promoter by human T-cell leukemia virus type I and type II Tax proteins. *Blood* **87**: 3410–3417.
66. AN Shakhov, MA Collart, P Vassalli, SA Nedospasov, CV Jongeneel (1990) *K* B-type enhancers are involved in lipopolysaccharide-mediated transcriptional activation of the tumor necrosis factor α gene in primary macrophages. *J Exp Med* **171**: 35–47.

67. MA Collart, P Baeuerle, P Vassalli (1990) Regulation of tumor necrosis factor α transcription in macrophages: Involvement of four κ B-like motifs and of constitutive and inducible forms of NF-κ B. *Mol Cell Biol* **10**: 1498–1506.
68. E Langholz, P Munkholm, M Davidsen, V Binder (1992) Colorectal cancer risk and mortality in patients with ulcerative colitis. *Gastroenterology* **103**: 1444–1451.
69. J Chen, XF Huang (2009) The signal pathways in azoxymethane-induced colon cancer and preventive implications. *Cancer Biol Ther* **8**: 1313–1317.
70. FR Greten, L Eckmann, TF Greten, JM Park, ZW Li, LJ Egan, MF Kagnoff, M Karin (2004) IKKβ links inflammation and tumorigenesis in a mouse model of colitis-associated cancer. *Cell* **118**: 285–296.
71. S Grivennikov, E Karin, J Terzic, D Mucida, GY Yu, S Vallabhapurapu, J Scheller, S Rose-John, H Cheroutre, L Eckmann, M Karin (2009) IL-6 and Stat3 are required for survival of intestinal epithelial cells and development of colitis-associated cancer. *Cancer Cell* **15**: 103–113.
72. C Becker, MC Fantini, C Schramm, HA Lehr, S Wirtz, A Nikolaev, J Burg, S Strand, R Kiesslich, S Huber, H Ito, N Nishimoto, K Yoshizaki, T Kishimoto, PR Galle, M Blessing, S Rose-John, MF Neurath (2004) TGF-β suppresses tumor progression in colon cancer by inhibition of IL-6 trans-signaling. *Immunity* **21**: 491–501.
73. TA Libermann, D Baltimore (1990) Activation of interleukin-6 gene expression through the NF-κ B transcription factor. *Mol Cell Biol* **10**: 2327–2334.
74. H Isshiki, S Akira, O Tanabe, T Nakajima, T Shimamoto, T Hirano, T Kishimoto (1990) Constitutive and interleukin-1 (IL-1)-inducible factors interact with the IL-1-responsive element in the IL-6 gene. *Mol Cell Biol* **10**: 2757–2764.
75. H Shimizu, K Mitomo, T Watanabe, S Okamoto, K Yamamoto (1990) Involvement of a NF-κ B-like transcription factor in the activation of the interleukin-6 gene by inflammatory lymphokines. *Mol Cell Biol* **10**: 561–568.
76. NC Tebbutt, AS Giraud, M Inglese, B Jenkins, P Waring, FJ Clay, S Malki, BM Alderman, D Grail, F Hollande, JK Heath, M Ernst (2002) Reciprocal regulation of gastrointestinal homeostasis by SHP2 and STAT-mediated trefoil gene activation in gp130 mutant mice. *Nat Med* **8**: 1089–1097.
77. H Yu, R Jove (2004) The STATs of cancer—new molecular targets come of age. *Nat Rev Cancer* **4**: 97–105.
78. J Yang, X Liao, MK Agarwal, L Barnes, PE Auron, GR Stark (2007) Unphosphorylated STAT3 accumulates in response to IL-6 and activates transcription by binding to NFκB. *Genes Dev* **21**: 1396–1408.
79. K Hagihara, T Nishikawa, Y Sugamata, J Song, T Isobe, T Taga, K Yoshizaki (2005) Essential role of STAT3 in cytokine-driven NF-κB-mediated serum amyloid A gene expression. *Genes Cells* **10**:1051–1063.

80. M Guma, D Stepniak, H Shaked, ME Spehlmann, S Shenouda, H Cheroutre, I Vicente-Suarez, L Eckmann, MF Kagnoff, M Karin (2011) Constitutive intestinal NF-κB does not trigger destructive inflammation unless accompanied by MAPK activation. *J Exp Med* **208**: 1889–1900.
81. JL Luo, S Maeda, LC Hsu, H Yagita, M Karin (2004) Inhibition of NF-κB in cancer cells converts inflammation- induced tumor growth mediated by TNF-α to TRAIL-mediated tumor regression. *Cancer Cell* **6**: 297–305.
82. E Pikarsky, RM Porat, I Stein, R Abramovitch, S Amit, S Kasem, E Gutkovich-Pyest, S Urieli-Shoval, E Galun, Y Ben-Neriah (2004) NF-κB functions as a tumour promoter in inflammation-associated cancer. *Nature* **431**: 461–466.
83. H Jing, J Kase, JR Dorr, M Milanovic, D Lenze, M Grau, G Beuster, S Ji, M Reimann, P Lenz, M Hummel, B Dorken, G Lenz, C Scheidereit, CA Schmitt, S Lee (2011) Opposing roles of NF-κB in anti-cancer treatment outcome unveiled by cross-species investigations. *Genes Dev* **25**: 2137–2146.
84. E Flossmann, PM Rothwell, British Doctors Aspirin Trail, UK-TIA Aspirin Trial.(2007) Effect of aspirin on long-term risk of colorectal cancer: Consistent evidence from randomised and observational studies. *Lancet* **369**: 1603–1613.
85. J Burn, AM Gerdes, F Macrae, JP Mecklin, G Moeslein, S Olschwang, D Eccles, DG Evans, ER Maher, L Bertario, ML Bisgaard, MG Dunlop, JW Ho, SV Hodgson, A Lindblom, J Lubinski, PJ Morrison, V Murday, R Ramesar, L Side, RJ Scott, HJ Thomas, HF Vasen, G Barker, G Crawford, F Elliott, M Movahedi, K Pylvanainen, JT Wijnen, R Fodde, HT Lynch, JC Mathers, DT Bishop, C Investigators (2011) Long-term effect of aspirin on cancer risk in carriers of hereditary colorectal cancer: An analysis from the CAPP2 randomised controlled trial. *Lancet* **378**: 2081–2087.
86. MJ Thun, MM Namboodiri, CW Heath, Jr. (1991) Aspirin use and reduced risk of fatal colon cancer. *N Engl J Med* **325**: 1593–1596.
87. R Newton, LM Kuitert, M Bergmann, IM Adcock, PJ Barnes (1997) Evidence for involvement of NF-κB in the transcriptional control of COX-2 gene expression by IL-1β. *Biochem Biophys Res Commun* **237**: 28–32.
88. HR Herschman, ST Reddy, W Xie (1997) Function and regulation of prostaglandin synthase-2. *Adv Exp Med Biol* **407**: 61–66.
89. G Steinbach, PM Lynch, RK Phillips, MH Wallace, E Hawk, GB Gordon, N Wakabayashi, B Saunders, Y Shen, T Fujimura, LK Su, B Levin, L Godio, S Patterson, MA Rodriguez-Bigas, SL Jester, KL King, M Schumacher, J Abbruzzese, RN DuBois, WN Hittelman, S Zimmerman, JW Sherman, G Kelloff (2000) The effect of celecoxib, a cyclooxygenase-2 inhibitor, in familial adenomatous polyposis. *N Engl J Med* **342**: 1946–1952.

90. A Rossi, P Kapahi, G Natoli, T Takahashi, Y Chen, M Karin, MG Santoro (2000) Anti-inflammatory cyclopentenone prostaglandins are direct inhibitors of IκB kinase. *Nature* **403**: 103–108.
91. JH Egberts, V Cloosters, A Noack, B Schniewind, L Thon, S Klose, B Kettler, C von Forstner, C Kneitz, J Tepel, D Adam, H Wajant, H Kalthoff, A Trauzold (2008) Anti-tumor necrosis factor therapy inhibits pancreatic tumor growth and metastasis. *Cancer Res* **68**: 1443–1450.
92. S Madhusudan, M Foster, SR Muthuramalingam, JP Braybrooke, S Wilner, K Kaur, C Han, S Hoare, F Balkwill, DC Talbot, TS Ganesan, AL Harris (2004) A phase II study of etanercept (Enbrel), a tumor necrosis factor α inhibitor in patients with metastatic breast cancer. *Clin Cancer Res* **10**: 6528–6534.
93. A Devin, A Cook, Y Lin, Y Rodriguez, M Kelliher, Z Liu (2000) The distinct roles of TRAF2 and RIP in IKK activation by TNF-R1: TRAF2 recruits IKK to TNF-R1 while RIP mediates IKK activation. *Immunity* **12**: 419–429.
94. D Bai, L Ueno, PK Vogt (2009) Akt-mediated regulation of NFκB and the essentialness of NFκB for the oncogenicity of PI3K and Akt. *Int J Cancer* **125**: 2863–2870.
95. MS Palanki, LM Gayo-Fung, GI Shevlin, P Erdman, M Sato, M Goldman, LJ Ransone, C Spooner (2002) Structure-activity relationship studies of ethyl 2-[(3-methyl-2,5-dioxo(3-pyrrolinyl))amino]-4-(trifluoromethyl)pyrimidine-5-carbo xylate: An inhibitor of AP-1 and NF-κB mediated gene expression. *Bioorg Med Chem Lett* **12**: 2573–2577.
96. D Wen, Y Nong, JG Morgan, P Gangurde, A Bielecki, J Dasilva, M Keaveney, H Cheng, C Fraser, L Schopf, M Hepperle, G Harriman, BD Jaffee, TD Ocain, Y Xu (2006) A selective small molecule IκB Kinase β inhibitor blocks nuclear factor κB-mediated inflammatory responses in human fibroblast-like synoviocytes, chondrocytes, and mast cells. *J Pharmacol Exp Ther* **317**: 989–1001.
97. N Kishore, C Sommers, S Mathialagan, J Guzova, M Yao, S Hauser, K Huynh, S Bonar, C Mielke, L Albee, R Weier, M Graneto, C Hanau, T Perry, CS Tripp (2003) A selective IKK-2 inhibitor blocks NF-κ B-dependent gene expression in interleukin-1 β-stimulated synovial fibroblasts. *J Biol Chem* **278**: 32861–32871.
98. C Frelin, V Imbert, E Griessinger, A Loubat, M Dreano, JF Peyron (2003) AS602868, a pharmacological inhibitor of IKK2, reveals the apoptotic potential of TNF-α in Jurkat leukemic cells. *Oncogene* **22**: 8187–8194.
99. K Ziegelbauer, F Gantner, NW Lukacs, A Berlin, K Fuchikami, T Niki, K Sakai, H Inbe, K Takeshita, M Ishimori, H Komura, T Murata, T Lowinger, KB Bacon (2005) A selective novel low-molecular-weight inhibitor of IκB kinase-β

(IKK-β) prevents pulmonary inflammation and shows broad anti-inflammatory activity. *Br J Pharmacol* **145**: 178–192.

100. G Takaesu, RM Surabhi, KJ Park, J Ninomiya-Tsuji, K Matsumoto, RB Gaynor (2003) TAK1 is critical for IκB kinase-mediated activation of the NF-κB pathway. *J Mol Biol* **326**: 105–115.
101. PG Richardson, T Hideshima, C Mitsiades, K Anderson (2004) Proteasome inhibition in hematologic malignancies. *Ann Med* **36**: 304–314.
102. CK Weber, S Liptay, T Wirth, G Adler, RM Schmid (2000) Suppression of NF-κB activity by sulfasalazine is mediated by direct inhibition of IκB kinases α and β. *Gastroenterology* **119**: 1209–1218.
103. S Majumdar, BB Aggarwal (2001) Methotrexate suppresses NF-κB activation through inhibition of IκBα phosphorylation and degradation. *J Immunol* **167**: 2911–2920.
104. I Strickland, S Ghosh (2006) Use of cell permeable NBD peptides for suppression of inflammation. *Ann Rheum Dis* **65** (Suppl 3): iii75–82.
105. DS Lind, SN Hochwald, J Malaty, S Rekkas, P Hebig, G Mishra, LL Moldawer, EM Copeland, 3rd, S Mackay (2001) Nuclear factor-kappa B is upregulated in colorectal cancer. *Surgery* **130**: 363–369.
106. AJ Schottelius, H Dinter (2006) Cytokines, NF-kappaB, microenvironment, intestinal inflammation and cancer. *Cancer Treat Res* **130**: 67–87.
107. MM Aranha, PM Borralho, P Ravasco, IB Moreira da Silva, L Correia, A Fernandes, ME Camilo, CM Rodrigues (2007) NF-kappaB and apoptosis in colorectal tumourigenesis. *Eur J Clin Invest* **37**: 416–424.
108. AP Sutter, M Zeitz, H Scherubl (2004) Recent results in understanding molecular pathways in the medical treatment of esophageal and gastric cancer. *Onkologie* **27**: 17–21.
109. BL Lee, HS Lee, J Jung, SJ Cho, HY Chung, WH Kim, YW Jin, CS Kim, SY Nam (2005) Nuclear factor-kappaB activation correlates with better prognosis and Akt activation in human gastric cancer. *Clin Cancer Res* **11**: 2518–2525.
110. MM Abdel-Latif, JM O'Riordan, N Ravi, D Kelleher, JV Reynolds (2005) Activated nuclear factor-kappa B and cytokine profiles in the esophagus parallel tumor regression following neoadjuvant chemoradiotherapy. *Dis Esophagus* **18**: 246–252.
111. MM Abdel-Latif, D Kelleher, JV Reynolds (2009) Potential role of NF-kappaB in esophageal adenocarcinoma: as an emerging molecular target. *J Surg Res* **153**: 172–180.
112. J Zhu, G Hu, Y Sun (2004) (Expression and significance of nuclear factor kappaB in laryngeal carcinoma). *Lin Chuang Er Bi Yan Hou Ke Za Zhi* **18**: 745–746, 766.

113. S Pan, Z Tao, L Wu, B Xiao, S Chen (2005) [Nuclear factor kappaB/p65 and cyclooxygenase-2 expression and clinic significance in human laryngeal squamous cell carcinoma]. *Lin Chuang Er Bi Yan Hou Ke Za Zhi* **19**: 535–537.
114. N Sasaki, T Morisaki, K Hashizume, T Yao, M Tsuneyoshi, H Noshiro, K Nakamura, T Yamanaka, A Uchiyama, M Tanaka, M Katano (2001) Nuclear factor-kappaB p65 (RelA) transcription factor is constitutively activated in human gastric carcinoma tissue. *Clin Cancer Res* **7**: 4136–4142.
115. L Wu, Z Pu, J Feng, G Li, Z Zheng, W Shen (2008) The ubiquitin-proteasome pathway and enhanced activity of NF-kappaB in gastric carcinoma. *J Surg Oncol* **97**: 439–444.

Chapter 10

Hypoxia-Inducible Factor-1α Modulation in Colorectal Carcinogenesis

Francesco Mariani, Stefano Mancini, Paola Sena, and Luca Roncucci

Abstract

Cells respond to hypoxia mainly by activating the transcription factor hypoxia-inducible factor-1α (HIF-1α) that is an oxygen-sensitive transcription factor. HIF-1α is overexpressed in various types of cancers, including colorectal, through mechanisms linked to the activation of oncogenes or inactivation of tumor suppressor genes. In colorectal carcinogenesis, the defect in frequently altered pathways, like Wnt and VHL, leads to the stabilization and activation of HIF-1α, both in preneoplastic lesions and in later stages of cancer development. HIF-1α regulates key genes involved in inflammation, cellular metabolism, and also angiogenesis and metastasis, conferring a more aggressive phenotype to colorectal tumors. Several compounds used in cancer therapy inhibit HIF-1α indirectly. Moreover, HIF-1α-regulated genes represent very attractive therapeutic targets. Indeed, recent advances in drug discovery point to the synthesis of more specific HIF-1α-targeting agents.

Introduction

Chronic inflammatory bowel diseases (IBD) such as Crohn disease and ulcerative colitis are characterized by microvascular abnormalities and tissue hypoxia. Thus, hypoxia is present in the inflammatory foci, and regulates both inflammation and resolution of IBD.[1,2] Hypoxia is also a feature of most solid tumors, driving a coordinated transcriptional response that increases the glycolytic metabolism and the angiogenic potential. Cells respond to hypoxia mainly by activating the transcription factor hypoxia-inducible factor-1 (HIF-1), which encompasses two subunits: HIF-1α that is oxygen-sensitive and HIF-1β that is constitutively expressed.[3] Both the subunits of HIF-1 are members of the family of transcription factors basic helix-loop-helix (bHLH) containing a PAS domain. HIF-1α dimerizes with HIF-1β through the bHLH domain and part of the PAS domain, where the bHLH domain is specifically required for DNA binding. The transcriptional activation and interaction with coactivators are mediated by two transactivation domains in the C-terminal half of HIF-1α, called N-terminal (N-TAD) and C-terminal (C-TAD).[4] The negative regulation of HIF in normoxic conditions is controlled by an oxygen-dependent degradation domain, called ODD.[5]

HIF-1 recruits a number of coactivators such as p300, Ref-1, Jab1, SCR-1, and TIF2[5] for the transactivation of specific hypoxia-responsive genes by binding to hypoxia response elements, located in the promoter regions of inducible genes.[6] HIF targets directly at least 800 genes and regulates indirectly transcription mechanisms by acting through genes encoding microRNAs and chromatin-modifying enzymes.[7,8] Also, transcribed-ultraconserved regions, long non-coding RNAs, transcribed from regions that exhibit extremely high conservation, acting as tissue-specific regulators of gene expression, can be upregulated by hypoxia and have been recently described as altered in colorectal cancer (CRC).[9]

HIF-1α Activation in Colorectal Cancer

Under normal oxygen tension, the HIF-1α protein is hydroxylated on two proline residues in the ODD domain from a family of prolyl-hydrolase (PHD1-3), becoming a substrate for ubiquitination by a protein complex containing the von Hippel–Lindau protein (pVHL). Under low oxygen tension, the PHD proteins are unable to modify HIF-1α; the non-hydroxylated protein escapes the binding to the VHL protein and the consequent degradation, leading to the hypoxic response.[5,10] Also, the factor inhibiting HIF-1, an HIF-1 asparaginil hydrolase, mediates the hydroxylation of a key residue of asparagine in the transactivation domain of *HIF1A*. Then, this hydroxylation blocks the interaction between HIF-1 and the transcriptional coactivator p300/CBP. Probably, there are other enzymes that regulate HIF-1 activation through phosphorylation on specific residues.[11]

The stabilization of the HIF-1α protein, however, is not limited to hypoxic conditions, and a so-called hypoxic response can also start with an appropriate oxygen tension. This response can result from a wide variety of possible genetic defects and malfunctions in signaling pathways, such as the deletion of tumor suppressor VHL, p53, PTEN, or by activation of oncogenic pathways related to the PI3K/Akt, Src, or the activation of growth factors (such as EGF or IGF).[10] It has been observed that the expression of VHL is restricted to the proliferative compartment on the bottom of the intestinal crypts. While there is an overexpression of VHL in the early stages of carcinogenesis, an inactivation mechanism by gene mutation has been suggested for this gene, leading to HIF-1α stabilization, mainly in the late stages of cancerogenesis both in patients with sporadic CRC and in patients with familial adenomatous polyposis.[12] Also the adenomatous polyposis coli (*APC*) gene, one of the most frequently mutated genes in CRC, represses HIF-1α, and the loss of function of *APC* leads to HIF-sustained survival.[13] Also *KRAS* and *BRAF* mutations seem to have different effects on the regulation of HIF-1α. Approximately, 30–50% of CRCs harbor the mutated gene. This mutation is associated with HIF-1α induction at the transcriptional level.[14]

Also, reactive oxygen species, nitric oxide, and the heat shock promote the expression of HIF-1α under normoxic conditions. Analysis of promoters has revealed that genes induced by HIF-1α under hypoxic conditions are similar to those induced under normoxic conditions.[15] Several studies have found an overexpression of HIF in most colorectal malignancies and in colonic adenomas. The highest expression of HIF has been observed at the front of infiltrating carcinoma, and it is associated with the most aggressive phenotype.[16]

HIF-1α and the Wnt pathway

There are several links between HIF-1 and the Wnt signal, a fundamental pathway in colonic physiology and cancerogenesis. It has been observed that β-catenin enhances the endogenous HIF-1 activity in hypoxic conditions, promoting survival of colonic tumor cells.[17] Some studies have also shown that HIF-1α and HIF-2α cooperate in reducing the levels of E-cadherin.[18] The network connecting HIF and β-catenin joins at the level of Akt. In fact, it has been reported that an activation of the latter helps increase the levels of HIF[19] and decrease those of GSK3β, the enzyme responsible for the degradation of cytosolic β-catenin.

HIF-1α and the MMR system

Some CRCs are characterized by mutations in the genes of the mismatch repair (MMR) system, which lead to the inability to recognize and repair errors made during DNA replication. These changes are inherited in the syndrome called hereditary non-polyposis colorectal cancer (HNPCC) or may occur sporadically in 10–15% of CRCs. The lack of a proficient MMR system leads to DNA microsatellite instability, often associated with hypoxia in tumors. It was shown that the expression of MLH1 is inhibited by hypoxia, resulting in a deficiency of the MMR system. It has also been reported that HIF-1α acts not only as a transcriptional repressor for MSH2 and MSH6, but also regulates the stability of these proteins. However, the link between the MMR system and HIF is still to be clarified, and some authors have recently ruled out a role for HIF in the repression of MSH2 and MLH1 for the creation of a high microsatellite instability (MSI) profile.[20]

HIF-1α and Modifications of Cellular Metabolism

Cancer cells exhibit multiple alterations in the structure and function of mitochondria activity and glycolytic enzymes. The imbalance in glucose uptake and in the production of lactic acid in cancer cells has been highlighted, when compared with non-cancerous cells.[21] The most commonly induced genes by hypoxia code for enzymes involved in the transport and metabolism of glucose, and other important biological processes.[10,17]

HIF-1α regulation of glycolysis

HIF-1 mediates adaptation to hypoxia by activating genes that increase glycolysis as the Glut-1 transporter of glucose. The overexpression of Glut-1, associated with the expression of HIF-1α, seems to characterize colorectal carcinomas with metastases in local lymph nodes, suggesting a more malignant phenotype.[22] A study on proteomics of colorectal carcinoma has shown the presence of hyperregulated glycolytic enzymes.[23] Enzymes such as aldolase, phosphoglycerate kinase (whose levels are increased already in the aberrant crypt foci (ACF) stage of carcinogenesis,[24] and enolase contain consensus sequences for HIF. Furthermore, it has been reported that HIF-1α induces the expression of an isoform of hexokinase (HK II, instead of the isoform HK IV) with a greater affinity for glucose. This hexokinase has been identified as a useful target for chemotherapy mediating both metabolic and antiapoptotic effects.[25] Moreover, both the lactate dehydrogenase A and the MCT4 lactate carriers are targets of HIF. Both these proteins are increased in cancer cells, stimulating the release of lactate from the cell. The lactate dehydrogenase A enzymatically favors the production of lactate from pyruvate, and the isoform is overexpressed in colorectal carcinomas.[26]

The increased induction of HIF target enzymes increases the acidity of the environment. HIF can also lead to adaptive responses such as the switching from the isoform II of carbonic anhydrase, the main isoform in the gastrointestinal tract, to the isoform IX. CA IX is important in sustaining cancer cell growth and survival by producing and maintaining a favorable intracellular pH. They act also by increasing the acidity of extracellular tumor microenvironment, thus enhancing cancer cell invasion. However, an overexpression of the isoform II in ACF, precursor lesions of CRC, has been reported, while CA IX is overexpressed in CRC, specifically in HNPCC.[27]

HIF-1α and oxidative phosphorylation

Pyruvate can enter the tricarboxylic acid cycle into the mitochondria via the pyruvate dehydrogenase. It is inhibited by pyruvate dehydrogenase kinase (PDK-1 and PDK-3), whose expression is induced by HIF.[28] In particular, high PDK3 expression is related to severity of CRC, and is negatively associated with disease-free survival, playing an important role both in the metabolic switch and in drug resistance of colon cancer cells. PDK inhibition has been proposed as a strategy for cancer treatment by reactivating enzymes of gluconeogenesis, leading to cancer cell death with high specificity.[29]

Moreover, HIF-1α is also implicated in the control of mitochondrial activity. It has been shown that HIF-1α controls the expression of the isoform 2 of Cytochrome C oxidase subunit IV (COX IV-2), which has a higher efficiency in conditions of deprivation of $O_{2,}$ through hypoxia responsive elements (HREs) present on the gene.[30] This could lead to a continuous production of ROS that can contribute to create mutations in mitochondrial DNA. The presence of these mutations has been indicated as a promoting factor of colorectal carcinogenesis.[31] However, HIF induces mitochondrial autophagy through BNIP3 and BNIP3L in order to prevent overproduction of mitochondrial reactive oxygen species with the generation of superoxide radicals that would cause cell death by DNA damage.[32]

HIF-1α as Modulator of Inflammation

During colonic inflammation, hypoxic foci are present throughout the mucosa. In these conditions, a dual effect of HIF has been reported, both as a protector of the mucosa in IBD by promoting the resolution of inflammation, and as a favoring factor in inflammation-induced neoplasia (Figure 1).

HIF-1α and mucosal protection

HIF-1α regulates several genes that are important in maintaining the barrier integrity of the intestinal epithelium, and genes that act as endogenous regulators of inflammation in the colonic mucosa, like the intestinal trefoil factor, the P-glycoprotein, and other involved in increased mucin production and modification, and in nucleotide signaling (the A2B adenosine receptor, and CD73).[33,34] Sites of mucosal inflammation are characterized by the generation of large amounts of adenine nucleotide metabolites. While ATP is considered a pro-inflammatory mediator and a danger signal, its enzymatic product adenosine has a role in the resolution of intestinal injury and inflammation.[35] In the extracellular compartment, AMP is converted to adenosine primarily by the ecto-enzyme CD73,[34,35] thus activating surface adenosine receptors that regulate endothelial and epithelial barrier functions. Moreover,

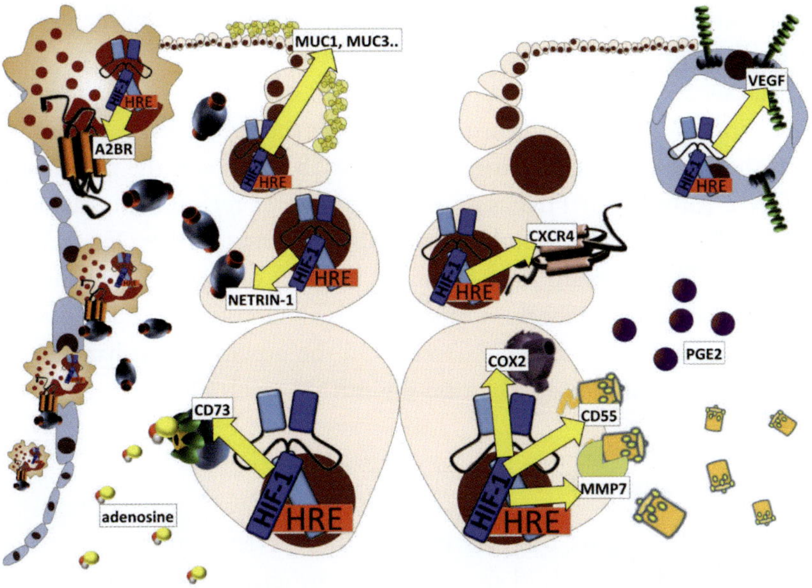

Figure 1. HIF-1 regulates both proresolving inflammation (left side of the figure) through Ntn1, CD73, A2BR, MUC) and a protumor inflammation (right side of the figure) by interacting with pathways like COX-2, CXCR4, CD55, and VEGF.

the induction of netrin-1 (Ntn1) in hypoxic epithelia drived by HIF-1, by engaging adenosine receptor expressed on neutrophils, attenuated neutrophil transmigration and inflammation at mucosal surfaces.[1]

HIF-1α and promotion of inflammation

The decay-accelerating factor (DAF or CD55), a regulatory protein of the complement, is a direct target of HIF-1, too. This protein has antiadhesive functions with respect to polymorphonuclear leukocytes, thus providing their release in inflammatory sites and their accumulation *in situ*.[36] An increased expression of CD55 was observed in 75% of CRC, and this increase has been associated with a worse prognosis, influencing immunotherapy, and encouraging the evasion of immune surveillance mechanisms.[37] The cyclooxygenases (COX) are among the most studied proteins involved in promotion, progression, and treatment of CRC. Prostaglandins modulate the immune functions in many ways: through the inhibition of the proliferation of T and B cells and by modulating the activity of antigen presenting cells. About 50% of adenomas and 80% of CRC expressed high levels of mRNA and COX-2 protein in the neoplastic tissues. Recently, it has been shown that HIF-1α, by binding with p300/CBP, activates the transcription of COX-2 through an HRE site on the promoter region, thus facilitating CRC development, survival of cancer cells, and angiogenesis. Furthermore, PGE_2 and PGI_2, the main products of COX-2 activation, enhance the activity of HIF-1α. This feedback mechanism may be important to maintain the overexpression of COX-2 in CRC cells. On the other hand, it has also been shown that COX inhibitors decrease the mRNA levels of HIF-1α.[38]

HIF-1α and Tumor Growth

Some evidence suggests that the increase of HIF levels in normal colonic epithelial cells does not lead to cancer, nor to an increased progression of early-stage tumors.[39] Nevertheless, one of the prominent roles of HIF-1α in carcinogenesis is related to the push to angiogenesis and metastasis formation, and to the resistance to radiotherapy and chemotherapy treatments conferred to hypoxic tumor cells.

HIF-1α and regulation of angiogenesis and metastasis

HIF-1α affects several steps of colon tumorigenesis, e.g. survival and proliferation, angiogenesis and invasion, by regulating proteins such as MMP2, cathepsin D, vimentin, TGFA, by inducing the expression of prosurvival genes (survivin, Bcl-XL, Mcl-1), and by decreasing proapoptotic signaling through decoy receptors, such as DcR2, that antagonize the apoptosis-inducing signaling from DR4 and DR5.[40] HIF-1 induces angiogenesis in CRC by controlling the expression of multiple target genes, like endotelin1 and nitric oxide synthase, involved in vasodilatation, vascular endothelial growth factor (VEGF), stromal-derived factor 1, placental growth factor, platelet-derived growth factor B, and angiopoietin 1 and 2. The HIF-1α/VEGF pathway in CRC has been associated with worse survival rates in CRC patients.[41]

HIF-1α also regulates hypoxia-induced autophagy activation in order to drive invasion and vascular remodeling.[42] Recent data link HIF to the mechanism of metastasis through the induction of the CXC chemokine receptor (CXCR4) and its ligand, stromal cell-derived factor-1 (CXCL12). It was hypothesized that this pathway is involved not only in chemotaxis of circulating multipotent stem cells for tissue repair, but also in the dissemination of individual tumor cells or micrometastases. The overexpression of this system has been associated with a poor prognosis in CRC.[43,44] The overexpression of CXCR4 together with VEGF is predictive of early distant relapse in stages II and III colon cancer.[45] HIF-1, by activating a large number of factors that can be linked to angiogenesis and metastasis, becomes an important target to control tumor growth.

HIF-1α and clinicopathological features

The expression of HIF-1α is higher in CRC compared to premalignant lesions, but is expressed also in adenomas.[46] HIF-1α expression is related to disease stages. Indeed, it is higher in patients with stage III than that in patients with stage I–II CRC. No correlation between HIF-1α and the metastatic status has been reported, suggesting a role for HIF-1α in the early acquisition of an angiogenetic and metastatic phenotype.[47]

A recent meta-analysis examined the prognostic effects of HIF-1α among 731 CRC patients. Important molecular signatures in CRC, as mutations in *KRAS, BRAF*, and *PIK3CA*, LINE-1 hypomethylation, MSI, and the CpG island methylator phenotype, were also evaluated. HIF-1α overexpression was associated with higher mortality, characterizing more aggressive CRC, and with overall and disease-free survival.[48] Hypoxia is also associated with tumor chemoresistance. Thus, it has been reported that HIF-1α can directly regulate the multidrug resistance (MDR1) gene expression.[49]

HIF-1α as a Therapeutic Target

Some studies have reported that the inhibition of HIF-1α can result in tumor regression, and many anti-cancer agents interfered indirectly with the HIF pathway. The absence of structural information makes it difficult to identify direct inhibitors of HIF-1. HIF-1 inhibitors derived by high throughput screening assays lack general specificity, indicating that HIF-1 inhibition cannot be separated from the inhibition of other multiple targets.[50] However, there are several ways for the inhibition of HIF-1.

1. *HIF-1α-mRNA expression*: Aminoflavone, a ligand of the arylhydrocarbon receptor (AhR), affects HIF-1α mRNA[51] YC-1; a stimulator of soluble guanylate cyclase inhibits the expression of HIF in a dose-dependent manner.[52] This is accompanied by reduced levels of HIF-inducible genes, reduction in tumor mass, and a significant decrease in angiogenesis and metastasis processes.
2. *HIF-1α protein translation*: From topotecan, that may affect HIF-1α -protein translation, EZN-2208 has been derived, a PEGylated form of SN38, and the active component of irinotecan. Another HIF-1 inhibitor in phase I clinical trial is PX-478, which inhibits HIF-1α at multiple levels. Also, mTOR inhibitors, including temsirolimus and everolimus, affect HIF-1α protein translation.[53–55]
3. *HIF-1α protein degradation*: Geldanamycin induces HIF-1α degradation under both hypoxic and normoxic conditions, by inhibiting Hsp90. The activation of Akt/PI3K pathway leads to decreased degradation of HIF. The inhibition of Akt is therefore another possible strategy to increase the degradation of HIF.[19–56]
4. *HIF-1α-DNA binding inhibition*: Small molecules may inhibit HIF-1 activity by targeting the DNA binding to the HRE. Echinomycin, a cyclic peptide of the family of quinoxaline antibiotics, has been shown to be a selective inhibitor of HIF-1 by binding DNA via recognition of a specific sequence.[57] However, echinomycin failed to show significant activity.
5. *HIF-1α transcriptional activity*: Chetomin, by interfering with the interaction of HIF-1α with the coactivator p300 is considered an inhibitor of HIF-1 transcriptional activity. However, its toxicity has precluded its clinical use. Also, menadione and ethacrynic acids were effective inhibitors of the interaction of HIF-1a with p300.[58] The dimerization of HIF-1α and HIF-1β is required for DNA binding and transcription activity. The heteroaromatic derivative acriflavine is an inhibitor of HIF-1 dimerization non-selectively inhibiting both HIF-1 and HIF-2. A new cyclic peptide (cyclo-CLLFVY) inhibits HIF-1 dimerization by binding to the PAS-B domain of HIF-1α, and disrupts HIF-1 dimerization.[59,60]
6. *Targeting hypoxia*: There are no drugs that radiosensitize the hypoxic tumor cells with the exception of nimorazole, used only in Denmark. Nitroaromatic compounds, quinones, or heterocyclic N-oxides act as

prodrugs and are activated via bioreduction in hypoxic environment, with a mechanism of action that is non-specific but selective for tumor environment.[61]

Targeting HIF-1α pathways in colorectal carcinoma

Regarding the molecules used against colon cancer, there are drugs designed for direct inhibition of HIF, and drugs that target HIF-regulated genes, critical for tumor growth. Among the drugs that inhibit the transcriptional or translational activity of HIF, there is PX-478, a drug effective in antitumor assays.[62] Chetomin, previously known as an antimicrobial drug, has been shown to inhibit the binding of p300 with HIF and the HIF-inducible transcription. It has been tested in CRC models, but its local toxicity precludes the use of this therapy;[63] SN38, the active component of irinotecan, affects HIF-1α protein translation, and thus overcomes chemoresistance under hypoxic conditions in colon cancer cells.[64]

Among the most important drugs that target HIF-regulated genes, inhibitors of VEGF are included. The bevacizumab, recombinant monoclonal antibody that inhibits the function of VEGF, is the only one belonging to this class currently approved for the treatment of CRC.[65] Also the inhibition of carbonic anhydrase (CA) activity by small molecules like sulphonamides and derivatives can lead to the inhibition of colorectal tumorigenesis. The CA inhibitors can concentrate in hypoxic tumors and thus target cancer cells.[66] The Hsp90 is also involved in the correct folding of HIF. The synergistic action of an inhibitor of COX associated with an inhibitor of Hsp90 has been evaluated on CRC cells.[67]

New strategies for HIF-1α targeting

Protein–protein interactions (PPIs) are essential for transcription factors like HIF-1α. Targeting PPIs is, however, a difficult process because the surface used as the inhibition target is more large and less well defined than the pockets used for the binding of classical small-molecules inhibitors. HIF-1α–p300 interaction is a valid target in the inhibition of HIF-1α function. However, the specificity of small molecules targeting this interaction is unclear, as they can act through other mechanisms. Thus, it has been reported that some α-helix mimetics compounds based on an oligoamide scaffold orthosterically and specifically inhibit this interaction by miming the C-terminal helix of the HIF-1α C-TAD. Although these compounds act as selective inhibitors of this interaction, they are less potent than HIF-1α. The result is interesting both for the use of peptidomimetics in allosteric PPIs inhibition, and because they reproduce only three of the 42 residues of HIF-1α C-TAD from which it is derived.[68]

The use of locked nucleic acid (LNA)-based oligonucleotides is a new antisense technology that markedly enhances base pairing to mRNA and resistance against degradation with respect to other oligonucleotides. LNA-based oligonucleotides are selective, potent, and long-lasting inhibitors of mRNA and microRNA targets and can act without a delivery vehicle. LNA-based oligonucleotides directed against HIF-1α (i.e. EZN-2968) that specifically downregulate HIF-1α and HIF-1α-regulated genes in experimental models[69] have been described.

Recently, promoter sequences containing several short runs of guanine nucleotides that can form complex structures, termed quadruplexes, have been described. The HIF-1α promoter contains a guanine-rich sequence, capable of forming a parallel, intramolecular G-quadruplex structure that modulates the activity of the HIF-1α promoter. An alteration of this region markedly reduces HIF-1α transcriptional activity. A di-substituted naphthalene compound (CL67) acting as G-quadruplex stabilizing agent has also been identified. CL67 inhibits HIF expression and downregulates the levels of downstream target genes.[70]

Conclusions

HIF-1α is overexpressed in various types of cancers, including colorectal, where it can drive COX-2 overexpression. It has been shown that the expression of HIF-1α gradually increases in the colorectal adenoma-adenocarcinoma sequence. A hyperregulation of VHL in preneoplastic lesions of CRC, presumably due to the activation of the Wnt pathway, has also been reported. In later stages, there is a reduction in the expression of VHL, which overlaps with the stabilization of HIF-1α. HIF-1α can be activated through mechanisms linked to the activation of oncogenes or inactivation of tumor suppressor genes, already in preneoplastic lesions. Thus, HIF-1 and its interactions with other relevant pathways have a prominent role in colorectal carcinogenesis, and both HIF-1 and its regulated genes represent very attractive therapeutic targets for cancers in the gastrointestinal tract.

References

1. YN Shah (2016) The role of hypoxia in intestinal inflammation. *Mol Cell Pediatr* **3**: 1 (Epub ahead of print Jan 26, 2016).
2. X Xue, S Ramakrishnan, E Anderson, M Taylor, EM Zimmermann, JR Spence, S Huang, JK Greenson, YM Shah (2013) Endothelial PAS domain protein 1 activates the inflammatory response in the intestinal epithelium to promote colitis in mice. *Gastroenterology* **145**: 831–41.
3. GL Wang, GL Semenza (1993) General involvement of hypoxia-inducible factor 1 in transcriptional response to hypoxia. *Proc Natl Acad Sci USA* **90**: 4304–4308.
4. F Dayan, D Roux, MC Brahimi-Horn, J Pouyssegur, NM Mazure (2006) The oxygen sensor factor-inhibiting hypoxia-inducible factor-1 controls expression of distinct genes through the bifunctional transcriptional character of hypoxia-inducible factor-1alpha. *Cancer Res* **66**: 3688–3698.
5. JI Bardos, M Ashcroft (2005) Negative and positive regulation of HIF-1: A complex network. *Biochim Biophys Acta* **1755**: 107–120.
6. J Schödel, S Oikonomopoulos, J Ragoussis, CW Pugh, PJ Ratcliffe, DR Mole (2011) High-resolution genome-wide mapping of HIF-binding sites by ChIP-seq. *Blood* **117**: e207–217.
7. ME Crosby, CM Devlin, PM Glazer, GA Calin, M Ivan (2009) Emerging roles of microRNAs in the molecular responses to hypoxia. *Curr Pharm Des* **15**: 3861–3866.
8. MZ Wu, YP Tsai, MH Yang, CH Huang, SY Chang, CC Chang, SC Teng, KJ Wu (2011) Interplay between HDAC3 and WDR5 is essential for hypoxia-induced epithelial-mesenchymal transition. *Mol Cell* **43**: 811–822.
9. J Ferdin, N Nishida, X Wu, MS Nicoloso, MY Shah, C Devlin, H Ling, M Shimizu, K Kumar, MA Cortez, M Ferracin, Y Bi, D Yang, B Czerniak, W Zhang, TD Schmittgen, MP Voorhoeve, MJ Reginato, M Negrini, RV Davuluri, T Kunej, M Ivan, GA Calin (2013) HINCUTs in cancer: hypoxia-induced noncoding ultraconserved transcripts. *Cell Death Differ* **20**: 1675–1687.
10. JT Chi, Z Wang, DS Nuyten, EH Rodriguez, ME Schaner, A Salim, Y Wang, GB Kristensen, A Helland, AL Borresen-Dale, A Giaccia, MT Longaker,

T Hastie, GP Yang, MJ van de Vijver, PO Brown (2006) Gene expression programs in response to hypoxia: Cell type specificity and prognostic significance in human cancers. *PLoS Med* **3**: e47.

11. DE Lancaster, LA McNeill, MA McDonough, RT Aplin, KS Hewitson, CW Pugh, PJ Ratcliffe, CJ Schofield (2004) Disruption of dimerization and substrate phosphorylation inhibit factor inhibiting hypoxia-inducible factor (FIH) activity. *Biochem J* **383**: 429–437.
12. RH Giles, MP Lolkema, CM Snijckers, M Belderbos, P van der Groep, DA Mans, M van Beest, M van Noort, R Goldschmeding, PJ van Diest, H Clevers, EE Voest (2006) Interplay between VHL/HIF1alpha and Wnt/beta-catenin pathways during colorectal tumorigenesis. *Oncogene* **25**: 3065–3070.
13. I Näthke, S Rocha (2009) Antagonistic crosstalk between APC and HIF-1α. *Cell Cycle* **10**: 1545–1547.
14. H Kikuchi, MS Pino, M Zeng, S Shirasawa, DC Chung (2009) Oncogenic KRAS and BRAF differentially regulate hypoxia-inducible factor-1alpha and -2alpha in colon cancer. *Cancer Res* **69**: 8499–8506.
15. M Lopez-Lazaro (2006) HIF-1: hypoxia-inducible factor or dysoxia-inducible factor? *FASEB J* **20**: 828–832.
16. H Zhong, AM De Marzo, E Laughner, M Lim, DA Hilton, D Zagzag, P Buechler, WB Isaacs, GL Semenza, JW Simons (2007) Overexpression of hypoxia-inducible factor 1alpha in common human cancers and their metastases. *Cancer Res* **59**: 5830–5835.
17. A Kaidi, AC Williams, C Paraskeva (2007) Interaction between beta-catenin and HIF-1 promotes cellular adaptation to hypoxia. *Nat Cell Biol* **9**: 210–217.
18. MA Esteban, MG Tran, SK Harten, P Hill, MC Castellanos, A Chandra, R Raval, TS O'brien, PH Maxwell (2006) Regulation of E-cadherin expression by VHL and hypoxia-inducible factor. *Cancer Res* **66**: 3567–3575.
19. N Pore, Z Jiang, HK Shu, E Bernhard, GD Kao, A Maity (2006) Akt1 activation can augment hypoxia-inducible factor-1alpha expression by increasing protein translation through a mammalian target of rapamycin-independent pathway. *Mol Cancer Res* **4**: 471–479.
20. M Koshiji, KK To, S Hammer, K Kumamoto, AL Harris, P Modrich, LE Huang (2005) HIF-1alpha induces genetic instability by transcriptionally downregulating MutSalpha expression. *Mol Cell* **17**: 793–803.
21. E Holm, E Hagmuller, U Staedt, G Schlickeiser, HJ Gunther, H Leweling, M Tokus, HB Kollmar (1995) Substrate balances across colonic carcinomas in humans. *Cancer Res* **55**: 1373–1378.
22. A Wincewicz, M Sulkowska, M Koda, S Sulkowski (2007) Clinicopathological significance and linkage of the distribution of HIF-1alpha and GLUT-1 in human primary colorectal cancer. *Pathol Oncol Res* **13**: 15–20.

23. X Bi, Q Lin, TW Foo, S Joshi, T You, HM Shen, CN Ong, PY Cheah, KW Eu, CL Hew (2006) Proteomic analysis of colorectal cancer reveals alterations in metabolic pathways: Mechanism of tumorigenesis. *Mol Cell Proteomics* **5**: 1119–1130.
24. OK Glebov, LM Rodriguez, P Soballe, J DeNobile, J Cliatt, K Nakahara, IR Kirsch (2006) Gene expression patterns distinguish colonoscopically isolated human aberrant crypt foci from normal colonic mucosa. *Cancer Epidemiol Biomarkers Prev* **15**: 2253–2262.
25. Q Peng, Q Zhou, J Zhou, D Zhong, F Pan, H Liang (2008). Stable RNA interference of hexokinase II gene inhibits human colon cancer LoVo cell growth in vitro and in vivo. *Cancer Biol Ther* **7**: 1128–11.
26. MS Ullah, AJ Davies, AP Halestrap (2006) The plasma membrane lactate transporter MCT4, but not MCT1, is up-regulated by hypoxia through a HIF-1alpha-dependent mechanism. *J Biol Chem* **281**: 9030–9037.
27. AM Niemelä, P Hynninen, JP Mecklin, T Kuopio, A Kokko, L Aaltonen, AK Parkkila, S Pastorekova, J Pastorek, A Waheed, WS Sly, TF Orntoft, M Kruhøffer, H Haapasalo, S Parkkila, AJ Kivelä (2007) Carbonic anhydrase IX is highly expressed in hereditary nonpolyposis colorectal cancer. *Cancer Epidemiol Biomarkers Prev* **16**: 1760–1766.
28. JW Kim, I Tchernyshyov, GL Semenza, CV Dang (2006) HIF-1-mediated expression of pyruvate dehydrogenase kinase: A metabolic switch required for cellular adaptation to hypoxia. *Cell Metab* **3**: 177–185.
29. CW Lu, SC Lin, CW Chien, SC Lin, CT Lee, BW Lin, JC Lee, SJ Tsai (2011) Overexpression of pyruvate dehydrogenase kinase 3 increases drug resistance and early recurrence in colon cancer. *Am J Pathol* **179**: 1405–1414.
30. R Fukuda, H Zhang, JW Kim, L Shimoda, CV Dang, GL Semenza (2007) HIF-1 regulates cytochrome oxidase subunits to optimize efficiency of respiration in hypoxic cells. *Cell* **129**: 111–122.
31. G Sui, S Zhou, J Wang, M Canto, EE Lee, JR Eshleman, EA Montgomery, D Sidransky, JA Califano, A Maitra (2006) Mitochondrial DNA mutations in preneoplastic lesions of the gastrointestinal tract: A biomarker for the early detection of cancer. *Mol Cancer* **5**: 73.
32. H Zhang, M Bosch-Marce, LA Shimoda, YS Tan, JH Baek, JB Wesley, FJ Gonzalez, GL Semenza (2008) Mitochondrial autophagy is an HIF-1-dependent adaptive metabolic response to hypoxia. *J Biol Chem* **283**: 10892–10903.
33. NA Louis, KE Hamilton, G Canny, LL Shekels, SB Ho, SP Colgan (2006) Selective induction of mucin-3 by hypoxia in intestinal epithelia. *J Cell Biochem* **99**: 1616–1627.
34. K Synnestvedt, GT Furuta, KM Comerford, N Louis, J Karhausen, HK Eltzschig, KR Hansen, LF Thompson, SP Colgan (2002) Ecto-5′-nucleotidase

(CD73) regulation by hypoxia-inducible factor-1 mediates permeability changes in intestinal epithelia. *J Clin Invest* **110**: 993–1002.
35. SP Colgan, HK Eltzschig (2012) Adenosine and hypoxia-inducible factor signaling in intestinal injury and recovery. *Annu Rev Physiol* **74**: 153–175.
36. NA Louis, KE Hamilton, T Kong, SP Colgan (2005) HIF-dependent induction of apical CD55 coordinates epithelial clearance of neutrophils. *FASEB J* **19**: 950–959.
37. LG Durrant, MA Chapman, DJ Buckley, I Spendlove, RA Robins, NC Armitage (2003) Enhanced expression of the complement regulatory protein CD55 predicts a poor prognosis in colorectal cancer patients. *Cancer Immunol Immunother* **52**: 638–642.
38. A Kaidi, D Qualtrough, AC Williams, C Paraskeva (2006) Direct transcriptional up-regulation of cyclooxygenase-2 by hypoxia-inducible factor (HIF)-1 promotes colorectal tumor cell survival and enhances HIF-1 transcriptional activity during hypoxia. *Cancer Res* **66**: 6683–6691.
39. X Xue, SK Ramakrishnan, YM Shah (2014) Activation of HIF-1? does not increase intestinal tumorigenesis. *Am J Physiol Gastrointest Liver Physiol* **307**: G187–195.
40. B Krishnamachary, S Berg-Dixon, B Kelly, F Agani, D Feldser, G Ferreira, N Iyer, J LaRusch, B Pak, P Taghavi, GL Semenza (2003) Regulation of colon carcinoma cell invasion by hypoxia-inducible factor 1. *Cancer Res* **63**: 1138–1143.
41. CQ Jiang, LF Fan, ZS Liu, Q Qian, D Xia, LM Diao, YM He, ZL Ai (2004) Expression levels and significance of hypoxia inducible factor-1 alpha and vascular endothelial growth factor in human colorectal adenocarcinoma. *Chin Med J (Engl)* **117**: 1541–1546.
42. S Rey, GL Semenza (2010) Hypoxia-inducible factor-1-dependent mechanisms of vascularization and vascular remodelling. *Cardiovasc Res* **86**: 236–242.
43. T Schioppa, B Uranchimeg, A Saccani, SK Biswas, A Doni, A Rapisarda, S Bernasconi, S Saccani, M Nebuloni, L Vago, A Mantovani, G Melillo, A Sica (2003) Regulation of the chemokine receptor CXCR4 by hypoxia. *J Exp Med* **198**: 1391–1402.
44. IS Zeelenberg, L Ruuls-Van Stalle, E Roos (2003) The chemokine receptor CXCR4 is required for outgrowth of colon carcinoma micrometastases. *Cancer Res* **63**: 3833–3839.
45. A Ottaiano, R Franco, A Aiello Talamanca, G Liguori, F Tatangelo, P Delrio, G Nasti, E Barletta, G Facchini, B Daniele, A Di Blasi, M Napolitano, C Ieranò, R Calemma, E Leonardi, V Albino, V De Angelis, M Falanga, V Boccia, M Capuozzo, V Parisi, G Botti, G Castello, R Vincenzo Iaffaioli, S Scala (2006) Overexpression of both CXC chemokine receptor 4 and vascular endothelial

growth factor proteins predicts early distant relapse in stage II–III colorectal cancer patients. *Clin Cancer Res* **12**: 2795–2803.

46. F Mariani, P Sena, L Marzona, M Riccio, R Fano, P Manni, C Di Gregorio, A Pezzi, M Ponz de leon, S Monni, A De Pol, L Roncucci (2009) Cyclooxygenase-2 and Hypoxia-Inducible Factor-1alpha protein expression is related to inflammation, and up-regulated since the early steps of colorectal carcinogenesis. *Cancer Lett* **279**: 221–229.
47. N Simiantonaki, M Taxeidis, C Jayasinghe, U Kurzik-Dumke, CJ Kirkpatrick (2008) Hypoxia-inducible factor 1 alpha expression increases during colorectal carcinogenesis and tumor progression. *BMC Cancer* **8**: 320.
48. Y Baba, K Nosho, K Shima, N Irahara, AT Chan, JA Meyerhardt, DC Chung, EL Giovannucci, CS Fuchs, S Ogino (2010) HIF1A overexpression is associated with poor prognosis in a cohort of 731colorectal cancers. *Am J Pathol* **176**: 2292–2301.
49. KM Comerford, TJ Wallace, J Karhausen, NA Louis, MC Montalto, SP Colgan (2002). Hypoxia-inducible factor-1-dependent regulation of the multidrug resistance (MDR1) gene. *Cancer Res* **62**: 3387–3394.
50. A Giaccia, BG Siim, RS Johnson (2003) HIF-1 as a target for drug development. *Nat Rev Drug Discov* **2**: 803–811.
51. E Terzuoli, M Puppo, A Rapisarda, B Uranchimeg, L Cao, AM Burger, M Ziche, G Melillo (2010) Aminoflavone, a ligand of the aryl hydrocarbon receptor, inhibits HIF-1alpha expression in an AhR-independent fashion. *Cancer Res* **70**: 6837–6848.
52. DH Shin, JH Kim, YJ Jung, KE Kim, JM Jeong, YS Chun, JW Park (2007) Preclinical evaluation of YC-1, a HIF inhibitor, for the prevention of tumor spreading. *Cancer Lett* **255**: 107–116.
53. P Sapra, P Kraft, F Pastorino, D Ribatti, M Dumble, M Mehlig, M Wang, M Ponzoni, LM Greenberger, ID Horak (2011) Potent and sustained inhibition of HIF-1? and downstream genes by a polyethyleneglycol-SN38 conjugate, EZN-2208, results in anti-angiogenic effects. *Angiogenesis* **14**: 245–253.
54. MY Koh, T Spivak-Kroizman, S Venturini, S Welsh, RR Williams, DL Kirkpatrick, G Powis (2008) Molecular mechanisms for the activity of PX-478, an antitumor inhibitor of the hypoxia-inducible factor-1alpha. *Mol Cancer Ther* 7: 90–100.
55. PK Majumder, PG Febbo, R Bikoff, R Berger, Q Xue, LM McMahon, J Manola, J Brugarolas, TJ McDonnell, TR Golub, M Loda, HA Lane, WR Sellers (2004) mTOR inhibition reverses Akt-dependent prostate intraepithelial neoplasia through regulation of apoptotic and HIF-1-dependent pathways. *Nat Med* **10**: 594–601.

56. JS Isaacs, YJ Jung, EG Mimnaugh, A Martinez, F Cuttitta, LM Neckers (2002) Hsp90 regulates a von Hippel Lindau-independent hypoxia-inducible factor-1 alpha-degradative pathway. *J Biol Chem* **277**: 29936–29944.
57. D Kong, EJ Park, AG Stephen, M Calvani, JH Cardellina, A Monks, RJ Fisher, RH Shoemaker, G Melillo (2005) Echinomycin, a small-molecule inhibitor of hypoxia-inducible factor-1 DNA-binding activity. *Cancer Res* **65**: 9047–9055.
58. YR Na, KC Han, H Park, EG Yang (2013) Menadione and ethacrynic acid inhibit the hypoxia-inducible factor (HIF) pathway by disrupting HIF-1? interaction with p300. *Biochem Biophys Res Commun* **434**: 879–884.
59. K Lee, H Zhang, DZ Qian, S Rey, JO Liu, GL Semenza (2009) Acriflavine inhibits HIF-1 dimerization, tumor growth, and vascularization. *Proc Natl Acad Sci USA* **106**: 17910–17915.
60. E Miranda, IK Nordgren, AL Male, CE Lawrence, F Hoakwie, F Cuda, W Court, KR Fox, PA Townsend, GK Packham, SA Eccles, A Tavassoli (2013) A cyclic peptide inhibitor of HIF-1 heterodimerization that inhibits hypoxia signaling in cancer cells. *J Am Chem Soc* **135**: 10418–10425.
61. H Nagasawa, Y Uto, KL Kirk, H Hori (2006) Design of hypoxia-targeting drugs as new cancer chemotherapeutics. *Biol Pharm Bull* **29**: 2335–2342.
62. GR Macpherson, WD Figg (2004) Small molecule-mediated anti-cancer therapy via hypoxia-inducible factor-1 blockade. *Cancer Biol Ther* **3**: 503–504.
63. M Lopez-Lazaro (2006) Hypoxia-inducible factor 1 as a possible target for cancer chemoprevention. *Cancer Epidemiol Biomarkers Prev* **15**: 2332–2335.
64. K Murono, NH Tsuno, K Kawai, K Sasaki, K Hongo, M Kaneko, M Hiyoshi, N Tada, T Nirei, E Sunami, K Takahashi, J Kitayama (2012) SN-38 overcomes chemoresistance of colorectal cancer cells induced by hypoxia, through HIF1alpha. *Anticancer Res* **32**: 865–872.
65. P Pfeiffer, C Qvortrup, JG Eriksen (2007) Current role of antibody therapy in patients with metastatic colorectal cancer. *Oncogene* **26**: 3661–3678.
66. AM Alafeefy, R Ahmad, M Abdulla, WM Eldehna, AM Al-Tamimi, HA Abdel-Aziz, O Al-Obaid, F Carta, AA Al-Kahtani, CT Supuran (2016) Development of certain new 2-substituted-quinazolin-4-yl-aminobenzenesulfonamide as potential antitumor agents. *Eur J Med Chem* **109**: 247–253.
67. S Kobayashi, R Nantz, T Kitamura, R Higashikubo, N Horikoshi (2005) Combined inhibition of extracellular signal-regulated kinases and HSP90 sensitizes human colon carcinoma cells to ionizing radiation. *Oncogene* **24**: 3011–3019.
68. GM Burslem, HF Kyle, AL Breeze, TA Edwards, A Nelson, SL Warriner, AJ Wilson (2014) Small-molecule proteomimetic inhibitors of the HIF-1α-p300 protein–protein interaction. *Chembiochem* **15**: 1083–1087.

69. LM Greenberger, ID Horak, D Filpula, P Sapra, M Westergaard, HF Frydenlund, C Albaek, H Schrøder, H Ørum (2008) A RNA antagonist of hypoxia-inducible factor-1alpha, EZN-2968, inhibits tumor cell growth. *Mol Cancer Ther* **7**: 3598–3608.
70. SJ Welsh, AG Dale, CM Lombardo, H Valentine, M de la Fuente, A Schatzlein, S Neidle (2013) Inhibition of the hypoxia-inducible factor pathway by a G-quadruplex binding small molecule. *Sci Rep* **3**: 2799.

Chapter 11

Therapeutic Approaches Targeting the Serrated Pathway of Colorectal Cancer Characterized by Mutation in the *BRAF* Gene and Overexpression of GTPase Rac1b

Paulo Matos, Vânia Gonçalves, and Peter Jordan

Abstract

Around 30% of all colorectal cancer cases are derived from the serrated polyp pathway and mostly carry a mutation in the *BRAF* gene. Here, we review the current knowledge about the association of this tumor subtype with the CpG island methylator and microsatellite instability phenotypes, immune cell infiltration, and overexpression of GTPase Rac1b. The corresponding therapeutic approaches for targeting these molecular characteristics are presented and critically discussed.

Introduction

Cancer of the colon and rectum (CRC) presents the third most common incidence worldwide (following lung and breast cancer) and the fourth most common mortality.[1,2]

The development of over 70% of sporadic CRCs is characterized by an adenoma-carcinoma sequence involving typical somatic mutations in the APC and p53 tumor suppressor genes or in the oncogene *KRAS*.[1,3–5] They further exhibit widespread chromosomal abnormalities, designated as the chromosomal instability phenotype (CIN) but possess an intact DNA mismatch repair mechanism so that repetitive nucleotide sequence stretches, such as the microsatellite markers, remain unchanged (microsatellite stability phenotype, or MSS). Another frequently observed genetic change in CRC is the overexpression of or activating mutation of the epidermal growth factor receptor (EGFR) gene.

A second major group of sporadic CRC includes about 15% of patients and is characterized by different molecular events. These tumors preferentially occur in the proximal colon, have a stable chromosome number, but show a high rate of DNA sequence mutations (microsatellite instability phenotype, or MSI) caused by deficient DNA mismatch repair.[3] The majority of these tumors further presents a serrated morphology[6,7] and derives from the group of hyperplastic polyps (HPs), as described in more detail below.

The Serrated Pathway to CRC

Molecular and morphological characteristics

Although the majority of sporadic CRCs are derived from adenomatous polyps, serrated carcinomas contribute to 30% of all CRC cases and were first described about 25 years ago. They evolve from serrated polyps mostly localized in the proximal colon. Morphologically, serrated polyps display a serrated folding of the crypt epithelium that is likely to result from increased epithelial mass due to a combination of hyperproliferation in the crypt and reduced apoptosis of differentiated cells. Serrated polyps form, however, a heterogeneous histological group composed of HPs, sessile serrated adenoma (SSA), and traditional serrated adenoma (TSA).[8–10] HPs represent around 30% of all detected colon polyps, they are the most frequent serrated polyps (75%) with an elongated symmetric architecture, and are mostly found in the distal colon. They are generally considered as benign when smaller than 5 mm, but clear distinction from other serrated polyp types is sometimes difficult. In particular, one HP subtype, the multivesicular HP (MVHP), shares morphologic and molecular features with serrated adenomas, especially when occurring in the proximal colon, and can progress to malignant carcinomas. SSAs grow as broad-based flat polyps on the mucosa surface of the proximal colon, represent up to 9% of all colon polyps but account for up to 25% of the serrated polyps. SSAs represent the main precursor lesion for about 12% of all sporadic CRC tumors and are characterized by a high level of MSI (MSI-H). Finally, TSAs appear usually in the distal colon and are rare (2–5% of all colorectal polyps) with distorted tubulovillous (filiform) architecture.[11,12]

Three molecular features that distinguish the serrated pathway deserve more detailed consideration: mitogen-activated protein kinase (MAPK) pathway activation, CpG island methylator phenotype (CIMP), and MSI. Two early tumor-initiating events are mutations in either the *KRAS* or *BRAF* genes as both stimulate proliferation downstream of the EGFR and along the same MAPK pathway. These mutations have already been detected when microdissected premalignant polyps or aberrant crypt foci were genotyped and revealed to be alternative events.

A highly significant association exists between the presence of mutated *BRAF* and genome-wide DNA hypermethylation at the CpG islands present in the majority of human gene promoters.[13] This tumor phenotype is called CIMP and results in epigenetic silencing of gene expression at the methylated promoters, for example, the genes encoding cell cycle inhibitor $p16^{INK4a}$, the p53 regulator $p14^{Arf}$, and the DNA repair factor MGMT.[14] The inhibition of apoptosis that is observed in serrated adenomas has been proposed to be a functional consequence of CIMP. Thus, CIMP represents a broad genome-wide change in epigenetic regulation.

Two distinct CIMP phenotypes have been recognized in the serrated pathway to CRC[13,15]: CIMP-high (CIMP-H) was initially defined by methylation in the majority of five or six selected CIMP marker gene promoters and is a characteristic feature of sporadic MSI-H tumors with *BRAF* mutation. These tumors occur preferentially in the proximal colon, and are responsible for 10–12% of all CRC cases and more prevalent in female patients. They derive from SSAs or sometimes MVHP.[16]

By contrast, a CIMP-low (CIMP-L) phenotype shows methylation in only few of the above CIMP markers and is associated with *KRAS* mutation and MSS or low-level MSI (MSI-L) status. Such tumors are mostly derived from TSAs with more adenomatous features and occur in the distal colon.[17] A recent genome-wide DNA methylation profiling has confirmed these two

CIMP classifications, and refined specific marker genes distinguish between CIMP-H and -L.[13] An additional, related subgroup of TSA with more serrated features is characterized by *BRAF* mutation and CIMP-H but retains mismatch repair function with an MSS or MSI-L status. Malignant progression of both these TSA groups involves TP53 mutation and Wnt pathway activation.[12,16] Altogether the serrated pathway is best characterized by the association between the CIMP and MAPK activation phenotypes, where CIMP can be high or low, and MAPK activation via gene mutation in *BRAF* or *KRAS*.[8]

In the majority of sporadic tumors that derive from CIMP-H/*BRAF* group of serrated polyps, CIMP eventually leads to methylation of the *hMLH1* gene promoter with subsequent mismatch repair deficiency. As a consequence, MSI-H tumors have a high prevalence of frameshift mutations in mononucleotide repeat regions, including those within the genes TGFBR2, ACVR2, BAX, and TCF7L2 (in 90%, 80%, 50%, or 30% of MSI-H tumors, respectively),[4] which causes their inactivation and promotes tumor progression.

Taken together, the above described molecular characteristics found in CRC were the basis for a classification into five subgroups, depending on the presence of CIN, MSI, or CIMP, and of mutation in the *KRAS* or *BRAF* genes[5] (see Table 1). A recent bioinformatics meta-analysis of gene expression profiles obtained from CRC has suggested a novel classification into four major consensus molecular subtypes (CMS)[18]: CMS1 corresponds to the MSI-H, CIMP-H, and *BRAF* mutant group of serrated adenomas in the proximal colon; CMS2 contains the canonical adenomatous polyp pathway with CIN and Wnt pathway activation; CMS3 can be MSI or CIN but show the presence of *KRAS* mutation and metabolic deregulation; CMS4 has CIN and strong activation of mesenchymal infiltrative characteristics. Overall, however, a clear-cut genotype–phenotype correlation to distinguish between the different CRC subtypes does not seem to exist.

Role of *BRAF* in colon cancer

BRAF is one of the three members of the RAF family of protein kinases (besides ARAF and CRAF (alias Raf-1)) that all operate as direct effector proteins recruited to activate GTP-loaded RAS proteins.

Table 1. Classification of CRC based on correlation of clinical, morphological, and molecular features.[5]

	Molecular and morphological characteristics	% of CCRC
1	CIMP-high, methylation of MLH1, MSI-H, BRAF mutation, chromosomally stable, origin in sessile serrated polyps (MVHP, SSA), known generally as sporadic MSI-H	12
2	CIMP-high, partial methylation of MLH1, MSS or MSI-L, BRAF mutation, TP53 alterations, chromosomally stable, origin in traditional serrated polyps (TSA)	8
3	CIMP-low, MGMT methylation, MSS or MSI-L, KRAS mutation, chromosomal instability, origin in traditional adenomas or serrated polyps (AP, TSA, HP)	20
4	CIMP-negative, mainly MSS, chromosomal instability, origin in traditional adenomas (may be sporadic or associated to FAP or MUTYH-polyposis (2%)	57
5	Lynch syndrome, CIMP-negative, MSI-H, BRAF mutation-negative, chromosomally stable	3

Mutations in the *BRAF* gene have been described in melanoma, thyroid, ovarian, and CRC, with a frequency of up to 70%, 45%, 30%, and 22%, respectively. The most frequently detected *BRAF* mutation is the V600E missense alteration, which alters the conformation of the catalytic domain and activates protein kinase activity.[19,20] As a consequence, the ERK/MAPK pathway is stimulated, promoting cell proliferation. Although *BRAF* was found as the main RAF kinase responsible for MEK/ERK activation; it also interacts with and activates CRAF, enabling activation of additional substrate proteins.[21]

A transgenic mouse model has been developed with a tissue-specific expression of mutant *BRAF* in colons[22,23] and revealed that transgenic mice show a proliferative response upon expression of BRAF-V600E; however, they induce a subsequent growth arrest program, termed oncogene-induced senescence (OIS). OIS is mediated through the upregulation of cell cycle inhibitory proteins such as $p16^{Ink4a}$ (see Ref. 24) and has been determined *in situ* in serrated colorectal adenomas.[25] Eventually, OIS is overcome by additional poorly understood alterations that occur in the initiated tumor cells and allow malignant progression.

Although mutation in the *BRAF* gene has been detected preferentially in MSI-H tumors of the proximal colon that show hMLH1 hypermethylation and account for about 12% of all CRC cases,[16] it can further be found in an additional 8% of CRCs that are characterized by CIMP-H but are MSS or MSI-L and mostly found in the distal colon. *BRAF* mutations confer poor prognosis when found in metastatic CRC with about a two-fold increase in mortality relative to patients with wild-type *BRAF*.[26] As with *KRAS* mutations, the presence of mutant *BRAF* is also used as an exclusion criterion for therapy with EGFR monoclonal antibodies, such as cetuximab.

Inflammation and *BRAF*-driven tumorigenesis

A further characteristic that distinguishes the CIMP-H/*BRAF*/MSI-H subgroup of CRC tumors is a high degree of infiltration by tumor-associated lymphocytes.[11] The presence of a local inflammatory process can provide survival and proliferative signals to initiated tumor cells: immune cells secrete corresponding mediators in their physiologic attempt to promote tissue repair or to fight against infection, and these mediators also act upon epithelial cells. They further activate stromal cells to secrete proteases that remodel the extracellular matrix, or pro-angiogenic factors that attract blood vessels.[27] Immune cells can also generate oxidative stress that may trigger further mutagenic events in initiated tumor cells. On the other hand, tumor immune surveillance can recognize tumor-associated or tumor-specific antigens and eliminate transformed cells and thus contain tumor development.[28]

The degree of immune cell infiltration and the corresponding immune response have been recognized as a positive factor for prognosis in MSI-H tumors. Infiltration is thought to be related to the high frequency of frameshift mutations throughout the cancer cell genome, which eventually affect also cell-surface proteins. This generates mutation-associated neoantigens, which then trigger an increased immune response.[29] However, MSI-H tumors also show a significant expression of cell-surface proteins involved in evasion of the immune response, such as PD-L1.[30]

Role of Rac1b overexpression in *BRAF*-driven tumorigenesis

About 80% of BRaf-V600E-positive, but not the *KRAS*-mutated, colorectal tumors also overexpress Rac1b, a highly activated splice variant of the signaling

GTPase Rac1.[31–34] A separate genetic pathway to CRC was proposed, which becomes initiated by a BRaf-V600E mutation but later selects for overexpression of hyperactive Rac1b allowing further tumor progression.[35] This model was based on the observations that, in contrast to Rac1, wild-type Rac1b exists predominantly in the GTP-bound active conformation *in vivo*. Active Rac1b promotes cell cycle progression and cell survival through activation of the transcription factor NF-κB.[36] Furthermore, colorectal tumor cells expressing BRaf-V600E and Rac1b were highly sensitive to combined depletion of both transcripts, leading to massive cell death.[31] Thus, Rac1b overexpression and BRaf-V600E functionally cooperate to sustain tumor cell survival and also correlate with poor patient prognosis.[37] This cooperation complements the observation that BRaf-V600E revealed a 50-fold lower oncogenic potential than mutant *KRAS* in cell transformation assays using fibroblasts.[21]

Colon inflammation can be a trigger for the increased Rac1b expression observed in colorectal cells. This was observed during experimentally induced acute colitis in mice but also in surgical samples from patients with inflammatory diseases of the colon.[38] The main morphological and molecular criteria distinguishing the serrated subtype of CRC are summarized in Figure 1.

Therapeutic Targets for the Serrated Pathway to CRC

As described in detail above, the main tumor type arising through the serrated pathway originates from sessile serrated adenomas in the proximal colon and bears several characteristics featured to be suitable for therapeutic

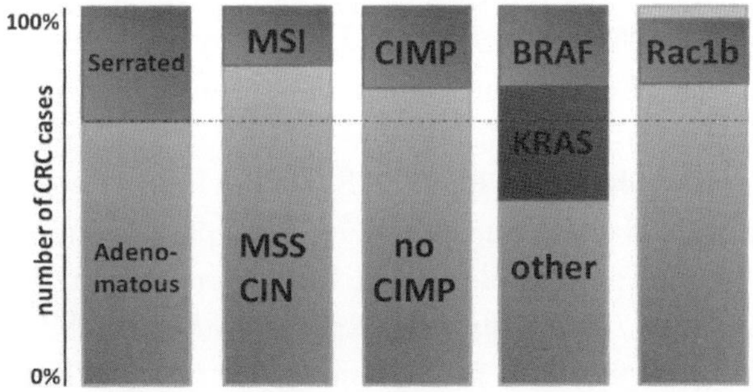

Figure 1. Main molecular criteria involved in the serrated subtypes of sporadic CRC. About 30% of all CRCs originate from serrated polyps, most of which share the MSI-H and CIMP-H phenotypes, present activating mutations in *BRAF* and overexpression of Rac1b.

targeting. These include mutation in *BRAF*, a CIMP-H and MSI-H phenotype, Rac1b overexpression, and immune cell infiltration. The suitability of these features for therapeutic targeting is discussed in the following.

Targeting *BRAF* with kinase inhibitors

As described, oncogenic *BRAF* mutations occur in ~20% of all CRCs, particularly in roughly 70% of the serrated tumors, and involve a single amino acid substitution at valine 600, mostly by glutamic acid (V600E). The corresponding stimulation of *BRAF* kinase activity leads to phosphorylation and activation of MEK kinases (MEK1 and MEK2), which in turn phosphorylate and activate ERK kinases (ERK1 and ERK2) responsible for the regulation of cytoplasmic and nuclear substrates, especially several transcription factors that control genes responsible for cell proliferation and survival.[21] The development of ATP-competitive small-molecule RAF inhibitors, such as vemurafenib and dabrafenib produced remarkable response rates of over 50% in *BRAF* mutant melanoma,[39,40] although tumor resistance usually occurs within 18 months of the initial treatment.[41,42]

In contrast to melanoma, *BRAF* inhibitor vemurafenib achieved no more than a 5% response rate in *BRAF* V600-mutant CRC.[42,43] The mechanism underlying this resistance to single-agent *BRAF* inhibition in CRC resides in rapid reactivation of MAPK signaling due to a release of an inhibitory feedback mechanism that controls receptor tyrosine kinase (RTK)-dependent activation of RAS signaling.[44,45] BRAF-V600E expressing cells show high levels of ERK activation and elevate ERK-dependent transcriptional output,[46] which activates the feedback suppression of signaling downstream of RTKs, including the EGF receptor,[45] and results in decreased RAS activation in the majority of *BRAF*-mutant tumors. Upon treatment with RAF inhibitors, the drug acts on BRAF-V600E and initially reduces ERK signaling. In consequence, the inhibitory RTK/RAS feedback is released, promoting MAPK signaling and thus drug resistance. This paradoxical MAPK activation involves an unexpected role of RAF heterodimerization and was identified when wild-type *BRAF* cells were exposed to *BRAF* inhibitors. In these cells, the RTK/RAS feedback mechanism is not in place so when BRAF–CRAF heterodimers are exposed to vemurafenib, binding of the drug to *BRAF* monomer induces a conformational change that results in allosteric transactivation of the other non-drug-bound CRAF monomer. Thus, although the drug-bound monomer is inactive in the heterodimer, the non-drug-bound CRAF is activated, resulting in increased ERK signaling and paradoxical activation of cell proliferation.[47–49] This allosteric CRAF activation depends on active RAS and may occur in normal tissues. Another implication is that RAF inhibitors are likely less effective in cell types with higher levels of RAS activation, which is often the case with CRC cells.[44,50]

Resistance to *BRAF* inhibitors can also result from primary amplification of the mutant *BRAF* gene,[44] or be acquired during treatment and involve either amplification of the *KRAS* or *BRAF* genes, or mutations in MEK1 or NRAS, or alternative splicing variants of *BRAF*.[41,51] Taken together, single-agent *BRAF* inhibition for the treatment of CRC did not result in the expected benefit due to the complex regulation of the MAPK pathway.

Combined therapeutic targeting of BRAF and EGFR

The identification of EGFR feedback activation as a major determinant in *BRAF* inhibitor resistance in CRC led to a rethinking of the pertinence of using EGFR inhibition in *BRAF*-mutant CRC tumors. Clinical trials were setup where *BRAF* inhibitors were combined with EGFR monoclonal antibodies in an effort to overcome resistance through feedback signals in CRCs.[26,52] While still in the pilot phase, these trials produced encouraging preliminary results, with the combined *BRAF*/EGFR inhibition being well tolerated and apparently more effective in inhibiting growth of BRAF V600-mutant CRC cells than *BRAF* inhibition alone. One of these ongoing trials recently reported that a combination of vemurafenib and the anti-EGFR monoclonal antibody panitumumab resulted in tumor regressions in over 60% of patients, of which 13% achieved stable disease lasting over 6 months.[52] Although only 15 patients were enrolled in this pilot study, the data suggest a potential outcome improvement through this approach. However, acquired drug resistance has still emerged.

Combined therapeutic targeting of BRAF and MEK1

It was shown *in vitro* that the combination of a *BRAF* inhibitor and an MEK inhibitor could induce a stronger and more prolonged inhibition of ERK activation in *BRAF* mutant CRC cells.[53] This also suggested that in patients the *BRAF*/MEK inhibitor combination could show increased efficacy over *BRAF* inhibition alone. The results of a phase I/II trial combining the inhibition of *BRAF* (dabrafenib) and MEK (trametinib) in 43 BRAF V600-mutant CRC patients were recently published.[54] Twelve percent of the patients achieved a partial response, or better, lasting over 36 months. Moreover, 56% of the patients achieved stable disease. The study supports that a subset of patients with BRAF V600-mutant CRC could benefit from a combined dabrafenib/trametinib therapy. Notably, the biopsies evaluated during treatment showed, on average, a 47% decrease in the levels of phosphorylated ERK, relative to pretreatment biopsies. However, the observed level of MAPK signaling inhibition is still beneath >75% decrease observed in *BRAF* mutant melanoma, which could account, among other factors, for the reduced efficacy of this treatment compared to dabrafenib alone in melanoma.[39]

Another recently published *in vitro* study described the use of pan-RAF inhibitors in combination with a MEK inhibitor to overcome resistance to *BRAF*-selective inhibitors in melanoma and CRC cell lines with RAS-activating events such as RTK activation, *KRAS* mutation, or NF1 loss-of-function mutations.[55] These results suggest that a dual pan-RAF and MEK inhibition could constitute a more effective therapeutic strategy for *BRAF*-mutant CRCs. However, in contrast to mutant *BRAF*-selective inhibitors, pan-RAF and MEK inhibitors will suppress ERK signaling in normal cells and tumor cells, irrespective of *BRAF* mutational status. Thus, by inhibiting ERK signaling in normal tissues, they have substantial off-target toxicities attributable to MAPK pathway inhibition that will probably limit their clinical efficacy. This may be also the case with the novel ERK inhibitors that are being developed for tumors refractory to upstream MAPK pathway inhibitors. One encouraging aspect is, however, that ERK inhibitors such as SCH772984 have nanomolar cellular potency in tumor cells with mutations in *BRAF*, *NRAS*, or *KRAS*.[56] Moreover, at tolerated doses this inhibitor was not only able to induce regression of tumor xenograft models bearing any of these oncogenic mutations but also in models resistant to *BRAF* or MEK inhibitor as well as to their combined administration.[56]

Other combination therapy strategies

One possible way to minimize off-target effects of MAPK inhibitors may be to target the main oncogenic event, such as mutations in *BRAF*, with specific inhibitors and avoid resistance by cotargeting non-oncogenic upstream and downstream pathway components, at tolerated doses. Consistent with this strategy, triple regimen trials combining anti-EGFR antibodies (e.g. panitumumab) with *BRAF* and MEK inhibitors are currently underway (https://clinicaltrials.gov/show/NCT01750918) with encouraging preliminary outputs.[57]

Another ongoing trial based on a triple inhibitor combination (https://clinicaltrials.gov/show/NCT01719380) is aligned with the observation that in a mouse model for BRAF-V600E CRC there was an upregulation of PI3K/mTOR signaling following *BRAF* inhibitor treatment.[44] This trial involves the combination of a PI3K specific inhibitor, alpelisib (BYL719), with the novel *BRAF* inhibitor encorafenib and the EGFR antibody cetuximab. The most recent report on the trial,[58] showed a comparable response rate between the dual (encorafenib and cetuximab alone) and triple (plus alpelisib) combinations (around 20–25%) arguing against a relevant clinical benefit being achieved through this triple combination. Nevertheless, a very recently published study assessed the effect of KRAS/BRAF/PI3K oncogenic pathways in CRC cells on the autophagic cell properties thought to promote cell survival.[59] The authors found evidence that oncogenic BRAF mutations induce the expression of key autophagic markers, such as LC3 and BECN1 in CRC cells. Moreover, they also report that PI3K/AKT/mTOR inhibitors induce autophagic tumor properties, whereas RAF/MEK/ERK inhibitors reduce expression of autophagic markers. They propose that the *BRAF*-related autophagic properties in CRC cells can be therapeutically exploited through a pretreatment with autophagy inhibitors followed by their combination with BRAF-V600E inhibitors, since, in their experimental settings, this can sensitize RAF/MEK/ERK inhibitor-resistant colorectal tumors.[59]

Other approaches can yet be predicted. For example, a recent genome-scale screen in a *BRAF*-mutant melanoma cell line has identified a number of candidate genes that appear to participate in the development of resistance to vemurafenib.[60] This suggests the feasibility of employing a similar approach in BRAF-mutant CRC. Such efforts may provide a way to identify additional therapeutic targets to exploit the critical dependence of CRCs on MAPK signaling but it can be anticipated that targeting BRAF-mutant CRC will always require combination therapy approaches.

Targeting CIMP

CIMP is a genome-wide epigenetic deregulation of DNA methylation at the CpG islands of gene promoters leading eventually to the silencing of tumor suppressor genes. At present, however, all available agents act in epigenetic modifications and have in common an indiscriminate genome-wide and unspecific action that causes severe side effects. In addition, it remains to be investigated whether the inhibition of the MAPK pathway can attenuate or revert CIMP given the reports that mutant *BRAF* or *KRAS* can drive CIMP development, as described above.

Targeting inflammation

The CRC subgroup of CIMP-H/BRAF/MSI-H tumors in the proximal colon can also be distinguished from other CRC subgroups through a high degree of infiltration by tumor-associated lymphocytes. This most likely reflects the generation of neoantigens due to mismatch repair deficiency in this tumor type; however, immune response checkpoint ligands, including PD-L1, inhibit tumor cell elimination.[30] A recently developed cancer immunotherapy approach exploited this property of the MSI-H tumor microenvironment by using anti-PD-1 antibodies, available under the trade name pembrolizumab. The antibody blocks the access of the inhibitory ligand PD-L1, expressed on tumor cells, to the PD-1 coreceptor, expressed on T lymphocytes, and thus reactivates the host immune response against cancer cells. Indeed, recent trials revealed that responsiveness of patients to anti-PD-1 therapy is significantly enhanced in patients with hereditary MSI-H colorectal tumors compared to MSS tumors.[61] This suggests that sporadic MSI-H/BRAF tumors with origin via the serrated pathway should also be a promising target group for anti-PD-1 therapy.

Inflammatory bowel disease patients are known to be at increased risk for CRC development, and the serrated pathway associated MSI subtypes appear with a frequency of 15%, such as in sporadic CRC. Interestingly, recent studies discovered that early-onset pediatric forms of IBD are frequently caused by monogenic defects. One key pathway identified by these monogenic diseases is the anti-inflammatory interleukin (IL) 10 pathway and mutations have been identified in both the IL10 ligand and its receptor genes IL10RA and IL10RB.[62] These defects identify candidate pathways involved in intestinal inflammation, which are likely to represent novel therapeutic targets to reduce tumor-associated inflammation and prevent tumor progression. IL10 receptor signaling, for example, stimulates the differentiation of M2 tolerogenic tumor-promoting macrophages, while receptor inhibition (or genetic loss of function) in the intestine favors generation of M1 antitumor macrophages[63] and also increases the antitumor response by cytotoxic T cells.[64] Infiltration of CRC tumors with M1 macrophages indicates better prognosis.[65]

Targeting Rac1b overexpression

A pharmacological approach to Rac1b overexpression was recently indicated by the finding that it responded specifically to the NSAID ibuprofen.[38] Treatment of the Rac1b-overexpressing colorectal cell line HT29 with ibuprofen markedly reduced the mRNA and protein levels of this variant. This effect was ibuprofen-specific and independent of the well-known inhibition of cyclooxygenase activity by NSAIDs, because neither aspirin nor related propionic acid-class NSAIDs, such as flurbiprofen or naproxen, were able to downregulate Rac1b. Although the underlying mechanism remains to be determined, this inhibitory effect of ibuprofen could be rescued by ectopic expression of wild-type Rac1b cDNA, which is not subjected to any mRNA splicing process.[38]

Ibuprofen not only reduced Rac1b levels in cultured cells, but also inhibited the growth of HT29 cells when implanted as tumor xenografts in mice that received ibuprofen treatment through drinking water. Similarly, experimentally induced acute colitis in mice drinking ibuprofen water was no longer able to increase Rac1b expression.[38] Notably, these effects were obtained using low, pain-management dosages of ibuprofen (100 μM).

The chemopreventive effect of Ibuprofen against colon cancer in general has been well documented at a dose of 200 mg/day, when taken for at least

10 years. Therefore, when targeted specifically to patients at risk for or after being diagnosed with SSAs in the proximal colon, adjuvant treatment with ibuprofen should be double effective: first, by reducing overall inflammation by suppressing cyclooxygenase activity required for prostaglandin synthesis, and second, because these adenomas are strongly associated with *BRAF* mutation and, thus, have a high probability for Rac1b overexpression. By contrast, treatment with piroxicam needs to be avoided because this drug promoted Rac1b overexpression[38] and may further stimulate malignant progression. There is, however, a clear need for clinical validation of the benefit of ibuprofen in patients with SSAs, the main group where *BRAF* mutation and Rac1b overexpression are expected to be associated.

An alternative approach to inhibit the Rac1b overexpression is to target the alternative splicing step directly. In general, aberrant splicing events may be therapeutically corrected by the overexpression or silencing of required splicing factors, by trans-splicing approaches (spliceosome-mediated trans-splicing between the endogenous transcript and a delivered cDNA copy), by using sequence-adapted U1 snRNAs (to promote or disturb exon recognition during spliceosome assembly), or by supplying short antisense oligonucleotides (ASOs).[66,67] Of these, ASOs represent the most promising splice-modulating therapeutic strategy to correct overexpression of a splice variant such as Rac1b, because they hybridize to a selected site in the pre-mRNA, and sterically hinder its recognition by the spliceosomal machinery. This strategy has been used to modify alternative splicing in diseases such as spinal muscular atrophy (SMN2 gene), allergic inflammation (IL-5 receptor gene), and cancer (Bcl-x and c-myc genes).[68–70] In the case of Duchenne muscular dystrophy, ASOs are already being tested in phase 3 clinical trials in patients carrying specific deletions for their ability to force exon skipping and restore the open reading frame to recover translation of a partially functional dystrophin protein.[71]

For the case of Rac1b, a perfect-match 25mer oligonucleotide can be designed that targets the splice junction between intron 3 and exon 3b including the exonic splice enhancer sequence for SRSF1 binding, which was previously identified to promote exon 3b inclusion and thus Rac1b protein overexpression.[72] Initial experiments, however, revealed that the designed Rac1b ASO only marginally decreased Rac1b transcripts when transfected into colorectal HT29 cell and was not able to inhibit cell viability, although the recommended manufacturer's guidelines for designing morpholino oligonucleotides (http://www.gene-tools.com/) had been followed (Gonçalves and Jordan, unpublished data). In contrast, previously described Rac1b-specific small interfering RNA (siRNA) oligonucleotides[31] efficiently depleted Rac1b transcript and diminished cell proliferation. Thus, rules for obtaining therapeutically efficient ASOs do not seem to be predictable based on simple sequence homology. Indeed, the identification of a potent and therapeutically active ASO that blocks an *SMN2* intronic splicing silencer element and efficiently promotes exon 7 inclusion, required systematic comparison of hundreds of ASOs that sometimes just differed in size by one nucleotide.[73] This ASO-tiling approach strongly suggests that secondary RNA structures with positive or negative effects contribute to exon recognition and add a strong empirical component to ASO design. Bearing this in mind, therapeutic correction of alternative Rac1b splicing will probably have to follow a similar tiling approach in order to find the most effective ASO to induce skipping exon 3b and thus decrease Rac1b protein and tumor cell survival.

Meanwhile, alternative chemical modifications of the nucleotide furanose ring have generated new types of ASOs such as phosphoroamidate morpholino oligomers, peptide nucleic acids, and locked nucleic acids, with improved target affinity, biostability, and pharmacokinetics.[74] Alternatively, tumor-cell targeted nanoparticles were described as carriers for the systemic administration of siRNAs in animal models[75] and human clinical trials[76] and produced a gene-specific inhibition via the expected an RNAi mechanism.[77] Also, the coupling of *KRAS*-specific siRNAs to anti-EGFR antibodies has been presented as a promising approach in CRC[78] and could be applied to target Rac1b.

Acknowledgments

We apologize that the reduced number of cited references allowed for this book chapter did not allow citing all relevant contributions published in the field. Work in the authors' laboratory was supported by Fundação para a Ciência e Tecnologia (FCT) (through center grant UID/MULTI/04046/2013 to BioISI, contract 'FCT Investigator' to PM, and fellowship SFRH/BPD/63395/2009 to VG) and the Portuguese association Maratona da Saúde — Cancro 2014 to PJ.

References

1. H Brenner, M Kloor, CP Pox (2014) Colorectal cancer. *The Lancet* **383**: 1490–1502.
2. J Ferlay, I Soerjomataram, R Dikshit, S Eser, C Mathers, M Rebelo, DM Parkin, D Forman, F Bray (2015) Cancer incidence and mortality worldwide: sources, methods and major patterns in GLOBOCAN 2012. *Int J Cancer* **136**: E359–386.
3. Cancer Genome Atlas Network (2012) Comprehensive molecular characterization of human colon and rectal cancer. *Nature* **487**: 330–337.
4. ER Fearon (2011) Molecular genetics of colorectal cancer. *Annu Rev Pathol Mech Dis* **6**: 479–507.
5. JR Jass (2007) Classification of colorectal cancer based on correlation of clinical, morphological and molecular features. *Histopathology* **50**: 113–130.
6. T Kambara (2004) BRAF mutation is associated with DNA methylation in serrated polyps and cancers of the colorectum. *Gut* **53**: 1137–1144.
7. DC Snover, JR Jass, C Fenoglio-Preiser, KP Batts (2005) Serrated polyps of the large intestine: A morphologic and molecular review of an evolving concept. *Am J Clin Pathol* **124**: 380–391.
8. M Bettington, N Walker, A Clouston, I Brown, B Leggett, V Whitehall (2013) The serrated pathway to colorectal carcinoma: Current concepts and challenges. *Histopathology* **62**: 367–386.
9. DK Rex, DJ Ahnen, JA Baron, KP Batts, CA Burke, RW Burt, JR Goldblum, JG Guillem, CJ Kahi, MF Kalady, MJ O'Brien, RD Odze, S Ogino, S Parry, DC Snover, EE Torlakovic, PE Wise, J Young, J Church (2012) Serrated lesions of the colorectum: Review and recommendations from an expert panel. *Am J Gastroenterol* **107**: 1315–1329.
10. HM Yang, JM Mitchell, JL Sepulveda, AR Sepulveda (2015) Molecular and histologic considerations in the assessment of serrated polyps. *Arch Pathol Lab Med* **139**: 730–741.
11. ML Bettington, R Chetty (2015) Traditional serrated adenoma: An update. *Hum Pathol* **46**: 933–938.
12. R Chetty (2016) Traditional serrated adenoma (TSA): Morphological questions, queries and quandaries. *J Clin Pathol* **69**: 6–11.
13. T Hinoue, DJ Weisenberger, CPE Lange, H Shen, HM Byun, D van Den Berg, S Malik, F Pan, H Noushmehr, CM van Dijk, RAEM Tollenaar, PW Laird (2012) Genome-scale analysis of aberrant DNA methylation in colorectal cancer. *Genome Res* **22**: 271–282.
14. SM Dong, EJ Lee, ES Jeon, CK Park, KM Kim (2005) Progressive methylation during the serrated neoplasia pathway of the colorectum. *Mod Pathol* **18**: 170–178.

15. H Suzuki, E Yamamoto, R Maruyama, T Niinuma, M Kai (2014) Biological significance of the CpG island methylator phenotype. *Biochem Biophys Res Commun* **455**: 35–42.
16. M Bettington, N Walker, C Rosty, I Brown, A Clouston, D McKeone, SA Pearson, B Leggett, V Whitehall (2015) Clinicopathological and molecular features of sessile serrated adenomas with dysplasia or carcinoma. *Oncotarget* 7(2016): 9188–9221.
17. R Chetty, S Hafezi-Bakhtiari, S Serra, R Colling, LM Wang (2015) Traditional serrated adenomas (TSAs) admixed with other serrated (so-called precursor) polyps and conventional adenomas: A frequent occurrence. *J Clin Pathol* **68**: 270–273.
18. J Guinney, R Dienstmann, X Wang, A de Reyniès, A Schlicker, C Soneson, L Marisa, P Roepman, G Nyamundanda, P Angelino, BM Bot, JS Morris, IM Simon, S Gerster, E Fessler, F De Sousa E Melo, E Missiaglia, H Ramay, D Barras, K Homicsko, D Maru, GC Manyam, B Broom, V Boige, B Perez-Villamil, T Laderas, R Salazar, JW Gray, D Hanahan, J Tabernero, R Bernards, SH Friend, P Laurent-Puig, JP Medema, A Sadanandam, L Wessels, M Delorenzi, S Kopetz, L Vermeulen, S Tejpar (2015) The consensus molecular subtypes of colorectal cancer. *Nat Med* **21**: 1350–1356.
19. H Davies, GR Bignell, C Cox, P Stephens, S Edkins, S Clegg, J Teague, H Woffendin, MJ Garnett, W Bottomley, N Davis, E Dicks, R Ewing, Y Floyd, K Gray, S Hall, R Hawes, J Hughes, V Kosmidou, A Menzies, C Mould, A Parker, C Stevens, S Watt, S Hooper, R Wilson, H Jayatilake, BA Gusterson, C Cooper, J Shipley, D Hargrave, K Pritchard-Jones, N Maitland, G Chenevix Trench, GJ Riggins, DD Bigner, G Palmieri, A Cossu, A Flanagan, A Nicholson, JWC Ho, SY Leung, ST Yuen, BL Weber, HF Seigler, TL Darrow, H Paterson, R Marais, CJ Marshall, R Wooster, MR Stratton, PA Futreal (2002) Mutations of the BRAF gene in human cancer. *Nature* **417**: 949–954.
20. PTC Wan, MJ Garnett, SM Roe, S Lee, D Niculescu-Duvaz, VM Good, CM Jones, CJ Marshall, CJ Springer, D Barford, R Marais (2004) Mechanism of activation of the RAF-ERK signaling pathway by oncogenic mutations of B-RAF. *Cell* **116**: 855–867.
21. C Wellbrock, M Karasarides, R Marais (2004) The RAF proteins take centre stage. *Nat Rev Mol Cell Biol* **5**: 875–885.
22. LAS Carragher, KR Snell, SM Giblett, VSS Aldridge, B Patel, SJ Cook, DJ Winton, R Marais, CA Pritchard (2010) V600EBraf induces gastrointestinal crypt senescence and promotes tumour progression through enhanced CpG methylation of p16INK4a. *EMBO Mol Med* **2**: 458–471.
23. R Rad, J Cadiñanos, L Rad, I Varela, A Strong, L Kriegl, F Constantino-Casas, S Eser, M Hieber, B Seidler, S Price, MF Fraga, V Calvanese, G Hoffman, H Ponstingl, G Schneider, K Yusa, C Grove, RM Schmid, W Wang, G Vassiliou,

T Kirchner, U McDermott, P Liu, D Saur, A Bradley (2013) A genetic progression model of Braf(V600E)-induced intestinal tumorigenesis reveals targets for therapeutic intervention. *Cancer Cell* **24**: 15–29.
24. M Collado, M Serrano (2006) The power and the promise of oncogene-induced senescence markers. *Nat Rev Cancer* **6**: 472–476.
25. L Kriegl, J Neumann, M Vieth, FR Greten, S Reu, A Jung, T Kirchner (2011) Up and downregulation of p16(Ink4a) expression in BRAF-mutated polyps/adenomas indicates a senescence barrier in the serrated route to colon cancer. *Mod Pathol* **24**: 1015–1022.
26. RB Corcoran (2015) New therapeutic strategies for BRAF mutant colorectal cancers. *J Gastrointest Oncol* **6**: 650–659.
27. JA DiDonato, F Mercurio, M Karin (2012) NF-κB and the link between inflammation and cancer. *Immunol Rev* **246**: 379–400.
28. SI Grivennikov, FR Greten, M Karin (2010) Immunity, inflammation, and cancer. *Cell* **140**: 883–899.
29. Y Schwitalle, M Kloor, S Eiermann, M Linnebacher, P Kienle, HP Knaebel, M Tariverdian, A Benner, M von Knebel Doeberitz (2008) Immune response against frameshift-induced neopeptides in HNPCC patients and healthy HNPCC mutation carriers. *Gastroenterology* **134**: 988–997.
30. NJ Llosa, M Cruise, A Tam, EC Wicks, EM Hechenbleikner, JM Taube, RL Blosser, H Fan, H Wang, BS Luber, M Zhang, N Papadopoulos, KW Kinzler, B Vogelstein, CL Sears, RA Anders, DM Pardoll, F Housseau (2015) The vigorous immune microenvironment of microsatellite instable colon cancer is balanced by multiple counter-inhibitory checkpoints. *Cancer Discov* **5**: 43–51.
31. P Matos, C Oliveira, S Velho, V Gonçalves, LT da Costa, MP Moyer, R Seruca, P Jordan (2008) B-Raf(V600E) cooperates with alternative spliced Rac1b to sustain colorectal cancer cell survival. *Gastroenterology* **135**: 899–906.
32. D Fiegen, L-C Haeusler, L Blumenstein, U Herbrand, R Dvorsky, IR Vetter, MR Ahmadian (2004) Alternative splicing of Rac1 generates Rac1b, a self-activating GTPase. *J Biol Chem* **279**: 4743–4749.
33. P Matos, JG Collard, P Jordan (2003) Tumor-related alternatively spliced Rac1b is not regulated by Rho–GDP dissociation inhibitors and exhibits selective downstream signaling. *J Biol Chem* **278**: 50442–50448.
34. A Singh, AE Karnoub, TR Palmby, E Lengyel, J Sondek, CJ Der (2004) Rac1b, a tumor associated, constitutively active Rac1 splice variant, promotes cellular transformation. *Oncogene* **23**: 9369–9380.
35. R Seruca, S Velho, C Oliveira, M Leite, P Matos, P Jordan (2009) Unmasking the role of KRAS and BRAF pathways in MSI colorectal tumors. *Expert Rev Gastroenterol Hepatol* **3**: 5–9.

36. P Matos, P Jordan (2005) Expression of Rac1b stimulates NF-kappaB-mediated cell survival and G1/S progression. *Exp Cell Res* **305**: 292–299.
37. V Alonso-Espinaco, M Cuatrecasas, V Alonso, P Escudero, M Marmol, C Horndler, J Ortego, R Gallego, J Codony-Servat, X Garcia-Albeniz, P Jares, A Castells, JJ Lozano, R Rosell, J Maurel (2014) RAC1b overexpression correlates with poor prognosis in KRAS/BRAF WT metastatic colorectal cancer patients treated with first-line FOLFOX/XELOX chemotherapy. *Eur J Cancer* **50**: 1973–1981.
38. P Matos, L Kotelevets, V Goncalves, A Henriques, P Zerbib, MP Moyer, E Chastre, P Jordan (2013) Ibuprofen inhibits colitis-induced overexpression of tumor-related Rac1b. *Neoplasia* **15**: 102–111.
39. KT Flaherty, I Puzanov, KB Kim, A Ribas, GA McArthur, JA Sosman, PJ O'Dwyer, RJ Lee, JF Grippo, K Nolop, PB Chapman (2010) Inhibition of mutated, activated BRAF in metastatic melanoma. *N Engl J Med* **363**: 809–819.
40. JA Sosman, KB Kim, L Schuchter, R Gonzalez, AC Pavlick, JS Weber, GA McArthur, TE Hutson, SJ Moschos, KT Flaherty, P Hersey, R Kefford, D Lawrence, I Puzanov, KD Lewis, RK Amaravadi, B Chmielowski, HJ Lawrence, Y Shyr, F Ye, J Li, KB Nolop, RJ Lee, AK Joe, A Ribas (2012) Survival in BRAF V600-mutant advanced melanoma treated with vemurafenib. *N Engl J Med* **366**: 707–714.
41. W Fiskus, N Mitsiades (2016) B-Raf Inhibition in the clinic: Present and future. *Annu Rev Med* **67**: 29–43.
42. DM Hyman, I Puzanov, V Subbiah, JE Faris, I Chau, J-Y Blay, J Wolf, NS Raje, EL Diamond, A Hollebecque, R Gervais, ME Elez-Fernandez, A Italiano, R-D Hofheinz, M Hidalgo, E Chan, M Schuler, SF Lasserre, M Makrutzki, F Sirzen, ML Veronese, J Tabernero, J Baselga (2015) Vemurafenib in multiple nonmelanoma cancers with BRAF V600 mutations. *N Engl J Med* **373**: 726–736.
43. S Kopetz, J Desai, E Chan, JR Hecht, PJ O'Dwyer, D Maru, V Morris, F Janku, A Dasari, W Chung, J-PJ Issa, P Gibbs, B James, G Powis, KB Nolop, S Bhattacharya, L Saltz (2015) Phase II pilot study of Vemurafenib in patients with metastatic BRAF-mutated colorectal cancer. *J Clin Oncol* **33**: 4032–4038.
44. RB Corcoran, H Ebi, AB Turke, EM Coffee, M Nishino, AP Cogdill, RD Brown, P Della Pelle, D Dias-Santagata, KE Hung, KT Flaherty, A Piris, JA Wargo, J Settleman, M Mino-Kenudson, JA Engelman (2012) EGFR-mediated re-activation of MAPK signaling contributes to insensitivity of BRAF mutant colorectal cancers to RAF inhibition with vemurafenib. *Cancer Discov* **2**: 227–235.
45. P Lito, CA Pratilas, EW Joseph, M Tadi, E Halilovic, M Zubrowski, A Huang, WL Wong, MK Callahan, T Merghoub, JD Wolchok, E de Stanchina, S Chandarlapaty, PI Poulikakos, JA Fagin, N Rosen (2012) Relief of profound feedback inhibition of mitogenic signaling by RAF inhibitors attenuates their activity in BRAFV600E melanomas. *Cancer Cell* **22**: 668–682.

46. EW Joseph, CA Pratilas, PI Poulikakos, M Tadi, W Wang, BS Taylor, E Halilovic, Y Persaud, F Xing, A Viale, J Tsai, PB Chapman, G Bollag, DB Solit, N Rosen (2010) The RAF inhibitor PLX4032 inhibits ERK signaling and tumor cell proliferation in a V600E BRAF-selective manner. *Proc Natl Acad Sci USA* **107**: 14903–14908.
47. G Hatzivassiliou, K Song, I Yen, BJ Brandhuber, DJ Anderson, R Alvarado, MJC Ludlam, D Stokoe, SL Gloor, G Vigers, T Morales, I Aliagas, B Liu, S Sideris, KP Hoeflich, BS Jaiswal, S Seshagiri, H Koeppen, M Belvin, LS Friedman, S Malek (2010) RAF inhibitors prime wild-type RAF to activate the MAPK pathway and enhance growth. *Nature* **464**: 431–435.
48. SJ Heidorn, C Milagre, S Whittaker, A Nourry, I Niculescu-Duvas, N Dhomen, J Hussain, JS Reis-Filho, CJ Springer, C Pritchard, R Marais (2010) Kinase-dead BRAF and oncogenic RAS cooperate to drive tumor progression through CRAF. *Cell* **140**: 209–221.
49. PI Poulikakos, C Zhang, G Bollag, KM Shokat, N Rosen (2010) RAF inhibitors transactivate RAF dimers and ERK signalling in cells with wild-type BRAF. *Nature* **464**: 427–430.
50. CB Meador, W Pao (2015) Old habits die hard: Addiction of BRAF-mutant cancer cells to MAP kinase signaling. *Cancer Discov* **5**: 348–350.
51. LG Ahronian, EM Sennott, EM Van Allen, N Wagle, EL Kwak, JE Faris, JT Godfrey, K Nishimura, KD Lynch, CH Mermel, EL Lockerman, A Kalsy, JM Gurski, S Bahl, K Anderka, LM Green, NJ Lennon, TG Huynh, M Mino-Kenudson, G Getz, D Dias-Santagata, AJ Iafrate, JA Engelman, LA Garraway, RB Corcoran (2015) Clinical acquired resistance to RAF inhibitor combinations in BRAF-mutant colorectal cancer through MAPK pathway alterations. *Cancer Discov* **5**: 358–367.
52. R Yaeger, A Cercek, EM O'Reilly, DL Reidy, N Kemeny, T Wolinsky, M Capanu, MJ Gollub, N Rosen, MF Berger, ME Lacouture, E Vakiani, LB Saltz (2015) Pilot trial of combined BRAF and EGFR inhibition in BRAF-mutant metastatic colorectal cancer patients. *Clin Cancer Res* **21**: 1313–1320.
53. RB Corcoran, D Dias-Santagata, K Bergethon, AJ Iafrate, J Settleman, JA Engelman (2010) BRAF gene amplification can promote acquired resistance to MEK inhibitors in cancer cells harboring the BRAF V600E mutation. *Sci Signal* **3**: ra84.
54. RB Corcoran, CE Atreya, GS Falchook, EL Kwak, DP Ryan, JC Bendell, O Hamid, WA Messersmith, A Daud, R Kurzrock, M Pierobon, P Sun, E Cunningham, S Little, K Orford, M Motwani, Y Bai, K Patel, AP Venook, S Kopetz (2015) Combined BRAF and MEK Inhibition with dabrafenib and trametinib in BRAF V600-mutant colorectal cancer. *J Clin Oncol* **33**: 4023–4031.

55. SR Whittaker, GS Cowley, S Wagner, F Luo, DE Root, LA Garraway (2015) Combined Pan-RAF and MEK inhibition overcomes multiple resistance mechanisms to selective RAF inhibitors. *Mol Cancer Ther* **14**: 2700–2711.
56. EJ Morris, S Jha, CR Restaino, P Dayananth, H Zhu, A Cooper, D Carr, Y Deng, W Jin, S Black, B Long, J Liu, E Dinunzio, W Windsor, R Zhang, S Zhao, MH Angagaw, EM Pinheiro, J Desai, L Xiao, G Shipps, A Hruza, J Wang, J Kelly, S Paliwal, X Gao, BS Babu, L Zhu, P Daublain, L Zhang, BA Lutterbach, MR Pelletier, U Philippar, P Siliphaivanh, D Witter, P Kirschmeier, WR Bishop, D Hicklin, DG Gilliland, L Jayaraman, L Zawel, S Fawell, AA Samatar (2013) Discovery of a novel ERK inhibitor with activity in models of acquired resistance to BRAF and MEK inhibitors. *Cancer Discov* **3**: 742–750.
57. JC Bendell, CE Atreya, T André, J Tabernero, MS Gordon, R Bernards, E Van Cutsem, S Tejpar, R Sidhu, WY Go, A Allred, M Motwani, BB Suttle, Y Wu, A Hoos, KW Orford, RB Corcoran, JHM Schellens (2014) Efficacy and tolerability in an open-label phase I/II study of MEK inhibitor trametinib (T), BRAF inhibitor dabrafenib (D), and anti-EGFR antibody panitumumab (P) in combination in patients (pts) with BRAF V600E mutated colorectal cancer (CRC). *J Clin Oncol* **325s**: Abstract No. 3515.
58. R van Geel, E Elez, JC Bendell, JE Faris, MPJK Lolkema, F Eskens, A Spreafico, P Kavan, JP Delord, MH Schuler, ZA Wainberg, Y Yamada, T Yoshino, T Demuth, E Avsar, A Chatterjee, P Zhu, R Bernards, J Tabernero, JHM Schellens (2014) Phase I study of the selective BRAFV600 inhibitor encorafenib (LGX818) combined with cetuximab and with or without the α-specific PI3K inhibitor BYL719 in patients with advanced BRAF-mutant colorectal cancer. *J Clin Oncol* **325s**: Abstract No. 3514.
59. M Goulielmaki, E Koustas, E Moysidou, M Vlassi, T Sasazuki, S Shirasawa, G Zografos, E Oikonomou, A Pintzas (2016) BRAF associated autophagy exploitation: BRAF and autophagy inhibitors synergise to efficiently overcome resistance of BRAF mutant colorectal cancer cells. *Oncotarget,* 7(2016) 9: 188–221.
60. O Shalem, NE Sanjana, E Hartenian, X Shi, DA Scott, TS Mikkelsen, D Heckl, BL Ebert, DE Root, JG Doench, F Zhang (2014) Genome-scale CRISPR-Cas9 knockout screening in human cells. *Science* **343**: 84–87.
61. DT Le, JN Uram, H Wang, BR Bartlett, H Kemberling, AD Eyring, AD Skora, BS Luber, NS Azad, D Laheru, B Biedrzycki, RC Donehower, A Zaheer, GA Fisher, TS Crocenzi, JJ Lee, SM Duffy, RM Goldberg, A de la Chapelle, M Koshiji, F Bhaijee, T Huebner, RH Hruban, LD Wood, N Cuka, DM Pardoll, N Papadopoulos, KW Kinzler, S Zhou, TC Cornish, JM Taube, RA Anders, JR Eshleman, B Vogelstein, LA Diaz (2015) PD-1 Blockade in Tumors with mismatch-repair deficiency. *N Engl J Med* **372**: 2509–2520.

62. HH Uhlig, T Schwerd, S Koletzko, N Shah, J Kammermeier, A Elkadri, J Ouahed, DC Wilson, SP Travis, D Turner, C Klein, SB Snapper, AM Muise (2014) The diagnostic approach to monogenic very early onset inflammatory bowel disease. *Gastroenterology* **147**: 990–1007.
63. DS Shouval, A Biswas, JA Goettel, K McCann, E Conaway, NS Redhu, ID Mascanfroni, Z Al Adham, S Lavoie, M Ibourk, DD Nguyen, JN Samsom, JC Escher, R Somech, B Weiss, R Beier, LS Conklin, CL Ebens, FGMS Santos, AR Ferreira, M Sherlock, AK Bhan, W Müller, JR Mora, FJ Quintana, C Klein, AM Muise, BH Horwitz, SB Snapper (2014) Interleukin-10 receptor signaling in innate immune cells regulates mucosal immune tolerance and anti-inflammatory macrophage function. *Immunity* **40**: 706–719.
64. T Chanmee, P Ontong, K Konno, N Itano (2014) Tumor-associated macrophages as major players in the tumor microenvironment. *Cancers* **6**: 1670–1690.
65. S Edin, ML Wikberg, AM Dahlin, J Rutegård, Å Öberg, P-A Oldenborg, R Palmqvist (2012) The distribution of macrophages with a M1 or M2 phenotype in relation to prognosis and the molecular characteristics of colorectal cancer. *PLoS ONE* **7**: e47045.
66. MA Havens, DM Duelli, ML Hastings (2013) Targeting RNA splicing for disease therapy. *Wiley Interdiscip Rev RNA* **4**: 247–266.
67. R Kole, AR Krainer, S Altman (2012) RNA therapeutics: Beyond RNA interference and antisense oligonucleotides. *Nat Rev Drug Discov* **11**: 125–140.
68. Y Hua, TA Vickers, HL Okunola, CF Bennett, AR Krainer (2008) Antisense masking of an hnRNP A1/A2 intronic splicing silencer corrects SMN2 splicing in transgenic mice. *Am J Hum Genet* **82**: 834–848.
69. JG Karras, RA McKay, NM Dean, BP Monia (2000) Deletion of individual exons and induction of soluble murine interleukin-5 receptor-α chain expression through antisense oligonucleotide-mediated redirection of pre-mRNA splicing. *Mol Pharmacol* **58**: 380–387.
70. HS Sekhon, CA London, M Sekhon, PL Iversen, GR Devi (2008) c-MYC antisense phosphosphorodiamidate morpholino oligomer inhibits lung metastasis in a murine tumor model. *Lung Cancer* **60**: 347–354.
71. T Koo, MJ Wood (2013) Clinical trials using antisense oligonucleotides in duchenne muscular dystrophy. *Hum Gene Ther* **24**: 479–488.
72. V Gonçalves, P Matos, P Jordan (2009) Antagonistic SR proteins regulate alternative splicing of tumor-related Rac1b downstream of the PI3-kinase and Wnt pathways. *Hum Mol Genet* **18**: 3696–3707.
73. Y Hua, TA Vickers, BF Baker, CF Bennett, AR Krainer (2007) Enhancement of SMN2 exon 7 inclusion by antisense oligonucleotides targeting the exon. *PLoS Biol* **5**: e73.

74. JHP Chan, S Lim, WSF Wong (2006) Antisense oligonucleotides: From design to therapeutic application. *Clin Exp Pharmacol Physiol* **33**: 533–540.
75. TS Zimmermann, ACH Lee, A Akinc, *et al.* (2006) RNAi-mediated gene silencing in non-human primates. *Nature* **441**: 111–114.
76. ME Davis, JE Zuckerman, CHJ Choi, D Seligson, A Tolcher, CA Alabi, Y Yen, JD Heidel, A Ribas (2010) Evidence of RNAi in humans from systemically administered siRNA via targeted nanoparticles. *Nature* **464**: 1067–1070.
77. Y Wang, Z Li, Y Han, LH Liang, A Ji (2010) Nanoparticle-based delivery system for application of siRNA *in vivo*. *Curr Drug Metab* **11**: 182–196.
78. S Bäumer, N Bäumer, N Appel, L Terheyden, J Fremerey, S Schelhaas, E Wardelmann, F Buchholz, WE Berdel, C Müller-Tidow (2015) Antibody-mediated delivery of anti-KRAS-siRNA *in vivo* overcomes therapy resistance in colon cancer. *Clin Cancer Res* **21**: 1383–1394.

Chapter 12

The "Yin" and "Yang" of Target-Oriented Anticancer Phytochemicals Derived from Herbal Medicines

Kathy K. Auyeung and Joshua K. S. Ko

Abstract

Contemporary chemotherapy has encountered many challenges including variable treatment outcomes and low therapeutic index of conventional cytotoxic drugs. There is an increasing trend to explore effective medicinal herbal products and the phytochemicals derived from them that have the potential to be developed as useful therapeutic adjuvants. Alternatively, concerns have also been raised regarding the lack of scientific evidence on action mechanisms and possibility of herb–drug interactions with the increased use of anticancer herbal medicinal compounds. The present review attempts to provide information to account for both positive (Yang) and negative (Yin) sides of the use of herbal medicinal products and their active constituents in daily clinical practice as well as the advancement of experimental works in target-oriented anticancer treatment. This chapter begins with a few examples of typical herb–drug interactions and to suggest several ways to prevent these from happening in future practice. Following this, the benefits of using herbal medicinal agents and the concepts behind will be introduced, allowing readers to envisage the rationale and potential of developing active phytochemicals as effective and well-tolerated chemotherapeutics in modern treatment approach of human cancers. The discovery of a series of anticancer herbal medicinal agents in the last 10 years that undergo precise mechanisms of action with known molecular targets will be discussed in details. The knowledge acquired during the identification and investigation of these potential herbal medicinal compounds could help oncologists to establish effective and safer chemotherapeutic adjuvants in the treatment of human cancers.

Introduction

Medicinal herbs and their derived active phytochemicals have been used as useful complementary treatments for cancer. Herbal supplements are popular nowadays but not too many people are willing to give up the mainstream Western medicine. There are still concerns such as the lack of scientific studies on medicinal herbs and the possibility of a herb–drug interaction. Nonetheless, increasing evidence has been provided over the years to demonstrate the beneficial effects of herbal medicines in enhancing the quality of life, prolonging life span, and boosting the immune system of cancer patients when they are used in combination with conventional chemotherapy. In spite of this, it remains controversial whether concurrent use of herbal medicine will increase or oppose the effectiveness of chemotherapy. In the view of possible herb–drug interactions, both pharmacokinetic and pharmacodynamic mechanisms of the prescribed drugs should be considered. The clinical importance of herb–drug interactions depends on many factors including the use of specific herbs, drugs, and patients (especially for those with pre-existing conditions). There are pros and cons when we use both herbal and Western medicines concomitantly. However, due to the lack of well-designed and properly conducted clinical trials as well as the limited research in the field of the herb–drug interaction, herbal medicine still cannot be widely used as first-line chemotherapeutics. In everyday life, polypharmacy is common in actual clinical settings, of which in addition to the medications being prescribed by physicians, patients would take some over-the-counter drugs, vitamins, or herbal medicines. Unfortunately, interactions may result among all the consumed substances. In a large-scale study, it was reported that 538 out of 1000 elderly patients were susceptible to 1087 drug–drug interactions, resulting in 189 side effects being observed in 130 patients.[1] Nonetheless, there has not been sufficient information on the cases of herb–drug interactions in the world being available so far. A meta-analysis on herb–drug interactions had been conducted by reviewing both English and Chinese database such as Ovid, Medline, EMBase, SciFinder Scholar, and CNKI. The keywords used in literature search include Western medicine, Chinese medicine, herbal medicine, plants and drug interaction. Over 80 commonly used chemotherapy drugs including cisplatin, carboplatin, doxorubicin, and fluorouracil have been searched. From the literature, over 10,000 papers contained information that may be related to interactions between anti-cancer drugs and/or herbs. Among these, only less than 900 papers were found to report actual cases of herb–drug interactions. Unfortunately, many of these papers lacked crucial documentation on time-based relations or concomitant drug/herb use, and thus failed to come up with a definite conclusion. For thorough coverage of the principles behind and the cases of herb–drug interactions, one should refer to the book written by Chan and Cheung in 2000.[2] In the present review, we aimed to illustrate both "Yin" (referring to the dark side or negative events) and "Yang" (referring to the bright side or positive events) aspects of the use of herbal medicines in cancer treatment. A good balance of the two sides could facilitate the development of effective herbal medicinal compounds or related phytochemicals as potential chemotherapeutic adjuvants.

Adverse Effects Resulting from the Use of Herbal Medicines or Phytochemical in Cancer Patients

Regarding the herb–drug interaction, it should be noted that the cytochrome P-450 (CYP) enzymes responsible for metabolizing both entities could be a major source of variability in their pharmacokinetics and tissue responses.[3] The use of herbal products that will affect CYP metabolism may result in the alteration of drug/herb bioavailability. Any inhibitory effect on CYP may cause enhancement in plasma concentration, leading to toxicity. In contrast, CYP enzyme induction may lead to reduced drug concentration and hence reduced drug/herb efficacy.[4]

Pharmacokinetic interaction involving CYP metabolizing enzymes

The concomitant use of herbal medicine and anti-cancer drug could result in safety concern in cancer patients since the active ingredients of herbal medicine may have the potential to affect both the pharmacokinetic and pharmacodynamic mechanisms of the prescribed anti-cancer drugs to affect drug efficacy. Among all commonly used health supplements, St. John's Wort (SJW) is one of the top 10 used herbal products for cancer patients,[5] and thus serves as a good example to illustrate the adverse effects from pharmacokinetic interactions between herbal and anti-cancer drugs. Many *in vitro* studies have revealed that SJW or its active components (hyperforin and hypericin) will alter the activity of CYP3A4 in a panel of cells including human colon carcinoma-derived cell line (LS180),[6] human hepatocytes,[7] human liver microsomes,[8] and supersomes.[9] From these studies, it was found that SJW or its main components could either induce or inhibit CYP3A4 mRNA or protein expression. It is believed that the induction and inhibition on CYP enzymes are associated with the duration of SJW treatment. Generally speaking, induction of CYP enzymes would be expected after prolonged treatment of SJW because hyperforin could activate pregnane X receptor (PXR), an orphan nuclear receptor that regulates the expression of the cytochrome P450 (CYP) 3A4 monooxygenase.[10] Therefore, according to the interaction between SJW and CYP3A4, it is expected that there are pharmacokinetic interactions between SJW and anti-cancer drugs metabolized by the same enzyme system. So far it has been identified that SJW would affect the drug metabolism of irinotecan[11] and imatinib.[12] However, these effects may not apply to all herbal products. Alternatively, both milk thistle and ginseng caused *in vitro* CYP3A4 inhibition but such an inhibition was not observed in clinical studies.[13]

The herb–drug interaction via modulation of drug transporter expression

A number of anti-cancer drugs and their metabolites have been identified as substrates of P-glycoprotein (P-gp), breast cancer resistance protein, multidrug resistance protein 1, and multidrug resistance protein 9, and/or other transporters.[14] Among all, P-gp plays an essential role in drug disposition. An *in vitro* study had demonstrated that LS-180 intestinal carcinoma cells treated with SJW or hypericin showed an increase in the expression of P-gp by 4–7 folds, while about 4-fold increase in intestinal P-gp expression was observed in rats after 14 days of SJW administration.[15] Another study had also revealed a 1.4-fold increase in P-gp expression in healthy volunteers after 14 days of oral administration of SJW.[16] Besides, it was reported that the coadministration of garlic supplement in women with advanced breast cancer reduced the clearance of docetaxel by 23.1–35.1%.[14] Results from these studies have indicated that the modulation of drug transporter expression by herbal products could be a crucial mechanism for herb–drug interactions.

Approach to avoid potential risk of the herb–drug interaction

The consumption of herbal supplements by the general public is an uprising trend, particularly in Asian countries where there is higher prevalence in the use of herbal medicine.[17] The percentage of population using complementary and alternative medicine (CAM) was reported to be about 76% in Japan,[18] whereas over 90% of cancer patients had used CAM in China.[19] A more recent review had analyzed about 3000 clinical studies (including both randomized controlled trials and non-randomized controlled trials); among those, 72% of cancer patients were found to be using Traditional Chinese Medicine (TCM) along with active conventional cancer therapies.[20] There is no doubt that TCM is effective in improving the quality of life of cancer patients. Some of the interactions may even exert beneficial effects by enhancing drug efficacy or reducing potential side effects. A summary of the selected phytochemicals being found to be effective in the treatment of cancers is listed in Table 1. However, people are still worried about the quality control and quality assurance of herbal medicines.

Quality control of herbal medicines

In order to maintain the safe use of herbs, we have to be aware of the standardization of herbal medicine, which includes the authentication, taxonomic assignment (DNA fingerprinting), identification of bioactive ingredients, as well as assessment of biological and pharmacological activities. Other than this, other factors like environmental contaminations (including air pollution, soil contaminations, and heavy metals), cultivation practices (such as the use of pesticides, fungicides, heavy metals, microorganisms, and endotoxins), as well as manufacture processing and handling (including storage, additives, microorganisms, endotoxins, and human adulteration) are also

Table 1. Beneficial effects of phytochemicals in *in vitro* cancer models.

Phytochemical	**Anti-carcinogenic activities in human cancer cells**
Silibinin	Synergistic effect with mitoxantrone to inhibit cell growth and induce apoptosis in human prostate cancer cells
Hyperforin	Induce docetaxel metabolism in human hepatocyte cultures
Epigallocatechin-3-gallate	Suppress cell proliferation, provoke apoptosis, and disturb cell-cell adhesion in MCF-7 cells
Curcumin	Suppress proliferation and migration of MDA-MB-231 breast cancer cells through autophagy-dependent Akt degradation
Baicalein	Exhibit dose-dependent growth-inhibitory effect in human prostate cancer cells
Formononetin	Downregulate the expression of key pro-angiogenic factors and decrease the cell invasiveness of metastatic colon cancer cells
Berberine	Inhibit hepatocellular carcinoma cell growth through NSAID-activated gene activation
Amorfrutin C	Induce apoptosis and inhibits proliferation of colon cancer cells by targeting mitochondria
Calycosin	Suppress A549 cell proliferation and metastasis via inhibition of the PKC-α/ERK1/2 pathway
Dihydrotanshinone I	Induce apoptosis and autophagy through caspase-dependent pathway in colon cancer

important for the safe use of herbal medicines.[21] Many cases of fatal herb–drug interactions have been reported when doctors have no information about their patients' concurrent use of drug/herb supplements. As shown in Table 2, many popular and common herbal medicines have been reported to cause adverse effects when being used along with orthodox drugs that could lead to severe consequences. Furthermore, more attention should be paid on the intrinsic toxicities of some herbal medicinal products on the renal, liver, cardiovascular. and nervous systems.[22,23] Besides, it is known that some herbal species such as *Aristolochiaceae* and *Aconitum* have been documented to possess high toxicity.[21] A recent clinical study in Taiwan had reported that aristolochic acid, the key component of all Aristolochia-based herbal medicines, would induce upper urinary tract urothelial carcinoma. This study also revealed that all patients with similar clinical predisposition had

Table 2. Adverse effects of herbal medicines being used in cancer patients.

Herbal medicines	Adverse effects
St John's wort	Increase imatinib clearance in healthy subjects by 43% Decrease the maximum plasma concentration of docetaxel
Schisandra sphenanthera extract	Increase the oral bioavailability of tacrolimus in healthy volunteers
Mistletoe	Induce hyper-eosinophilia in a patient with pancreatic carcinoma
Phytoestrogen	Induce breast cancer in a man
Baicalin	Reduce the clearance of midazolam by increasing its pharmacokinetics
Ginseng	Interact with warfarin by reducing the plasma level of warfarin and the anticoagulant effect in ischemic stroke patients
Gingko biloba	Inhibit paclitaxel metabolism in human hepatocytes
Allium sativum L. (Garlic)	Reduce apoptotic activity of etoposide, paclitaxel, vinblastine, and vincristine in healthy volunteers
Ganoderma lucidum (Reishi)	Generate multidrug-resistant leukemic cell line
Curcuma longa L. (Turmeric)	Facilitate cisplatin resistance in cisplatin-resistant lung cancer cells by inhibiting the FA/BRCA pathway

aristolactam–DNA adducts.[24] Based on these concerns, a well-established database with essential information on the properties of herbal products and the contraindications of concomitant use with conventional therapeutic drugs should be developed to facilitate the safe use of herbal medicines with orthodox medicines.

Awareness of the safety of herbal medicine

The herb–drug interaction has long been considered as an essential factor to consider its practicality in combined use with one or more types of medications. Understanding of the use of specific herbal medicines as adjuvants to conventional chemotherapy may help to avoid the occurrence of a potential adverse interaction. In addition, better communication and coordination between physicians and/or other health care providers and patients are necessary. It has been suggested that a proper label should be put on herbal medicinal products to alert consumers/patients on their potential interactions when concomitantly used with orthodox drugs. Other than this, the manufacturer also has the responsibility to ensure herbal drug safety before their products are marketed in countries without proper licensing legislation. For patients' own benefits, it is always a good practice to tell their doctors about the herbal supplements which they are currently taking before commencement of drug prescription. In turn, physicians are advised to check with their patients about the use of any health supplements including herbal medicines. Proper communications between doctors and patients as well as between orthodox physicians of Western medicine and TCM practitioners could ensure a good pharmacovigilance of herbal medicinal products.[25] On the other hand, it would always be an asset to carry out evidence-based study to support the use of herbal medicines. It is a reality that even though TCM has been used for thousands of years and mainly derived from daily use in mankind, most of them have not been tested in well-designed double-blinded and placebo-controlled clinical trials. In general, it is suggested to establish a better practical approach to advise both physicians and patients about the use of herbal medicines. On the side of physician, they should make a detailed record of all the herbal medicines concurrently taken by their patients. As for the patients, they should cooperate with the physician by voluntarily providing information about their use of herbal medicines. In the case of significant herb–drug interaction, the use of such herbal products must be discontinued at once and to report the incidence to any health professional, where information about the herbal drugs and/or any leftover of the products should be provided for detailed analysis. Taken together, an effective model of safety monitoring and risk management of TCM drugs would be essential to ensure a good pharmacovigilance practice.[26]

Beneficial Effects of Herbal Medicines or Phytochemicals in the Treatment of Cancer

The inhibition of cancer growth by a variety of human nutrients derived from plants as well as of non-nutritive plant-derived constituents (phytochemicals) has been confirmed in different tumor animal models, with an increased emphasis on cancer prevention strategies in which these dietary factors are utilized. Herbal medicines are generally used in combination with first-line chemotherapy or radiotherapy to improve the efficacy of cancer therapy and reduce the drug-induced side effects and complications. A better understanding of the use and action mechanisms of specific herbal medicines as adjuvants to conventional therapy may help to offset the negative impact of individual herb/drug or herb–drug interactions and hence prevent any unwanted adverse body reactions and toxicities.

Beneficial effects of TCM in cancer patients

A clinical study has revealed the use of *Ping Xiao* capsules (PXC, a commercial anti-cancer product commonly used in Mainland China) in the treatment of late stage mammary cancer (LSMC). Results have shown that PXC could improve the quality of life and prolong the progression time in patients with LSMC with fewer side effects.[27] Another clinical trial attempted to investigate the anti-cancer effects of Rg3, the active ingredient of ginseng in treating advanced non-small-cell lung cancer. A total of 115 patients were enrolled and Rg3 was used in a combination with a chemotherapy regimen NP (vinorelbine+cisplatin). Results indicate that there were improvements in both response rate and survival time (median and mean) in patients of the Rg3 treatment group.[28] These experiences have marked the beginning of vigorous standardized herbal drug testing in contemporary cancer research.

Therapeutic effects of PHY906 in gastrointestinal cancers

We have mentioned earlier that a lot of TCM drug products have not been tested in well-designed studies like double-blind and placebo-controlled clinical trials, which are essential to prove the efficacy of the herbal drugs and to identify the potential adverse drug reactions, and if possible to unveil the unique mechanism of action. One of the good examples is the study on PHY906, a TCM formulation that has been used for over 1800 years to treat gastrointestinal disorders. It is a medicinal mixture of four herbs: *Glycyrrhiza uralensis Fisch*, *Paeonia lactiflora Pall*, *Scutelleria baicalensis Georgi*, and *Ziziphus jujuba Mill.* Cheng and his research team had provided lots of scientific evidences for the use of PHY906. Preclinical animal models were used to confirm that PHY906 could improve the effectiveness of conventional chemotherapies by attenuation of their systemic side effects.[29] By establishing both experimental and early-phase clinical trials, it was found that the combination of PHY906 and chemotherapeutic drug produced promising treatment outcomes in patients with advanced hepatocellular carcinoma (HCC), pancreatic cancer, and other gastrointestinal malignancies.[30] This is one of a few examples of herbal medicines that have obtained extensive scientific data and comprehensive platform to support its clinical use.

Identification of potential anti-cancer herbal medicinal compounds: The experience in the past decade

Because of the low response rate and high toxicity of orthodox anti-cancer drugs, there are increasing needs to acquire chemotherapeutic agents that have higher antitumor efficacy and reduced systemic side effects. Many herbal medicines contain a large amount of polysaccharides and thousands of phenolic and terpenoid compounds that have demonstrated anti-inflammatory and anti-carcinogenic properties in the gastrointestinal tract. Research studies in recent years have proven the use of herbal extracts and compounds that undergo antitumor activities. However, the precise mechanisms of actions underlying their pharmacological activities need to be unveiled to evaluate drug efficacy and safety. Several herbal mixtures and medicinal compounds have been tested in the past decade for their potential to be established as effective chemotherapeutic adjuvants in the treatment of gastrointestinal cancers.

Triptolide and pseudolaric acid B

Terpenoids from plant origin have demonstrated excellent antineoplastic functions by the suppression of tumor proliferation and induction of apoptosis. The diterpene triepoxide triptolide isolated from the herb *Tripterygium wilfordii* hook f. has received supporting evidences for being a potential antineoplastic agent. It was found that triptolide could inhibit the growth and metastasis of various solid tumors and is capable of acting synergistically with conventional chemotherapeutic drugs.[31] Pseudolaric acid B (PAB) is another natural diterpenoid extracted from the root bark of the tree

Pseudolarix kaempferi Gordon, which has been used in Chinese folk medicine for the treatment of fungal infections. Crude extract of the herb as well as purified PAB had both demonstrated potent cytotoxicity against several tumor cells, including those in the colon. It was proposed that the subtypes of the nuclear peroxisome proliferator-activated receptor (PPAR) are cellular targets of PAB in its action. Study had demonstrated that both triptolide and PAB induced growth inhibition and apoptosis in HT-29 colonic cancer cells, which were associated with cell cycle arrest at the G_2/M phase, modulation of cyclin expression, and downregulation of the proto-oncogene c-*myc*, with more pronounced and consistent effects being brought forth by PAB.[32] In addition, they also inhibited the expression of bcl-x_L and the resulting induction of caspase-3 activation together with cleavage of its substrate poly(ADP-ribose) polymerase (PARP). These events brought the promotion of apoptosis, which involved induction of the proapoptotic protein non-steroidal anti-inflammatory drug (NSAID)-activated gene (NAG-1) along with cyclooxygenase-2 inhibition. Nevertheless, due to the high toxicity in the human body and the narrow therapeutic index of triptolide, the comparatively safer drug PAB would have a higher value for further development in prospective study as effective antitumor adjuvant.

Herbal isoprenoids

Isoprenoids belong to a large and diverse class of naturally occurring organic chemicals similar to terpenes that are derived from five-carbon isoprene units assembled and modified in many ways. They play a certain role in traditional herbal remedies and are under investigation for antibacterial, antineoplastic, and other pharmaceutical effects. There are two main pathways for creating terpenoids: the mevalonic acid pathway and 2-C-methyl-D-erythritol 4-phosphate pathway. IPP, the common intermediate of two pathways, represents the activated building block for all other isoprenoids. Geranylgeraniol (GGOH; $C_{20}H_{34}O$), an acyclic isoprenoid, is the common precursor of all natural diterpenoids being biosynthesized via the terpenoid pathway, with the immediate precursor geranylgeranyl diphosphate. Sources of GGOH include the TCM herb *Munronia delavayi* Franch and byproducts from *Bixa orellana* seeds. Earlier studies had demonstrated pronounced apoptotic effects of GGOH in a variety of cancer cells. Farnesol (FOH; $C_{15}H_{26}O$), having three isoprene units, belongs to the family of sesquiterpenes. This 15-carbon isoprenoid alcohol is a naturally occurring phytochemical that exists in many flowers, leaves, and stems of plants, used in many Chinese traditional herbs and essential oils. It had been demonstrated that both FOH and GGOH could suppress growth and induce apoptosis in HT-29 and HCT 116 colon cancer cells by the modulation of various proapoptotic and antiapoptotic factors, including downregulation of the antiapoptotic proteins bcl-x_L and survivin.[33] Furthermore, it was also discovered that both FOH and GGOH markedly induced the transcriptional activation of peroxisome proliferator-activated receptor (PPAR)γ in a comparable way to that produced by the PPARγ ligand rosiglitazone. However, the use of a PPARγ antagonist GW9662 could not reverse the GGOH-induced growth inhibition and proapoptotic action as in the case of FOH-treated cells. It then recalls the fact that FOH had once been identified as a central regulatory component in the convergent effect of PPAR and RXR that leads to hepatocarcinogenesis.[34] Based on the above results, it appears that there is unique involvement of PPARγ in FOH-induced apoptosis, which does not seem to be a common effect of all isoprenoids.

Licorice and isoliquiritigenin

Licorice, the powder form of the dried root or rhizome of the European plant *Glycyrrhiza glabra* L. or the Chinese herb *Glycyrrhiza uralensis* Fisch., belongs to a member of legume and has been used both in Asia and Western countries since ancient times. Cytotoxic and radical scavenging activities of glycyrrhizae radix extract had been reported.[35] Essential constituents of licorice root include triterpenoids, such as glycyrrhizin and its aglycone glycyrrhizic acid, various polyphenols, and polysaccharides. Among these, glycyrrhizic acid (made up of 4–20% of the root) consists of a glucuronic acid moiety attached to a steroid-like triterpenoid glycyrrhetinic acid, which could be responsible for their antioxidation and anti-inflammatory effects. Beside its mild estrogenic effects, glycyrrhizin also facilitates the production of hormones such as hydrocortisone and inhibits COX-2, which may further explain its anti-inflammatory and anti-carcinogenic properties. Both licorice root and glycyrrhizin modulate immune activity and were found to induce interferon production. Glycyrrhizin had been reported to stimulate host resistance against solid tumors as well as to inhibit colon tumor cell activity.[36] Other than glycyrrhizin, about 300 different polyphenols (made up of about 5% of the root) also possess antioxidative ability and have antitumor potential. Many of them are flavonoids and isoflavonoids. Glabridine, a major isoflavan in licorice root, had been shown to possess some estrogen-like activities and a strong antiproliferative property in human breast cancer cells.

Isoliquiritigenin (2′,4′,4′-3-hydroxychalcone, $C_{15}H_{12}O_4$, ISL) is one of the natural flavonoids isolated from licorice. In the past, the main focus of research in licorice resided in glycyrrhizin, but recently ISL has received more attention in different therapeutic areas. It is known for its anti-inflammatory, anti-carcinogenic, and antihistaminic effects. It is recently used as an experimental drug for cancer treatment due to its pro-inflammatory and antioxidant properties, as well as the ability to suppress key intracellular enzymes and signaling cascades. In 2004, Takahashi had reported the inhibition of aberrant crypt foci development and a possible apoptotic effect of ISL via the reduction of prostaglandin E_2 and nitric oxide.[37] ISL can effectively suppress tumor cell proliferation, migration, and tube formation in human endothelial hybridoma (EAhy926) cells *in vitro*. Besides, it can also suppress tumor angiogenesis, specifically via the downregulation of mTOR-dependent VEGF production by adenoid cystic carcinoma cells, with concurrent activation of c-Jun NH2-terminal kinase and inhibition of extracellular signal-regulated kinase (ERK).[38] In a study, ISL had shown anti-carcinogenic activities in HCT 116 human colon cancer cells via promotion of caspase-dependent apoptosis and inhibition of cell growth, which was contributed by downregulation of the Bcl-2 family of antiapoptotic proteins.[39] It could also act by facilitation of G2 phase cycle arrest through the induction of a novel proapoptotic protein NAG-1 by upregulation of its upstream transcription factor EGR-1. In a pilot study, ISL had demonstrated significant growth inhibition in human pancreatic PANC-1 cells in a concentration-dependent manner. Its mode of action involves a dual stimulation of apoptosis and autophagy in the cancer cells. Isobologram analysis also indicated that combined treatment of ISL with other chemotherapeutic adjuvants such as the mTOR inhibitor rapamycin would generate synergistic effect. These findings have provided enough evidence to support ISL as the next generation of effective anti-cancer agent in treating gastrointestinal cancers.

Astragalus membranaceus and AST

Radix Astragali, the processed root of the plant *Astragalus membranaceus*, has a long history of medicinal use in Chinese herbal medicine. It is commonly used as an immunomodulating agent in mixed herbal decoctions to treat a variety of human diseases. In recent years, Radix astragalus has also been used to ameliorate the side effects of cytotoxic antineoplastic drugs. The active pharmacological constituents of *Astragalus membranaceus* include various polysaccharides, saponins, and flavonoids. Among the Astragalus saponins (AST), astragaloside IV, the quantitative marker of the herb, could increase murine B- and T-cell proliferation and thus received most attention.

It had been demonstrated that radix Astragali possesses strong anti-inflammatory action against the development of experimental colitis through inhibition of oxidants and adhesion molecules[40] as well as modulation of pro-inflammatory cytokines.[41] In recent years, investigation of the anti-carcinogenic properties of total AST in human gastrointestinal cancer cells and tumor xenograft, especially of the colon, had been focused (Table 3). It was first discovered that AST could inhibit cell proliferation through phase-specific cell cycle arrest and caspase-dependent apoptosis.[42] The reduction of tumor volume as well as proapoptotic and antiproliferative effects in HT-29 nude mice xenograft are comparable to that produced by 5-FU. In addition, the side effects associated with the drug combo 5-FU and oxaliplatin could be alleviated by AST. These results indicate that AST could be an effective chemotherapeutic agent in colon cancer treatment, which might also be used as an adjuvant in combination with other orthodox chemotherapeutic drugs to reduce the side effects of the latter compounds. Subsequent study using multiple human cancer cells has shown a universal growth-inhibitory and proapoptotic effects of AST in seven cell lines, including those of the colon, stomach, and liver. A strong correlation with the PI3K-Akt signaling pathway during the anti-cancer effects of AST had been proposed.[43] This information provides evidence that AST can be developed into a novel target-specific chemotherapeutic adjuvant with a known molecular mechanism. Other than colon cancer cells, anti-carcinogenic effects of AST have also exemplified in HepG2 hepatocellular carcinoma (HCC), with down-regulation of the HCC tumor marker α-fetoprotein through modulation of an ERK-independent NF-κB signaling.[44] In addition, it has been shown that AST could boost the effects of the microtubule inhibitor vinblastine on

Table 3. Anticancer mechanisms of herbal compounds/phytochemicals.

Herbal compound/ phytochemical	Anticancer mechanism	Cancer cell type
Triptolide/PAB (Diterpenoid)	• Growth inhibition • Apoptosis • Cell cycle arrest (modulation of cyclins) • Inhibition of c-myc expression • Inhibit caspase 3 activation and PARP cleavage • Inhibition of bcl-xL • NAG-1 induction • COX-2 inhibition	HT-29 (colon)
GGOH/FOH (Isoprenoids)	• Growth inhibition • Apoptosis • Inhibition of bcl-xL and survivin • PPAR activation (GGOH ??)	HT-29, HCT116 (colon)
ISL (Isoflavonoid)	• Growth inhibition • Apoptosis • Cell cycle arrest • Inhibit caspase 3 activation and PARP cleavage • Inhibition of bcl-xL and bcl-2 • NAG-1 induction • Synergistic effect with mTOR inhibitor rapamycin	HCT116 (colon) PANC-1 (pancreatic)

(Continued)

Table 3. (*Continued*)

Herbal compound/ phytochemical	**Anticancer mechanism**	**Cancer cell type**
AST (Saponins)	• Growth inhibition • Inhibition of colony formation • Apoptosis • Cell cycle arrest, inhibit cell proliferation • Inhibit caspase 3 activation and PARP cleavage • Inhibition of bcl-xL and bcl-2, induce cleavage of bid • Increase Bax expression • NAG-1 induction • Downregulate α-fetoprotein • Modulate NF-κB and IFN-β • Regulate PI3K-Akt-mTOR and MAPK pathways • COX-2 inhibition • Regulate ER stress and oxidative stress in the tumor microenvironment • Inhibition of angiogenesis and pro-angiogenic factors • Inhibition of invasiveness and migration and metastatic factors • Regulation of calpains, glucose-regulated proteins and calcium homeostasis • Synergistic effect with orthodox drugs 5-FU/oxaliplatin • Synergistic effect with inhibitors of PI3K, Akt and mTOR • Potentiate anticancer effect of the microtubule inhibitor vinblastine • Attenuate hematological toxicities of orthodox drugs • Enhance cytokine production in human peripheral blood mononuclear cells	HT-29, HCT116, DLD-1, LoVo (colon) AGS, MKN45 (gastric) HepG2 (liver)

colon tumor progression, including growth inhibition, cell proliferation, apoptotic activity, and antiangiogenesis in nude mice.[45] Treatment with the chemotherapeutic drug like 5-FU or the adjuvant vinblastine suppresses the immune system of Balb/c mice as observed by reduced white blood cell count and decreased hematocrit. Nonetheless, the combination of AST with 5-FU or vinblastine could reverse these hematologic toxicities. Additional experiments were performed to test the differential actions of AST on the viability of human leukemic cell lines and normal human peripheral blood mononuclear cells (PBMC). Results indicate that AST induces growth inhibition in the promyelocytic leukemic cell HL-60 and T-lymphocyte leukemic Jurkat cells, while no cytotoxic effect has been observed in normal human PBMC.[46] It was further demonstrated that AST could enhance the production of Th1 cytokines IFN-γ, IL-12, and TNF-α in human PBMC.

AST is capable of controlling the invasive behavior of LoVo, the metastatic colon cancer cell. Following this exciting discovery, the gene profile of HCT 116 colon adenocarcinoma cells following AST treatment had been displayed. By using a customized cDNA array, it was found that AST increases the gene expression of IFN-β and modulates the expression of a series of molecules that are related to angiogenesis.[47] These include upregulation of the inhibitor of angiogenesis as well as downregulation of both pro-angiogenic factors and genes that facilitate metastasis and invasion. Based on these results, it becomes evident that AST has significant effects on angiogenesis, tumor invasiveness, and metastasis. In order to further study the antimetastatic potential of AST *in vivo*, a modified liver metastasis model has been employed. After 35 days of intrasplenic injection of 2×10^6 LoVo cells in nude mice, a large cluster of tumor mass has been formed on both left and right liver lobes. In AST-treated animals, the size of the tumor mass has been reduced by more than 85%. It is the first time when the anti-invasive and antiangiogenic potential of AST was observed in AGS gastric adenocarcinoma cells.[48] Under $CoCl_2$ mimicked hypoxia, it was demonstrated that the oxidative stress-induced HIF-1α and VEGF expression in HCT 116 cells could be attenuated by AST and the effect was intensified with the cotreatment of rapamycin, a mTOR inhibitor.[49] These findings further confirm that AST may modulate tumor progression in colon cancer cells by inhibiting the angiogenic factors and invasion-related promoters. Glucose-regulated proteins (GRP) are induced to promote tumor survival, metastasis, and drug resistance. Recent findings have exemplified that calpains play a permissive role in the modulation of GRP78 and consequent regulation of ER stress-induced apoptosis caused by AST in the cancer microenvironment.[50]

Despite the vigorous research on AST, we are also interested to know if other Astragalus constituents may possess similar antitumorigenic activity as its saponins counterpart and can be used to treat human colon cancer. Dietary flavonoids are commonly found in a wide variety of plants, fruits, vegetables, and medicinal herbs. Many of them have been known to possess beneficial effects in the human body due to their antioxidative, tumor growth-inhibitory, and proapoptotic activities. Contemporary research has reported the potential anti-carcinogenic actions of flavonoids such as quercetin, nobiletin, and luteolin in treating colorectal cancer. Data show that total Astragalus isoflavonoids and its major constituent formononetin could both inhibit the growth and promote apoptosis of HCT 116 colon cancer cells.[39] These processes were accompanied by caspase activation and downregulation of the antiapoptotic proteins Bcl-2 and Bcl-x_L. Like ISL, the novel proapoptotic protein NAG-1 and its upstream regulator EGR-1 were also overexpressed in formononetin-treated cells. However, a close comparison between the growth-inhibitory and proapoptotic powers of Astragalus isoflavonoids and formononetin with AST indicate that AST remains a more efficacious anti-cancer agent with a diversified mechanism of action,[47] which could be developed further as a chemotherapeutic adjuvant. Other functional Astragalus flavonoids such as calycosin are currently under active investigation.

Conclusion

This book chapter provides concise accounts of the possible adverse effects of herbal medicinal compounds and cases of herb–drug interactions, as well as to display the prospects of using phytochemicals in the treatment of human cancers through various experimental works. The knowledge of the facts and principles behind the "Yin" and "Yang" of herbal medicines is essential for further development of effective phytochemicals into potential chemotherapeutic adjuvants. The low therapeutic index and increased drug resistance of conventional chemotherapeutic agents are the two major challenges that oncologists now urgently need to tackle with. The high accommodative power of herbal medicinal compounds by the human body and their relatively low toxicity make them suitable alternatives in contemporary cancer therapy. PHY906 is a good example to show how an effective traditional herbal remedy can be developed as cancer therapeutics by providing enough scientific evidence through experimental studies and well-designed randomized clinical trials. From our ongoing research, it is known that there are many functional phytochemicals derived from herbal source, including, but not exclusive to, flavonoids and terpenoids, that possess potential anti-carcinogenic activities through diversified but definite mechanisms of action. The identification of effective compounds from remedy like AST could enable us to establish prospective chemotherapeutic adjuvants in the treatment of human cancers that may synergistically work with conventional anti-cancer drugs.

References

1. J Doucet, P Chassagne, C Trivalle, I Landrin, MD Pauty, N Kadri, JF Menard, E Bercoff (1996) Drug-drug interactions related to hospital admissions in older adults: A prospective study of 1000 patients. *J Am Geriatr Soc* **44:** 944–948.
2. K Chan, L Cheung (2000) *Interactions Between Chinese Herbal Medicinal Products and Orthodox Drugs.* Singapore: Harwood Academic Publishers.
3. UM Zanger, M Schwab (2013) Cytochrome P450 enzymes in drug metabolism: Regulation of gene expression, enzyme activities, and impact of genetic variation. *Pharmacol Ther* **138:** 103–141.
4. C Colalto (2010) Herbal interactions on absorption of drugs: Mechanisms of action and clinical risk assessment. *Pharmacol Res* **62:** 207–227.
5. U Werneke, J Earl, C Seydel, O Horn, P Crichton, D Fannon (2004) Potential health risks of complementary alternative medicines in cancer patients. *Br J Cancer* **90:** 408–413.
6. H Gutmann, B Poller, KB Buter, A Pfrunder, W Schaffner, J Drewe (2006) Hypericum perforatum: Which constituents may induce intestinal MDR1 and CYP3A4 mRNA expression? *Planta Med* **72:** 685–690.
7. BJ Komoroski, RA Parise, MJ Egorin, SC Strom, R Venkataramanan (2005) Effect of the St. John's wort constituent hyperforin on docetaxel metabolism by human hepatocyte cultures. *Clin Cancer Res* **11:** 6972–6979.
8. J Hokkanen, A Tolonen, S Mattila, M Turpeinen (2011) Metabolism of hyperforin, the active constituent of St. John's wort, in human liver microsomes. *Eur J Pharm Sci* **42:** 273–284.

9. TS Hansen, OG Nilsen (2008) In vitro CYP3A4 metabolism: Inhibition by *Echinacea purpurea* and choice of substrate for the evaluation of herbal inhibition. *Basic Clin Pharmacol Toxicol* **103:** 445–449.
10. LB Moore, B Goodwin, SA Jones, GB Wisely, CJ Serabjit-Singh, TM Willson, JL Collins, SA Kliewer (2000) St. John's wort induces hepatic drug metabolism through activation of the pregnane X receptor. *Proc Natl Acad Sci USA* **97:** 7500–7502.
11. RH Mathijssen, J Verweij, P de Bruijn, WJ Loos, A Sparreboom (2002) Effects of St. John's wort on irinotecan metabolism. *J Natl Cancer Inst* **94:** 1247–1249.
12. RF Frye, SM Fitzgerald, TF Lagattuta, MW Hruska, MJ Egorin (2004) Effect of St John's wort on imatinib mesylate pharmacokinetics. *Clin Pharmacol Ther* **76:** 323–329.
13. AK Goey, KD Mooiman, JH Beijnen, JH Schellens, I Meijerman (2013) Relevance of in vitro and clinical data for predicting CYP3A4-mediated herb–drug interactions in cancer patients. *Cancer Treat Rev* **39:** 773–783.
14. AK Yang, SM He, L Liu, JP Liu, MQ Wei, SF Zhou (2010) Herbal interactions with anticancer drugs: Mechanistic and clinical considerations. *Curr Med Chem* **17:** 1635–1678.
15. D Durr, B Stieger, GA Kullak-Ublick, KM Rentsch, HC Steinert, PJ Meier, K Fattinger (2000) St John's Wort induces intestinal P-glycoprotein/MDR1 and intestinal and hepatic CYP3A4. *Clin Pharmacol Ther* **68:** 598–604.
16. GK Dresser, UI Schwarz, GR Wilkinson, RB Kim (2003) Coordinate induction of both cytochrome P4503A and MDR1 by St John's wort in healthy subjects. *Clin Pharmacol Ther* **73:** 41–50.
17. MZ Liu, YL Zhang, MZ Zeng, FZ He, ZY Luo, JQ Luo, JG Wen, XP Chen, HH Zhou, W Zhang (2015) Pharmacogenomics and herb-drug interactions: Merge of future and tradition. *Evid Based Comp Altern Med* **2015:** 321091.
18. S Hori, I Mihaylov, JC Vasconcelos, M McCoubrie (2008) Patterns of complementary and alternative medicine use amongst outpatients in Tokyo, Japan. *BMC Comp Altern Med* **8:** 14.
19. L Teng, K Jin, K He, C Bian, W Chen, K Fu, T Zhu, Z Jin (2010) Use of complementary and alternative medicine by cancer patients at Zhejiang University Teaching Hospital Zhuji Hospital, China. *Afr J Trad Comp Altern Med* **7:** 322–330.
20. X Li, G Yang, X Li, Y Zhang, J Yang, J Chang, X Sun, X Zhou, Y Guo, Y Xu, J Liu, A Bensoussan (2013) Traditional Chinese medicine in cancer care: A review of controlled clinical studies published in Chinese. *PLoS One* **8:** e60338.

21. SH Liu, WC Chuang, W Lam, Z Jiang, YC Cheng (2015) Safety surveillance of traditional Chinese medicine: Current and future. *Drug Safety* **38:** 117–128.
22. K Palmer (2004) Indications for anti-reflux surgery and endoscopic anti-reflux procedures. *Aliment Pharmacol Ther* **20** (Suppl 8)**:** 32–35.
23. D Shaw (2010) Toxicological risks of Chinese herbs. *Planta Med* **76:** 2012–2018.
24. CH Chen, KG Dickman, CY Huang, M Moriya, CT Shun, HC Tai, KH Huang, SM Wang, YJ Lee, AP Grollman, YS Pu (2013) Aristolochic acid-induced upper tract urothelial carcinoma in Taiwan: Clinical characteristics and outcomes. *Int J Cancer* **133:** 14–20.
25. S Debbie, L Graeme, D Pierre, W Elizabeth, K Chan (2012) Pharmacovigilance of herbal medicine. *J Ethnopharmacol* **140:** 513–518.
26. L Zhang, J Yan, X Liu, Z Ye, X Yang, R Meyboom, K Chan, D Shaw, P Duez (2012) Pharmacovigilance practice and risk control of Traditional Chinese Medicine drugs in China: Current status and future perspective. *J Ethnopharmacol* **140:** 519–525.
27. QY Zhang, WH Zhao, YJ Lai (2005) [Effect on late-stage mammary cancer treated by endocrinotherapy or chemotherapy combined with pingxiao capsule]. *Zhongguo Zhong Xi Yi Jie He Za Zhi* **25:** 1074–1076 (in Chinese).
28. Y Sun, H Lin, Y Zhu, J Feng, Z Chen, G Li, X Zhang, Z Zhang, J Tang, M Shi, X Hao, H Han (2006) [A randomized, prospective, multi-centre clinical trial of NP regimen (vinorelbine+cisplatin) plus Ginseng Rg3 in the treatment of advanced non-small cell lung cancer patients]. *Zhongguo Fei Ai Za Zhi* **9:** 254–258 (in Chinese).
29. W Lam, S Bussom, F Guan, Z Jiang, W Zhang, EA Gullen, SH Liu, YC Cheng (2010) The four-herb Chinese medicine PHY906 reduces chemotherapy-induced gastrointestinal toxicity. *Sci Transl Med* **2:** 45ra59.
30. MW Saif, F Lansigan, S Ruta, L Lamb, M Mezes, K Elligers, N Grant, ZL Jiang, SH Liu, YC Cheng (2010) Phase I study of the botanical formulation PHY906 with capecitabine in advanced pancreatic and other gastrointestinal malignancies. *Phytomedicine* **17:** 161–169.
31. S Yang, J Chen, Z Guo, XM Xu, L Wang, XF Pei, J Yang, CB Underhill, L Zhang (2003) Triptolide inhibits the growth and metastasis of solid tumors. *Mol Cancer Ther* **2:** 65–72.
32. JKS Ko, WC Leung, WK Ho, P Chiu (2007) Herbal diterpenoids induce growth arrest and apoptosis in colon cancer cells with increased expression of the nonsteroidal anti-inflammatory drug-activated gene. *Eur J Pharmacol* **559:** 1–13.

33. KK Auyeung, P Liu, C Chan, W Wu, SS Lee, JKS Ko (2008) Herbal isoprenols induce apoptosis in human colon cancer cells through transcriptional activation of PPARγ. *Cancer Invest* **26:** 708–717.
34. N Takahashi, T Kawada, T Goto, T Yamamoto, A Taimatsu, N Matsui, K Kimura, M Saito, M Hosokawa, K Miyashita, T Fushiki (2002) Dual action of isoprenols from herbal medicines on both PPARgamma and PPARalpha in 3T3-L1 adipocytes and HepG2 hepatocytes. *FEBS Lett* **514:** 315–322.
35. Y Nemoto, K Satoh, K Toriizuka, Y Hirai, T Tobe, H Sakagami, H Nakashima, Y Ida. Cytotoxic and radical scavenging activity of blended herbal extracts. *In Vivo* **16:** 327–332.
36. JG Chung, HL Chang, WC Lin, HH Wang, CC Yeh, CF Hung, YC Li (2000) Inhibition of N-acetyltransferase activity and DNA-2-aminofluorene adducts by glycyrrhizic acid in human colon tumour cells. *Food Chem Toxicol* **38:** 163–172.
37. T Takahashi, N Takasuka, M Iigo, M Baba, H Nishino, H Tsuda, T Okuyama (2004) Isoliquiritigenin, a flavonoid from licorice, reduces prostaglandin E2 and nitric oxide, causes apoptosis, and suppresses aberrant crypt foci development. *Cancer Sci* **95:** 448–453.
38. ZJ Sun, G Chen, W Zhang, X Hu, CF Huang, YF Wang, J Jia, YF Zhao (2010) Mammalian target of rapamycin pathway promotes tumor-induced angiogenesis in adenoid cystic carcinoma: Its suppression by isoliquiritigenin through dual activation of c-Jun NH2-terminal kinase and inhibition of extracellular signal-regulated kinase. *J Pharmacol Exp Ther* **334:** 500–512.
39. KKW Auyeung, JKS Ko (2010) Novel herbal flavonoids promote apoptosis but differentially induce cell cycle arrest in human colon cancer cell. *Invest New Drugs* **28:** 1–13.
40. JKS Ko, FYL Lam, APL Cheung (2005) Amelioration of experimental colitis by *Astragalus membranaceus* through anti-oxidation and inhibition of adhesion molecule synthesis. *World J Gastroenterol* **11:** 5787–5794.
41. JKS Ko, CWS Chik (2009) The protective action of *radix Astragalus membranaceus* against hapten-induced colitis through modulation of cytokines. *Cytokine* **47:** 85–90.
42. MMY Tin, CH Cho, K Chan, AE James, JKS Ko (2007) *Astragalus* saponins induce growth inhibition and apoptosis in human colon cancer cells and tumor xenograft. *Carcinogenesis* **28:** 1347–1355.
43. KK Auyeung, CH Cho, JKS Ko (2009) A novel anticancer effect of *Astragalus* saponins: Transcriptional activation of NSAID-activated gene. *Int J Cancer* **125:** 1082–1091.

44. KKW Auyeung, PC Law, JKS Ko (2009) *Astragalus* saponins induces apoptosis via an ERK-independent NF-κB signaling pathway in the human hepatocellular HepG2 cell line. *Int J Mol Med* **23:** 189–196.
45. KKW Auyeung, PC Law, JKS Ko (2014) Combined therapeutic effects of vinblastine and Astragalus saponins (AST) in human colon cancer cells and tumor xenograft via inhibition of tumor growth and proangiogenic factors. *Nutr Cancer* **66:** 662–674.
46. LC Zheng, TJ Ren, HB Chen, JKS Ko, & KKW Auyeung (2016) Astragalus saponins inhibits lipopolysaccharide-induced inflammation in mouse macrophages. *Am J Chin Med*, in press.
47. KKW Auyeung, Q Han, JKS Ko (2016) Astragalus membranaceus: A review of its protection against inflammation and gastrointestinal cancers. *Am J Chin Med* **44:** 1–22.
48. KKW Auyeung, PK Woo, PC Law, JKS Ko (2012) Astragalus saponins modulate cell invasiveness and angiogenesis in human gastric adenocarcinoma cells. *J Ethnopharmacol* **141:** 635–641.
49. KKW Auyeung, PC Law, LY Chan, JKS Ko (2012) Astragalus saponins downregulate hypoxia-induced VEGF induction in colon cancer cells. *BMC Comp Altern Med* **12:** 160.
50. Y Wang, KKW Auyeung, X Zhang, JKS Ko (2014) AST modulates colon cancer development by regulating calpain-mediated glucose-regulated protein expression. *BMC Comp Altern Med* **14:** 401.

Chapter 13

The Degradation System of Prostaglandin E_2 in Gastrointestinal Cancer

Tetsuya Tanigawa, Toshio Watanabe, Shogo Takeda, Hiroshi Tatsuwaki, Masatsugu Shiba, Kazunari Tominaga, Yasuhiro Fujiwara, and Tetsuo Arakawa

Abstract

Prostaglandin (PG) E_2 (PGE_2) promotes gastrointestinal carcinogenesis and tumor progression. The total amount of biologically active PGE_2 in tissues is determined by a balance between PG biosynthesis and degradation pathways. PGE_2 is transported out of and into cells by two transport proteins: multidrug resistance-associated protein 4 and PG transporter, respectively, which modulate PGE_2 signaling by increasing or decreasing the levels of PGE_2 available to cells, respectively. In the cytoplasm, 15-hydroxyprostaglandin dehydrogenase metabolizes PGE_2 and thereby inactivates its biological function. The purpose of this chapter is to summarize recent advances in the understanding of the importance of the PGE_2 transport system and degradation pathways in gastrointestinal tumor biology, with an emphasis on the roles of the relevant proteins in gastric adenocarcinomas.

Introduction

Prostaglandins (PGs), synthesized by cyclooxygenase (COX) from arachidonic acid liberated from membrane phospholipids, have a variety of biological functions. In gastrointestinal carcinogenesis and tumor progression, PGs, especially PGE_2, play important roles in tumor cell proliferation, inhibition of apoptosis, tumor angiogenesis, and immunosuppression.[1] Much attention to clarify the significance of PGE_2 in gastrointestinal tumors has been paid on the COX-2 enzyme, an inducible isoform of COX. The overexpression of COX-2 has been detected in many solid tumors, including gastric cancer, in clinical studies, and epidemiological studies have shown that COX inhibitors, such as aspirin and non-steroidal anti-inflammatory drugs (NSAIDs), have antitumor effects.[2–5] Although NSAIDs and aspirin show preventive activity against a variety of carcinogenesis and tumor progression, the long-term use of these drugs is known to increase the risk of severe adverse effects such as gastrointestinal mucosal injury and bleeding.[6–8] Therefore, new therapeutic and chemopreventive targets need to be identified in this oncogenic pathway for further advance in therapy and chemoprevention against gastrointestinal cancer.

The transporter and degradation enzyme of PGE_2 regulate the intracellular and extracellular levels of PGE_2 available for cell signaling. Multidrug resistance-associated protein 4 (MRP4) and PG transporter (PGT) modulate PGE_2 signaling by respectively increasing or decreasing the levels of extracellular PGE_2 available to cells. 15-hydroxyprostaglandin dehydrogenase (15-PGDH) metabolizes PGE_2 into an inactive form, 15-keto PGE_2, and terminates the signaling pathway (Figure 1). This chapter summarizes the current knowledge about the PGE_2 transport and degradation system in relation to gastrointestinal tumor biology, with a focus on our more limited understanding of the role of PGT and 15-PGDH in gastric cancer and our recent research.

Multidrug Resistance-Associated Protein 4 (MRP4)

This protein is the fourth member of the C subfamily of ATP-binding cassette (ABC) proteins.[9] MRP4 was identified because of its role in the modulation of chemotherapeutic drug resistance in several tumor types. MRP4 exports a variety of exogenous compounds, including camptothecins,

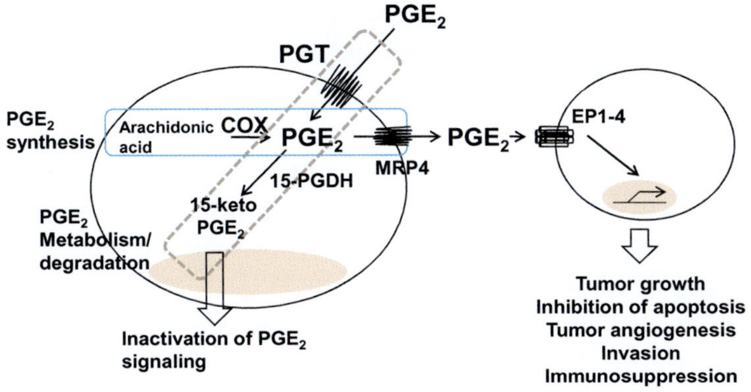

Figure 1. Degradation system of PGE_2 in gastrointestinal cancer. PG: prostaglandin, 15-PGDH: 15-hydroxyprostaglandin dehydrogenase, PGT: prostaglandin transporter, COX: cyclooxygenase, MRP4: multidrug resistance protein 4.

methotrexate, ceftins, and antiretroviral compounds, including anti-HIV compounds.[10,11] Endogenous substrates of MRP4 include PGs, leukotrienes, cyclic nucleotides (cAMP and cGMP), and glutathione-conjugated molecules such as bile acids and steroid hormones.[12]

The overexpression of MRP4 has been observed in several types of tumors, including neuroblastoma, prostate cancer, pancreatic cancer, and acute myeloid leukemia; this overexpression is associated with a poor prognosis.[11,12,13–15] It is possible that the alteration of expression or activity of MRP4 in gastrointestinal cancer affects the tumorigenic effect of PGE_2 via an increase in PGE_2 concentration in the extracellular environment.[12,16]

Prostaglandin Transporter (PGT)

Although PGE_2 is non-specifically exported to the extracellular space via MRP4, this PG is imported from the extracellular environment into the cytoplasm by a specific transporter, that is, PGT.[17] The latter is also known as a solute carrier organic anion transporter family member 2A1 (*SLCO2A1*).[17] PGT functions as an antiporter for PGE_2, $PGF_2\alpha$, and PGD_2 by exchanging a lactate anion, which is negatively charged at physiological pH.[18] Importing PGE_2 from the pericellular into intracellular space attenuates PGE_2-dependent signaling by preventing PGE_2 from binding to E prostanoid (EP) receptors on the cell surface. Several studies suggest the importance of PGT in physiological conditions. It is reported that mutations in the *SLCO2A1* gene, which encodes PGT, are associated with the pathogenesis of chronic non-specific multiple ulcers of the small intestine,[19] primary hypertrophic osteoarthropathy,[20] and pachydermoperiostosis with myelofibrosis.[21] The hyperglycemia induce PGT expression in human dermal microvascular endothelial cells accompanied by impairment of its migration. PGT expression is also induced by wounding and diabetes *in vivo*.[22] The inhibition of PGT with T26A, a recently developed inhibitor of PGT, promotes wound healing in a dose-dependent manner.[22]

15-Hydroxyprostaglandin Dehydrogenase (15-PGDH)

This protein is a key prostaglandin-catabolic enzyme catalyzing the oxidation of the 15(S)-hydroxyl group of PGs, thus forming 15-keto-PGs, which show greatly reduced biological activities.[23] The regulation of 15-PGDH is important for the regulation of inflammation. The downregulation of 15-PGDH is observed in the inflamed colonic mucosa of patients with Crohn's disease and ulcerative colitis,[24] and a small-molecule inhibitor of 15-PGDH (SW033291) has been found to promote tissue regeneration in mouse models of inflammatory bowel disease.[25] After ultraviolet (UV) irradiation, elevated levels of PGs accompanied by the downregulation of 15-PGDH have been detected in human skin.[26] *Helicobacter pylori* (*H. pylori*)-positive gastric mucosa has two-fold lower 15-PGDH mRNA levels and significantly lesser 15-PGDH protein than *H. pylori*-negative samples.[27] PGE_2 plays an important role in the maintenance of gastrointestinal mucosal integrity and wound healing via several mechanisms including the regulation of gastrointestinal mucosal blood flow, enhancement of epithelial cell proliferation, synthesis of mucus, and immunosuppressive properties that contribute to the resolution phase of acute inflammation. The above findings suggest that the downregulation of 15-PGDH protects from tissue damage in some inflammatory conditions such as *H. pylori*-induced gastritis and inflammatory bowel diseases, but it may also be associated with inflammation-related carcinogenesis such as colitis- and *H. pylori*-induced gastrointestinal carcinogenesis.

Expression of 15-PGDH and PGT in Gastrointestinal Cancer and Its Significance

The gastrointestinal mucosa is a major source of PGE_2; therefore, it is logical that the constitutive expression of 15-PGDH and PGT maintains the cellular homeostasis of PGE_2 via the degradation of excess PGE_2. In the colonic mucosa and small intestinal mucosa, 15-PGDH and PGT are expressed in mucosal epithelial cells.[28] In our recent study, both 15-PGDH and PGT were found to be constitutively expressed, mainly in gastric mucosal epithelial cells and inflammatory cells in the lamina propria.[29,30]

Recent research showed that the downregulation of 15-PGDH is accompanied by an aggressive phenotype and unfavorable prognostic factors in breast cancer,[31] prostate cancer,[32] lung cancer,[33] bladder cancer,[34] esophageal cancer,[35] and medullary thyroid cancer.[36] In the gastrointestinal tract, the downregulation of 15-PGDH is observed in colorectal[37] and gastric cancers.[38,39] In our recent study, we found that the expression of 15-PGDH decreased in ~50% of the gastric adenocarcinomas examined and that the reduction in the 15-PGDH protein expression was correlated with the unfavorable prognosis of gastric adenocarcinoma.[29]

In contrast to 15-PGDH, limited information is available on PGT expression patterns in cancer. Holla *et al.* showed that the PGT expression in human colorectal cancer specimens is lower than the expression noted in the healthy mucosa.[40] Our recent study revealed that the downregulation of PGT relative to that in the healthy mucosa is observed in 32.3% of gastric adenocarcinomas and that the absence of detectable PGT expression is an independent negative prognostic factor.[30]

Biological Significance of Downregulation of 15-PGDH and PGT in Gastrointestinal Cancer

PGE_2 is closely involved in gastrointestinal carcinogenesis via the stimulation of cell migration, proliferation, inhibition of apoptosis, suppression of immune responses, and tumor-associated neovascularization with the inhibition of cell death.[1] Therefore, the significance of the downregulation of PGT and 15-PGDH is related to PGE_2-associated molecular carcinogenesis.

In our recent study, we demonstrated that the 15-PGDH expression is reduced in ~50% of the gastric adenocarcinomas examined and that the low expression of 15-PGDH is associated with the enhanced proliferation of cancer cells in tumor tissue, as was shown in an empirical study on a gastric cancer cell line.[29] In line with our findings, it was reported that the overexpression of 15-PGDH via transfection of a plasmid encoding 15-PGDH suppresses cell growth in glioblastoma[41] and in a breast cancer cell line.[31] The knockdown of the *15-PGDH* gene markedly sensitizes normally resistant C57BL/6J mice to colon tumor induction by azoxymethane.[42] The knockdown of 15-PGDH by small interfering RNA stimulates the proliferation of human medullary thyroid carcinoma[36] and breast cancer cells,[31] increases motility of bladder cancer cells,[34] and promotes cell cycle entry of breast cancer cells.[31]

We also showed that PGT is an independent prognostic factor of poor survival in gastric cancer, and that decreased PGT expression is associated with increased tumor angiogenesis in clinical samples obtained from patients with gastric adenocarcinoma.[30] In addition, we found that the downregulation of PGT in gastric cancer cells results in an increase in PGE_2-induced vascular endothelial growth factor (VEGF) production.[30] To confirm this result, we examined the expression patterns of PGT and VEGF in gastric tumor tissue and found that gastric adenocarcinomas with a reduced expression of PGT show an increased expression of VEGF; in contrast, in gastric adenocarcinomas with normal expression levels of PGT, the expression level of VEGF was relatively low immunohistochemically (Figure 2).

Regulation of PGT and 15-PGDH in Gastrointestinal Cancer

Epigenetic modulation

Genetic silencing by methylation or histone deacetylation of the *15-PGDH* promoter has been proposed as a possible mechanism underlying the reduced expression of 15-PGDH in human breast cancer.[31] Similarly, Thiel *et al.* also demonstrated that in a gastric cancer cell line which shows negligible 15-PGDH expression (TMK-1), the *15-PGDH* promoter was methylated, and that treatment with the demethylating agent 5-aza-2′-deoxycytidine restored 15-PGDH expression.[39]

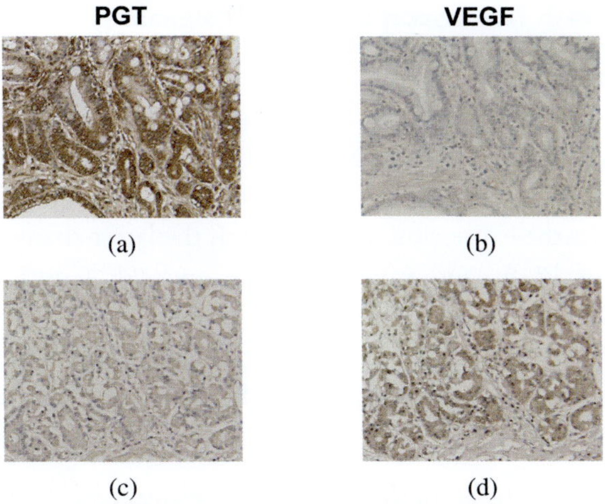

Figure 2. Relationships between the PGT expression and the VEGF expression in gastric adenocarcinoma tissues. (a) In tumor tissues with positive immunoreactivity for PGT protein, (b) immunoreactivity for VEGF protein is weak. In contrast, (c) in tumor tissues with negative immunoreactivity for PGT protein, (d) immunoreactivity for VEGF protein is strong. Original magnification, ×200.

As is the case for 15-PGDH, the expression of PGT is induced by treatment with 5-aza-2′-deoxycytidine and with the histone deacetylase inhibitor trichostatin A[40] in colorectal cancer cell lines in which the PGT expression is lower than that in healthy cells. These results indicate that the expression of 15-PGDH and PGT is suppressed in cancer via an epigenetic mechanism in a direct or indirect manner.

β-catenin

Aberrant *β*-catenin signaling is found in many solid tumors and contributes to proliferative and migratory phenotypes observed in aggressive cancers. Some reports indicate that the *β*-catenin signaling pathway decreases 15-PGDH[43] and PGT expression[28] in colorectal cancer. It has already been shown that the Wnt/*β*-catenin signaling pathway plays an important role in gastric adenocarcinomas.[44] Therefore, it is possible that the Wnt/*β*-catenin signaling pathway suppresses PGT expression in gastric adenocarcinomas.

Epidermal growth factor receptor (EGFR) signaling

Epidermal growth factor receptor (EGFR) signaling pathway is involved in pathophysiology of a variety of malignancies. The expression of EGFR is known to be associated with poor survival in patients with colorectal cancer[45] and breast cancer.[46] It is reported that the activation of the EGFR signaling pathway inhibits the expression of 15-PGDH; the latter change results in the upregulation of PGE_2 and cancer progression.[37,47,48] Consistently, EGFR tyrosine kinase inhibitor, erlotinib, upregulates the expression of 15-PGDH.[37,47,48] These results suggest that downregulation of 15-PGDH is involved in part in oncogenic effect of EGFR signaling pathway.

Transforming growth factor-β (TGF-β) signaling

TGF-β is a multifunctional cytokine that regulates diverse cellular processes, including proliferation, apoptosis, and differentiation. TGF-β is known as a tumor suppressor, and TGF-β signaling is commonly inactivated in colon cancers via mutations in type II receptor or in a downstream Smad signaling element. TGF-β is known to induce 15-PGDH in colon cancer cells[49] and lung adenocarcinoma cells.[50] These observations suggest that the tumor suppressor action of TGF-β is in part due to the upregulation of 15-PGDH.

Interleukin (IL)-1β

IL-1β is a key pro-inflammatory cytokine that has been implicated in gastric carcinogenesis.[51] Thiel *et al.* discovered that IL-1β downregulates 15-PGDH in gastric cancer cells.[39]

microRNAs

These are a group of small non-coding RNAs that modulate translation of genes by binding to specific sites in a target mRNA.

Lu *et al.* reported that miR-21 directly targets 15-PGDH and promotes cholangiocarcinoma growth.[52] Yao *et al.* showed that ω-3 polyunsaturated fatty acids (ω-3 PUFAs) upregulate 15-PGDH by inhibiting miR-26a and miR-26b possibly via the inhibition of c-myc — a transcription factor that regulates miR-26a/b expression — thereby contributing to ω-3 PUFA-induced inhibition of human cholangiocarcinoma cell growth.[53]

Perspectives

Accumulating evidence suggests that 15-PGDH and PGT are downregulated in cancer; these phenomena represent another mechanism of PGE_2-related gastrointestinal carcinogenesis aside from COX-2. Thus, 15-PGDH and PGT may act as tumor suppressors via inactivation of the oncogenic effect of PGE_2. Calcitriol[32], apricoxib[54], and ω-3 PUFAs[53] have already been proposed as chemopreventive agents for targeting 15-PGDH and PGT in cancer. Recent advances in this field indicate that these molecules could be prognostic biomarkers of gastrointestinal cancer and may serve as targets for the treatment and chemoprevention of PGE_2-related gastrointestinal cancers.

Acknowledgment

This work was supported by a grant-in-aid from the Japanese Society of Gastroenterology and grant-in-aid from the Ministry of Education, Science and Culture of Japan.

References

1. WK Wu, JJ Sung, CW Lee, J Yu, CH Cho (2010) Cyclooxygenase-2 in tumorigenesis of gastrointestinal cancers: An update on the molecular mechanisms. *Cancer Lett* **295**: 7–16.
2. H Ishikawa, M Mutoh, S Suzuki, S Tokudome, Y Saida, T Abe, *et al.* (2014) The preventive effects of low-dose enteric-coated aspirin tablets on the development of colorectal tumours in Asian patients: A randomised trial. *Gut* **63**: 1755–1759.
3. CC Abnet, ND Freedman, F Kamangar, MF Leitzmann, AR Hollenbeck, A Schatzkin (2009) Non-steroidal anti-inflammatory drugs and risk of gastric and oesophageal adenocarcinomas: Results from a cohort study and a meta-analysis. *Br J Cancer* **100**: 551–557.
4. AT Chan, S Ogino, CS Fuchs (2007) Aspirin and the risk of colorectal cancer in relation to the expression of COX-2. *New Engl J Med* **356**: 2131–2142.

5. J Cuzick, F Otto, JA Baron, PH Brown, J Burn, P Greenwald, *et al.* (2009) Aspirin and non-steroidal anti-inflammatory drugs for cancer prevention: An international consensus statement. *Lancet Oncol* **10**: 501–507.
6. DL Bhatt, J Scheiman, NS Abraham, EM Antman, FK Chan, CD Furberg, *et al.* (2008) ACCF/ACG/AHA 2008 expert consensus document on reducing the gastrointestinal risks of antiplatelet therapy and NSAID use. *Am J Gastroenterol* **103**: 2890–2907.
7. T Tanigawa, T Watanabe, Y Nadatani, K Otani, H Machida, H Okazaki, *et al.* (2011) Gastrointestinal bleeding after percutaneous coronary intervention. *Digestion* **83**: 153–160.
8. Y Nadatani, T Watanabe, T Tanigawa, M Sogawa, H Yamagami, M Shiba, *et al.* (2013) Incidence and risk factors of gastrointestinal bleeding in patients on low-dose aspirin therapy after percutaneous coronary intervention in Japan. *Scand J Gastroenterol* **48**: 320–325.
9. M Dean, A Rzhetsky, R Allikmets (2001) The human ATP-binding cassette (ABC) transporter superfamily. *Genome Res* **11**: 1156–1166.
10. FG Russel, JB Koenderink, R Masereeuw (2008) Multidrug resistance protein 4 (MRP4/ABCC4): A versatile efflux transporter for drugs and signalling molecules. *Trends Pharmacol Sci* **29**: 200–207.
11. T Huynh, MD Norris, M Haber, MJ Henderson (2012) ABCC4/MRP4: A MYCN-regulated transporter and potential therapeutic target in neuroblastoma. *Front Oncol* **2**: 178.
12. JI Fletcher, M Haber, MJ Henderson, MD Norris (2010) ABC transporters in cancer: More than just drug efflux pumps. *Nat Rev Cancer* **10**: 147–156.
13. A Rasmuson, A Kock, OM Fuskevag, B Kruspig, J Simon-Santamaria, V Gogvadze, *et al.* (2012) Autocrine prostaglandin E2 signaling promotes tumor cell survival and proliferation in childhood neuroblastoma. *PloS One* 7: e29331.
14. M Montani, T Hermanns, M Muntener, P Wild, T Sulser, G Kristiansen (2013) Multidrug resistance protein 4 (MRP4) expression in prostate cancer is associated with androgen signaling and decreases with tumor progression. *Virchows Arch* **462**: 437–443.
15. S Copsel, C Garcia, F Diez, M Vermeulem, A Baldi, LG Bianciotti, *et al.* (2011) Multidrug resistance protein 4 (MRP4/ABCC4) regulates cAMP cellular levels and controls human leukemia cell proliferation and differentiation. *J Biol Chem* **286**: 6979–6988.
16. L Chen, J Gu, L Xu, C Qu, Y Zhang, W Zhang (2014) RNAi-mediated silencing of ATP-binding cassette C4 protein inhibits cell growth in MGC80-3 gastric cancer cell lines. *Cell Mol Biol* (*Noisy-le-Grand*) **60**: 1–5.

17. VL Schuster (2002) Prostaglandin transport. *Prostaglandins Other Lipid Mediat* **68–69**: 633–647.
18. BS Chan, S Endo, N Kanai, VL Schuster (2002) Identification of lactate as a driving force for prostanoid transport by prostaglandin transporter PGT. *Am J Physiol Renal Physiol* **282**: F1097–1102.
19. J Umeno, T Hisamatsu, M Esaki, A Hirano, N Kubokura, K Asano, *et al.* (2015) A hereditary enteropathy caused by mutations in the SLCO2A1 gene, encoding a prostaglandin transporter. *PLoS Genet* **11**: e1005581.
20. Z Zhang, W Xia, J He, Z Zhang, Y Ke, H Yue, *et al.* (2012) Exome sequencing identifies SLCO2A1 mutations as a cause of primary hypertrophic osteoarthropathy. *Am J Hum Genet* **90**: 125–132.
21. CP Diggle, DA Parry, CV Logan, P Laissue, C Rivera, CM Restrepo, *et al.* (2012) Prostaglandin transporter mutations cause pachydermoperiostosis with myelofibrosis. *Hum Mutat* **33**: 1175–1181.
22. MM Syeda, X Jing, RH Mirza, H Yu, RS Sellers, Y Chi (2012). Prostaglandin transporter modulates wound healing in diabetes by regulating prostaglandin-induced angiogenesis. *Am J pathology* **181**: 334–346.
23. CM Ensor, HH Tai (1995) 15-Hydroxyprostaglandin dehydrogenase. *J Lipid Mediat Cell Signal* **12**: 313–319.
24. T Otani, K Yamaguchi, E Scherl, B Du, HH Tai, M Greifer, *et al.* (2006) Levels of NAD(+)-dependent 15-hydroxyprostaglandin dehydrogenase are reduced in inflammatory bowel disease: Evidence for involvement of TNF alpha. *Am J Physiol Gastrointest Liver Physiol* **290**: G361–368.
25. Y Zhang, A Desai, SY Yang, KB Bae, MI Antczak, SP Fink, *et al.* (2015) TISSUE REGENERATION. Inhibition of the prostaglandin-degrading enzyme 15-PGDH potentiates tissue regeneration. *Science* **348**: aaa2340.
26. BL Judson, A Miyaki, VD Kekatpure, B Du, P Gilleaudeau, M Sullivan-Whalen, *et al.* (2010) UV radiation inhibits 15-hydroxyprostaglandin dehydrogenase levels in human skin: Evidence of transcriptional suppression. *Cancer Prev Res* (*Phila*) **3**: 1104–1111.
27. YM Ryu, SJ Myung, YS Park, DH Yang, HJ Song, JY Jeong, *et al.* (2013) Inhibition of 15-hydroxyprostaglandin dehydrogenase by *Helicobacter pylori* in human gastric carcinogenesis. *Cancer Prev Res* (*Phila*) **6**: 349–359.
28. HJ Smartt, A Greenhough, P Ordonez-Moran, M Al-Kharusi, TJ Collard, JM Mariadason, *et al.* (2012) Beta-catenin negatively regulates expression of the prostaglandin transporter PGT in the normal intestinal epithelium and colorectal tumour cells: A role in the chemopreventive efficacy of aspirin? *Br J Cancer* **107**: 1514–1517.

29. H Tatsuwaki, T Tanigawa, T Watanabe, H Machida, H Okazaki, H Yamagami, *et al.* (2010) Reduction of 15-hydroxyprostaglandin dehydrogenase expression is an independent predictor of poor survival associated with enhanced cell proliferation in gastric adenocarcinoma. *Cancer Sci* **101**: 550–558.
30. S Takeda, T Tanigawa, T Watanabe, H Tatsuwaki, Y Nadatani, K Otani, *et al.* (2016) Reduction of prostaglandin transporter predicts poor prognosis associated with angiogenesis in gastric adenocarcinoma. *J Gastroentrol Hepatol* **31**: 376–383.
31. I Wolf, J O'Kelly, T Rubinek, M Tong, A Nguyen, BT Lin, *et al.* (2006) 15-hydroxyprostaglandin dehydrogenase is a tumor suppressor of human breast cancer. *Cancer Res* **66**: 7818–7823.
32. S Swami, AV Krishnan, J Moreno, RB Bhattacharyya, DM Peehl, D Feldman (2007) Calcitriol and genistein actions to inhibit the prostaglandin pathway: Potential combination therapy to treat prostate cancer. *J Nutr* **137**: 205s–210s.
33. Y Ding, M Tong, S Liu, JA Moscow, HH Tai (2005) NAD+-linked 15-hydroxyprostaglandin dehydrogenase (15-PGDH) behaves as a tumor suppressor in lung cancer. *Carcinogenesis* **26**: 65–72.
34. S Tseng-Rogenski, J Gee, KW Ignatoski, LP Kunju, A Bucheit, HJ Kintner, *et al.* (2010) Loss of 15-hydroxyprostaglandin dehydrogenase expression contributes to bladder cancer progression. *Am J Pathol* **176**: 1462–1468.
35. GT Yang, J Wang, TZ Xu, XF Sun, ZY Luan (2015) Expression of PGDH correlates with cell growth in both esophageal squamous cell carcinoma and adenocarcinoma. *Asian Pac J Cancer Prev* **16**: 997–1000.
36. V Quidville, N Segond, S Lausson, M Frenkian, R Cohen, A Jullienne (2006) 15-Hydroxyprostaglandin-dehydrogenase is involved in anti-proliferative effect of non-steroidal anti-inflammatory drugs COX-1 inhibitors on a human medullary thyroid carcinoma cell line. *Prostaglandins Other Lipid Mediat* **81**: 14–30.
37. MG Backlund, JR Mann, VR Holla, FG Buchanan, HH Tai, ES Musiek, *et al.* (2005) 15-Hydroxyprostaglandin dehydrogenase is down-regulated in colorectal cancer. *J Biol Chem* **280**: 3217–3223.
38. SH Seo, MS Kang, KH Kim, MS An, TK Ha, KB Bae, *et al.* (2015) Correlation of 15-prostagladin dehydrogenase expression with clinicopathological factors and survival rate in gastric adenocarcinoma. *Int J Surg* **13**: 96–101.
39. A Thiel, A Ganesan, J Mrena, S Junnila, A Nykanen, A Hemmes, *et al.* (2009) 15-hydroxyprostaglandin dehydrogenase is down-regulated in gastric cancer. *Clin Cancer Res* **15**: 4572–4580.
40. VR Holla, MG Backlund, P Yang, RA Newman, RN DuBois (2008) Regulation of prostaglandin transporters in colorectal neoplasia. *Cancer Prevent Res* **1**: 93–99.

41. N Wakimoto, I Wolf, D Yin, J O'Kelly, T Akagi, L Abramovitz, *et al.* (2008) Nonsteroidal anti-inflammatory drugs suppress glioma via 15-hydroxyprostaglandin dehydrogenase. *Cancer Res* **68**: 6978–6986.
42. SJ Myung, RM Rerko, M Yan, P Platzer, K Guda, A Dotson, *et al.* (2006) 15-Hydroxyprostaglandin dehydrogenase is an *in vivo* suppressor of colon tumorigenesis. *Proc Natl Acad Sci USA* **103**: 12098–12102.
43. HJ Smartt, A Greenhough, P Ordonez-Moran, E Talero, CA Cherry, CA Wallam, *et al.* (2012) beta-catenin represses expression of the tumour suppressor 15-prostaglandin dehydrogenase in the normal intestinal epithelium and colorectal tumour cells. *Gut* **61**: 1306–1314.
44. K Ganesan, T Ivanova, Y Wu, V Rajasegaran, J Wu, MH Lee, *et al.* (2008) Inhibition of gastric cancer invasion and metastasis by PLA2G2A, a novel beta-catenin/TCF target gene. *Cancer Res* **68**: 4277–4286.
45. A Mayer, M Takimoto, E Fritz, G Schellander, K Kofler, H Ludwig (1993) The prognostic significance of proliferating cell nuclear antigen, epidermal growth factor receptor, and mdr gene expression in colorectal cancer. *Cancer* **71**: 2454–2460.
46. DJ Slamon, W Godolphin, LA Jones, JA Holt, SG Wong, DE Keith, *et al.* (1989) Studies of the HER-2/neu proto-oncogene in human breast and ovarian cancer. *Science* **244**: 707–712.
47. L Yang, JM Amann, T Kikuchi, P Rorta, M Guix, A Gonzalez, *et al.* (2007) Inhibition of epidermal growth factor receptor signaling elevates 15-hydroxyprostaglandin dehydrogenase in non-small-cell lung cancer. *Cancer Res* **67**: 5587–5593.
48. JR Mann, MG Backlund, FG Buchanan, T Daikoku, VR Holla, DW Rosenberg, *et al.* (2006) Repression of prostaglandin dehydrogenase by epidermal growth factor and snail increases prostaglandin E2 and promotes cancer progression. *Cancer Res* **66**: 6649–6656.
49. M Yan, RM Rerko, P Platzer, D Dawson, J Willis, M Tong, *et al.* (2004) 15-Hydroxyprostaglandin dehydrogenase, a COX-2 oncogene antagonist, is a TGF-β-induced suppressor of human gastrointestinal cancers. *Proc Natl Acad Sci USA* **101**: 17468–17473.
50. M Tong, Y Ding, HH Tai (2006) Histone deacetylase inhibitors and transforming growth factor-beta induce 15-hydroxyprostaglandin dehydrogenase expression in human lung adenocarcinoma cells. *Biochem Pharmacol* **72**: 701–709.
51. EM El-Omar, M Carrington, WH Chow, KE McColl, JH Bream, HA Young, *et al.* (2000) Interleukin-1 polymorphisms associated with increased risk of gastric cancer. *Nature* **404**: 398–402.

52. L Lu, K Byrnes, C Han, Y Wang, T Wu (2014) miR-21 targets 15-PGDH and promotes cholangiocarcinoma growth. *Mol Cancer Res* **12**: 890–900.
53. L Yao, C Han, K Song, J Zhang, K Lim, T Wu (2015) Omega-3 polyunsaturated fatty acids upregulate 15-PGDH expression in cholangiocarcinoma cells by inhibiting miR-26a/b expression. *Cancer Res* **75**: 1388–1398.
54. MA St John, G Wang, J Luo, M Dohadwala, D Hu, Y Lin, *et al.* (2012) Apricoxib upregulates 15-PGDH and PGT in tobacco-related epithelial malignancies. *Br J Cancer* **107**: 707–712.

Chapter 14

Prostaglandin and Its Receptors: Potential Targets for Gastrointestinal Inflammation and Cancer

Vivian Y. Shin and Ava Kwong

Abstract

Prostaglandins (PGs) are critical mediators in inflammation and they also promote tumor cell proliferation, angiogenesis, and metastasis. Cyclooxygenase (COX) is an important component in the biosynthesis of PGs. It converts arachidonic acid to prostaglandin E_2 (PGE_2). On the one hand, constitutively expressed COX-1 was found in many tissues and it protects the gastrointestinal (GI) tract from mucosal injury. On the other hand, COX-2 was induced during inflammation and cancer progression. Preclinical and clinical studies have demonstrated that non-steroidal anti-inflammatory drugs and COX-2 inhibitors are promising therapeutic agents for GI cancer prevention and treatment. The prolonged use of COX-2 inhibitors, however, can cause renal and GI toxicities and increase cardiovascular risks. All these actions could limit their use as anti-cancer drugs. PGE_2 medicates its effect through binding to its receptors (EP1–EP4) that triggers different cellular signaling to incite tumor progression. This review recapitulates the important findings and signaling pathways of these EP receptors in inflammation and GI cancers; in particular, antagonism of

EP2 and EP4 receptors has been extensively studied *in vivo* and *in vitro* with encouraging results. They may serve as potential effective therapeutic agents in treating against GI cancers.

Introduction

Development of gastrointestinal (GI) cancers can be due to prolonged inflammation and genetic alternations. Activation of oncogenes and inactivation of tumor suppressor genes promote tumor growth through regulation of the cell cycle machinery. Cell proliferation and angiogenesis are important processes during tumorigenesis, in which activation of cyclooxygenase-2 (COX-2) and its downstream effectors mediate these events.[1,2] COX-2 and prostaglandins (PGs) have been extensively studied in their association with many solid tumors, and thus provides the rationale for the development of therapeutic compounds that suppress COX-2 expression. Non-steroidal anti-inflammatory drugs (NSAIDs) suppress PG production by inhibiting both COX-1 and COX-2 enzymes. Epidemiological studies revealed that there is an inverse correlation between the use of NSAIDs and incidence of colon cancer. Individuals who took NSAIDs had a 40% risk reduction of colorectal cancer than those who did not.[3] In view of the severe GI and renal toxicities upon long-term treatment with NSAIDs, selective COX-2 inhibitors have been developed to reduce GI complications. Treatment with selective COX-2 inhibitors improved the prognosis and clinical outcomes in patients with gastric and colon cancers. The incidence of new adenoma was significantly lowered in patients with selective COX-2 inhibitor than the control. However, there was an increase in cardiac disorders and renal/hypertension risk within 5 years of follow-up.[4] Despite the promising effects of NSAIDs or selective COX-2 inhibitors, various unwanted side effects (e.g. cardiovascular disorders and gastric ulceration) hindered the long-term use of these drugs.[5] Therefore, there is a pressing need for better alternatives for anti-inflammatory and anti-cancer drugs with fewer side effects. In recent years, many studies have been carried out to examine the efficacy of EP receptors as a potential drug target for inflammation and cancers. Preclinical studies demonstrated that EP receptors are implicated in tumorigenesis of GI cancers and other cancers. Therefore, antagonism of EP receptors has emerged as promising therapeutic targets for the development of anti-cancer agents in humans.

Cyclooxygenase (COX) metabolism

Prostaglandins (PGs) and leukotrienes are collectively termed eicosanoids, which contribute in many biological events such as inflammation, development, and cancer. Arachidonic acid (AA) is released from phospholipids from plasma membrane by phospholipase A_2. The biosynthesis of prostaglandins derived from AA by COX, lipoxygenase (LOX), and cytochrome P450 is illustrated in Figure 1. LOX enzymes (5-LOX, 8-LOX, 12-LOX, 15-LOX-1, and 15-LOX-2) convert AA into leukotrienes, lipoxins, and hydroxyeicosatetraenoic acids (HETEs). Cytochrome P450 pathway involves epoxygenases and ω-hydroxylases to form epoxyeicosatrienoic acid regioisomers and 20-HETE, respectively. COX enzymes (COX-1 and COX-2) convert AA into PGG_2 and then PGH_2. It is further converted into $PGF_{2\alpha}$, PGD_2, PGE_2, PGI_2, and thromboxane A_2 through different synthases. In particular, PGE synthase is responsible for the release of PGE_2 during inflammation and tumorigenesis. In response to stimuli, PGE_2 binds to its surface receptors to mediate various physiological effects. PGE_2 is the most abundant and

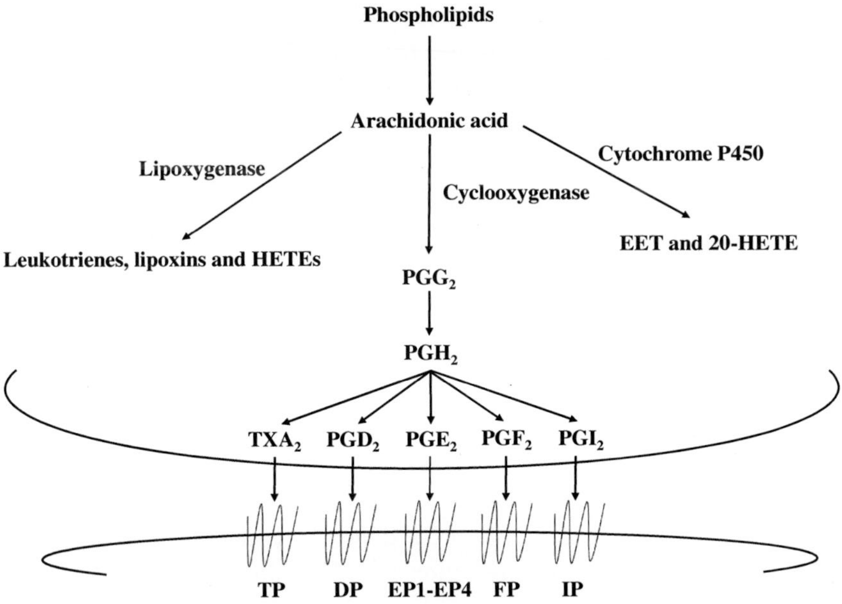

Figure 1. Biosynthesis of PGE_2.

well-studied PGs in human cancers, and yet both COX-2 expressed and PGE_2 levels are increased in most of the cancer tissues and cell lines; thus, targeting COX-2/PGE_2 pathway has been used in cancer therapy.

Roles of COX-2 in GI cancers

Chronic inflammation is one of the hallmarks of cancers particularly in GI cancers.[6] *Helicobacter pylori* infection is the major cause of inflammation in the gastric mucosa that leads to the development of gastric adenocarcinoma. *H. pylori* is classified as class I carcinogen by the World Health Organization and associated with increased risk of gastric cancer.[7] Enormous studies demonstrated that elevated COX-2 expression was induced by *H. pylori* to stimulate the release of PGE_2 for cell proliferation during gastric carcinogenesis. Intervention with celecoxib (a selective COX-2 inhibitor) decreased PGE_2 levels and delayed the progression of gastric carcinogenesis.[8] *H. pylori*-induced COX-2 expression has been positively correlated with signal transducer and activator of transcription 3 (STAT3) by binding to the COX-2 promoter, that contributed to poor prognosis in gastric cancer patients.[9] Crosstalk between epidermal growth factor receptor (EGFR) signaling and COX-2 activation was demonstrated in gastric epithelial cells and yet cag type IV secretion is crucial for the development of gastric cancer.[10] Many clinical studies reported that patients could benefit from NSAIDs with lower gastric cancer risk than those without NSAIDs.[11] Patients with precancerous lesions had a better regression in treatment with NSAIDs, implicating COX-2 is crucial in mediating gastric carcinogenesis.[12]

During inflammation, various pro-inflammatory cytokines (IL-1β, IL-8, IL-10, TNF, CSF) and growth factors (NF-κB, TGF-β, VEGFA, STAT3) are activated and trigger the synthesis of COX-2 in human tissues. The expression of COX-2 has been shown to be higher in colon cancer than normal tissues. This could contribute to tumor progression and metastasis. The recurrent rate of colon adenoma was greatly reduced in patients treated with NSAIDs in clinical trial.[13] Evidence showed that STAT3 induction during invasion and metastasis is in a COX-2 dependent manner.[14] However, the molecular mechanism of the interaction of COX-2 in inflammation-induced GI cancer is still undefined. Nevertheless, targeting COX-2 is a good candidate for chemoprevention of GI tumors.

NSAIDs are effective in suppression of COX activity and have been used in pain relief and inhibiting inflammation. By inhibiting both COX-1 and COX-2, the increased risk of cardiovascular events is one of the major drawbacks for long-term treatment with NSAIDs (VIOXX and BEXTRA). Selective COX-2 inhibitors are thereby developed to reduce the GI and other toxicities. Despite the promising antitumor effect of COX inhibitors, there is an urgent need for the other alternatives that target COX-2 pathway with smaller side effects. Indeed, PGE receptors are the downstream effectors of COX-2 pathway which is thought to be a better candidate and option for cancer treatment.[15]

PGE_2 signaling and its receptors

There are four distinct G-protein coupled plasma membrane receptors (EP1, EP2, EP3, and EP4). They participate in the PGE_2 signaling during the process of carcinogenesis.[16] The abundance of these receptors varied in different tissues or cell types, and the interaction with PGE_2 largely depends on its binding affinities. For example, EP1 and EP2 activation entail large amount of PGE_2 for mediation of cellular events, whereas EP3 and EP4 have a higher binding affinity to PGE_2. Activation of different receptors initiates different signaling cascades that lead to development of different disease states. EP2 and EP4 receptors activate PKA and GSK3β/β-catenin pathways through cAMP induction. Both EP1 and EP3 receptors increase intracellular Ca^{2+} through PKC and PLC, respectively.

EP1 receptor

Among the four EP receptors, EP1 receptor has the lowest binding affinity to PGE_2 and is activated when PGE_2 level is high. The contribution of EP1 receptor has been demonstrated in chemically induced colon malignancy in mice in which $EP1^{-/-}$ mice had a reduction in tumor formation. Similarly, the incidence of colon adenocarcinoma was also decreased when mice were treated with ONO-8711 (EP1 antagonist).[17] In addition, blockade of EP1 receptor showed similar tumor suppressive effect in breast and skin cancers.[18,19] The activation of EP1 receptor promoted cell invasion and migration with the induction of integrin expression. Another study showed that

EP1 receptor interacted with EGFR signaling and PKC pathway to initiate cell proliferation and migration. It is noted that survivin has been implicated in many cancers and associated with prognosis and recurrence. Previous study demonstrated that EP1 receptor agonist (17-P-T-PGE_2) upregulated survivin expression and increased EGFR and Akt phosphorylation.[20] The expression of EP1 receptor has been correlated with the ER status in breast cancer, which determines the management of such cancer. The use of EP1 antibody had a slight improvement in the sensitivity as SP2 antibody in determination of ER status, which could be an alternative for immunostaining in the clinical setting.[21]

Retinoic acid, an active metabolite of vitamin A, exhibits antitumor activities in colon cancer by inhibiting cell proliferation and inducing apoptosis through the suppression of COX-2 and EP1/EP4 receptors in cell lines, as well as in mice xenografts.[22] Retinoic acid morpholine amide suppressed Fas ligand (FasL) expression in colon cancer cells via COX-2 and EP1 receptor, but not EP2 and EP4 receptors.[23] The binding of FasL to its receptor is a key process in the regulation of immune response and apoptosis. Other study also showed that PGE_2-induced FasL expression is EP1 receptor dependent in colon cancer cells.[24] The upregulation of FasL expression is positively correlated with COX-2 expression in colon adenocarcinomas. On the other hand, the expression of EP1 receptor correlates well with good prognosis and reduction in metastasis.[25,26] Nevertheless, EP1 receptor is overexpressed in GI cancers and other cancers,[27] suggesting the therapeutic value of EP1 receptor in treating cancers. Further investigations of the antitumor efficacy through EP1 receptor in humans are warranted.

EP2 receptor

EP2 receptor couples to adenylyl cyclase to increase cAMP, which is the major second messenger of PEG_2 pathway contributing in the antitumor immune response.[28] Transcriptional activation of β-catenin is an important process in the COX-2/PGE_2 signaling, which affects the downstream mediators including IL-8 and VEGFR. The tumorigenic role of EP2 receptor was seen in 4-(methylnitrosamino)-1-(3-pyridyl)-1-butanone (NNK)-induced gastric cancer growth and angiogenesis.[29] In addition to being associated with tumor growth, the induction of VEGF and its receptor was mediated by p38 phosphorylation which was abrogated by p38 inhibitor (SB203580) and EP2 antagonist (AH6809). Study from anther group demonstrated that upregulated VEGF and p38 phosphorylation were important in gastric carcinogenesis by the PGE_2/EP2/EP4 pathway.[30] *H. pylori* stimulated the expression of urokinase-type plasminogen activator and its receptors were significantly inhibited by EP2 receptor antagonist in the process of invasion and angiogenesis.[31] Nuclear translocation of NF-κB in the upregulation of miR-16 and miR-21 was shown in the activation of COX-2/PGE_2 signaling, in which the signaling cascade was mediated through EP2 and EP4 receptors.[32]

PGE_2 contributes to cancer progression in mediating crosstalk between tumor cells and stromal cells in tumor microenvironment. Cancer-association fibroblast promoted tumor growth with increased IL-6 levels, and resulted in enhanced epithelial–mesenchymal transition and stemness in part through EP2 receptor.[33] During inflammation, TNFα, Wnt5A, and IL-6 expression were increased in wild-type mice for tumor formation. In contrast, EP2 receptor knockout mice had lower incidence of tumor formation and reduced expression of inflammatory genes and NF-κB activation. In colitis-associated colon cancer mouse model, the effect of EP2 antagonist (PF-04418948) on tumor formation was suppressed with reduced infiltration of inflammatory cells.[34]. In consistent with other studies, the release of PGE_2 coupled with EP2 receptor is commonly seen in colon carcinogenesis in mice and cell lines,[35,36] and yet treatment with NSAIDs reduces tumor formation via EP2 suppression.[37] In addition, genetic variation in EP2 4950G>A (odd ratio=0.71) has marginal significance with an increase of colon adenoma.[38]

EP3 receptor

The activation of EP3 receptor-mediated cellular events through suppression of adenylate cyclase, which is different from EP2 and EP4 receptors. There are three EP3 isoforms identified in mouse, namely EP3α, EP3β, and EP3γ, which are derived by alternative splicing from EP3 receptor gene. The contribution of EP3 receptor in carcinogenesis is still unclear. Study showed that the expression of EP3 receptor was lower in primary cancer tissues than normal colon mucosae, which is different from EP2 expression.[39] In view of the tumor forming ability, $EP3^{-/-}$ mice had a higher tumor incidence of colon tumors than wild-type mice. Cells treated with EP3 agonist (ONO-AE-248) reduced the cell viability in colon cancer cells that expressed EP3. It is suggested that the low expression of EP3 in colon tumors and cancer cells is probably due to hypermethylation in carcinogenesis. The tumor suppressive role of EP3 was not only seen in colon cancer but also in skin and breast cancers. However, inflammation was reduced in mice lacking EP3 receptor.[40] Late onset of tumor formation was seen in $EP3^{-/-}$ mice when compared with wild-type mice, probably due to reduction of inflammation with EP3 receptor deficiency.[41] Taken together, the exact role of EP3 receptor in cancer development warrants more studies to confirm.

EP4 receptor

EP4 receptor has been extensively studied for its tumorigenic role in various cancers. In colon cancer, the expression of EP4 receptors is present in the lateral crypt epithelia where cell migration and differentiation occur and facilitate tumor progression. The tumor stimulating effect of EP4 receptor has been reported to involve in many different pathways, in which one of them involves β-catenin/Tcf signaling that increases the level of COX-2 and survival in colon cancer.[42] Other study showed that agonists of EP2 or EP3 have no effect on COX-2 expression. The activation of EP4 receptors activate PI3K pathway and induce EGR-1 and phosphorylation of ERK. It has been shown that EP4 receptor antagonist (GW627368X) suppressed EGFR phosphorylation through Akt/MAPK pathway. The increased expression of cancer stem cell (CSC) markers (CD133, CD44, and LRG5) has been associated with tumor load in Apc(Min/+) mice. EP4 receptor promoted CSC formation and liver metastasis via NF-κB/ERK pathway.[43] The levels of HIF-1α increased cell density and regulated COX-2 and EP4 receptor expression in colon cancer cells. These findings suggest that cancer cell population is a contributing factor in mediating PEG_2/EP4 pathway.[44] Inflammation-induced EP4 receptor expression increases rapamycin complex 1 (mTORC1) expression to promote angiogenesis and colon cancer growth.[45] EP4 receptors on myeloid cells were induced by PGE_2 in stromal cells or tumor cells in a paracrine fashion, which could facilitate intestinal adenoma development. Interestingly, the depletion of myeloid cell EP4 receptors had similar effect as antagonism of EP4 causing polarization of protumorigenic M2 to antitumorigenic M1 phenotype. Maintaining M2 phenotypic macrophages favors the tumor–host interaction, and thus promotes colon cancer carcinogenesis.[46]

Our previous study showed that cigarette smoke could induce gastric cancer growth through the activation of EP4 receptors. This activation mediated through p38 phosphorylation to increase cyclin D1, cyclin-dependent kinases, and VEGF, thus promoting tumor growth and angiogenesis.[29] EP4 antagonist, CAY10598, induced apoptosis through p53 pathway in the mitochondria of colon cancer cells.[47] Consistent with other studies, EP4 receptor contributed in GI carcinogenesis by promoting cell proliferation, migration, invasion, and angiogenesis. Other mechanism involving EP4 receptor on gastric cancer progression was reported. PGE_2-induced EGFR transactivation by means of ectodomain shedding of EGFR ligands (e.g. epiregulin and ADAMS) could lead to tumor growth. Hence, dual treatment with COX-2 and EGFR inhibitors significantly retarded cancer growth in mice.[48] Infection with *H. pylori* increased the release of VEGF to promote angiogenesis through the MAPK-related pathway.[30] All these studies demonstrated that antagonism of EP4 is effective in reducing tumor formation both *in vivo* and *in vitro*, which may be useful as therapeutic drugs to combat GI cancers.

Conclusion and Future Direction

Enormous evidence demonstrates that COX-2 plays a significant role in inflammation and tumorigenesis including tumor growth, angiogenesis, invasion, and metastasis. Inhibitors of COX-2 have been shown to be effective in the prevention and treatment of cancer patients. However, long-term treatment with COX-2 inhibitors (Celebrex, Vioxx, Bextra) increases the risk of GI, renal, and cardiovascular side effects. This leads to the discovery of other promising and safer drugs to substitute COX inhibitors. Emerging evidence showed that the activation of EP receptors contributed to GI tumor development via multiple mechanisms. Our studies and majorities of other investigations also showed that EP2 and EP4 receptors are highly expressed in gastric and colon tumor tissues and elicit various signaling pathways (Figure 2), while EP1 and EP3 receptors have ambiguous results with limited published data. These four G-protein coupled receptors have different binding affinities to PGE_2 and yet it is anticipated that their expressions and functions are different depending on cell types or tissues they are expressed in.

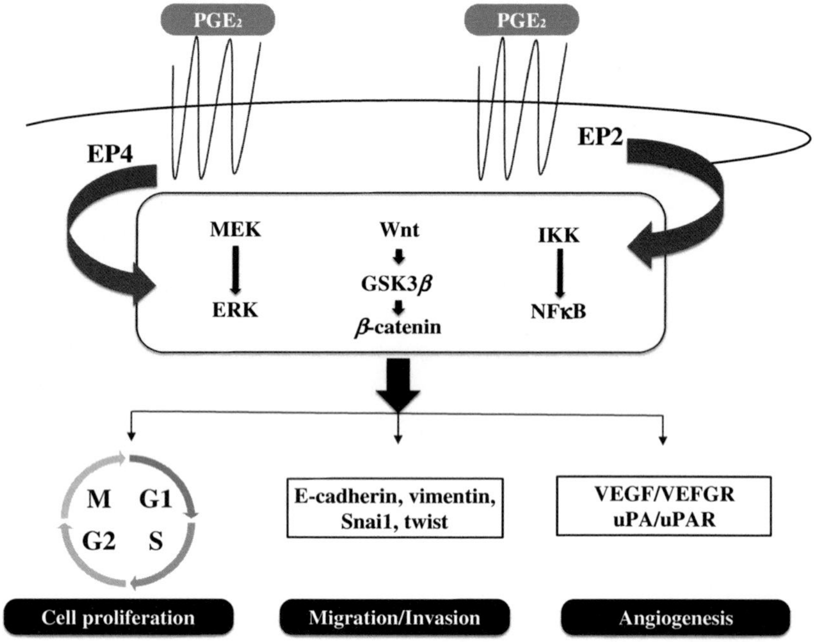

Figure 2. Signaling pathways activated by EP2 and EP4 receptors. PGE_2 binds to EP2 and EP4 receptors to activate mitogen-activated protein kinase (MAPK), Wnt/β-catenin, and NFkB pathways. All these signaling cascades promote cell proliferation, migration/invasion, and angiogenesis which are important processes for cancer progression.

With a better development of EP-related compounds becoming available, further investigations on the signal transduction mediated by EP receptors in GI cancers are warranted. The efficacy of EP4 antagonist (AAT-007) is now tested in phase II clinical trial in advanced prostate, breast, and lung tumors and is waiting for any published results. It is expected that more clinical trials are needed to ascertain the safety and efficacy of EP receptor modulators in the treatment of GI and other cancers in humans.

References

1. D Wang, RN Dubois (2006) Prostaglandins and cancer. *Gut* **55**: 115–122.
2. SI Grivennikov, FR Greten, M Karin (2010) Immunity, inflammation, and cancer. *Cell* **140**: 883–899.

3. C Dube, A Rostom, G Lewin, A Tsertsvadze, N Barrowman, C Code, *et al.* (2007) The use of aspirin for primary prevention of colorectal cancer: A systematic review prepared for the U.S. Preventive Services Task Force. *Ann Intern Med* **146**: 365–375.
4. N Arber, J Spicak, I Racz, M Zavoral, A Breazna, P Gerletti, *et al.* (2011) Five-year analysis of the prevention of colorectal sporadic adenomatous polyps trial. *Am J Gastroenterol* **106**: 1135–1146.
5. AT Chan, EL Giovannucci, JA Meyerhardt, ES Schernhammer, GC Curhan, CS Fuchs (2005) Long-term use of aspirin and nonsteroidal anti-inflammatory drugs and risk of colorectal cancer. *JAMA* **294**: 914–923.
6. D Wang, RN Dubois (2010) The role of COX-2 in intestinal inflammation and colorectal cancer. *Oncogene* **29**: 781–788.
7. RM Peek, Jr., JE Crabtree (2006) Helicobacter infection and gastric neoplasia. *J Pathol* **208**: 233–248.
8. Y Zhang, KF Pan, L Zhang, JL Ma, T Zhou, JY Li, *et al.* (2015) Helicobacter pylori, cyclooxygenase-2 and evolution of gastric lesions: Results from an intervention trial in China. *Carcinogenesis* **36**: 1572–1579.
9. H Xiong, W Du, TT Sun, YW Lin, JL Wang, J Hong, *et al.* (2014) A positive feedback loop between STAT3 and cyclooxygenase-2 gene may contribute to Helicobacter pylori-associated human gastric tumorigenesis. *Int J Cancer* **134**: 2030–2040.
10. JC Sierra, S Hobbs, R Chaturvedi, F Yan, KT Wilson, RM Peek, Jr., *et al.* (2013) Induction of COX-2 expression by Helicobacter pylori is mediated by activation of epidermal growth factor receptor in gastric epithelial cells. *Am J Physiol Gastrointest Liver Physiol* **305**: G196–G203.
11. CY Wu, MS Wu, KN Kuo, CB Wang, YJ Chen, JT Lin (2010) Effective reduction of gastric cancer risk with regular use of nonsteroidal anti-inflammatory drugs in Helicobacter pylori-infected patients. *J Clin Oncol* **28**: 2952–2957.
12. BC Wong, L Zhang, JL Ma, KF Pan, JY Li, L Shen, *et al.* (2012) Effects of selective COX-2 inhibitor and Helicobacter pylori eradication on precancerous gastric lesions. *Gut* **61**: 812–818.
13. JA Baron, RS Sandler, RS Bresalier, H Quan, R Riddell, A Lanas, *et al.* (2006) A randomized trial of rofecoxib for the chemoprevention of colorectal adenomas. *Gastroenterology* **131**: 1674–1682.
14. X Liu, Q Ji, N Ye, H Sui, L Zhou, H Zhu, *et al.* (2015) Berberine inhibits invasion and metastasis of colorectal cancer cells via COX-2/PGE2 mediated JAK2/STAT3 signaling pathway. *PLoS One* **10**: e0123478.
15. S Misra, K Sharma (2014) COX-2 signaling and cancer: New players in old arena. *Curr Drug Targets* **15**: 347–359.

16. U Yokoyama, K Iwatsubo, M Umemura, T Fujita, Y Ishikawa (2013) The prostanoid EP4 receptor and its signaling pathway. *Pharmacol Rev* **65**: 1010–1052.
17. N Niho, M Mutoh, T Kitamura, M Takahashi, H Sato, H Yamamoto, *et al.* (2005) Suppression of azoxymethane-induced colon cancer development in rats by a prostaglandin E receptor EP1-selective antagonist. *Cancer Sci* **96**: 260–264.
18. JL Lee, A Kim, L Kopelovich, DR Bickers, M Athar (2005) Differential expression of E prostanoid receptors in murine and human non-melanoma skin cancer. *J Invest Dermatol* **125**: 818–825.
19. T Kawamori, N Uchiya, S Nakatsugi, K Watanabe, S Ohuchida, H Yamamoto, *et al.* (2001) Chemopreventive effects of ONO-8711, a selective prostaglandin E receptor EP(1) antagonist, on breast cancer development. *Carcinogenesis* **22**: 2001–2004.
20. XM Bai, H Jiang, JX Ding, T Peng, J Ma, YH Wang, *et al.* (2010) Prostaglandin E2 upregulates survivin expression via the EP1 receptor in hepatocellular carcinoma cells. *Life Sci* **86**: 214–223.
21. C Diorio, D Furrer, A Michaud, S Laberge, I Popa, S Jacob, *et al.* (2016) Validation of EP1 Antibody Clone for Estrogen Receptor Immunohistochemistry for Breast Cancer. *Anticancer Res* **36**: 435–437.
22. C Jiang, Q Wang, Z Xu, WS Li, C Chen, XQ Yao, *et al.* (2015) Cyclooxygenase-2 knockdown using retinoic acid chalcone (RAC), a promising therapeutic strategy for colon cancer. *Am J Cancer Res* **5**: 2012–2021.
23. SX Chen, SY Du, YT Wang, HC Zhao, YL Zhang, L Yao (2015) Retinoic acid morpholine amide (RAMA) inhibits expression of Fas ligand through EP1 receptor in colon cancer cells. *Tumour Biol.*
24. G O'Callaghan, J Kelly, F Shanahan, A Houston (2008) Prostaglandin E2 stimulates Fas ligand expression via the EP1 receptor in colon cancer cells. *Br J Cancer* **99**: 502–512.
25. MA Thorat, A Morimiya, S Mehrotra, R Konger, SS Badve (2008) Prostanoid receptor EP1 expression in breast cancer. *Mod Pathol* **21**: 15–21.
26. X Ma, N Kundu, OB Ioffe, O Goloubeva, R Konger, C Baquet, *et al.* (2010) Prostaglandin E receptor EP1 suppresses breast cancer metastasis and is linked to survival differences and cancer disparities. *Mol Cancer Res* **8**: 1310–1318.
27. L Chen, SM Park, AV Tumanov, A Hau, K Sawada, C Feig, *et al.* (2010) CD95 promotes tumour growth. *Nature* **465**: 492–496.
28. P Kalinski (2012) Regulation of immune responses by prostaglandin E2. *J Immunol* **188**: 21–28.

29. VY Shin, HC Jin, EK Ng, CH Cho, WK Leung, JJ Sung, *et al.* (2011) 4-(Methylnitrosamino)-1-(3-pyridyl)-1-butanone promoted gastric cancer growth through prostaglandin E receptor (EP2 and EP4) in vivo and in vitro. *Cancer Sci* **102**: 926–933.
30. N Liu, Q Wu, Y Wang, H Sui, X Liu, N Zhou, *et al.* (2014) Helicobacter pylori promotes VEGF expression via the p38 MAPK-mediated COX2PGE2 pathway in MKN45 cells. *Mol Med Rep* **10**: 2123–2129.
31. J Iwamoto, Y Mizokami, K Takahashi, T Matsuoka, Y Matsuzaki (2008) The effects of cyclooxygenase2-prostaglandinE2 pathway on Helicobacter pylori-induced urokinase-type plasminogen activator system in the gastric cancer cells. *Helicobacter* **13**: 174–182.
32. VY Shin, H Jin, EK Ng, AS Cheng, WW Chong, CY Wong, *et al.* (2011) NF-kappaB targets miR-16 and miR-21 in gastric cancer: Involvement of prostaglandin E receptors. *Carcinogenesis* **32**: 240–245.
33. P Li, JX Shan, XH Chen, D Zhang, LP Su, XY Huang, *et al.* (2015) Epigenetic silencing of microRNA-149 in cancer-associated fibroblasts mediates prostaglandin E2/interleukin-6 signaling in the tumor microenvironment. *Cell Res* **25**: 588–603.
34. X Ma, T Aoki, T Tsuruyama, S Narumiya (2015) Definition of prostaglandin E2-EP2 signals in the colon tumor microenvironment that amplify inflammation and tumor growth. *Cancer Res* **75**: 2822–2832.
35. M Sonoshita, K Takaku, N Sasaki, Y Sugimoto, F Ushikubi, S Narumiya, *et al.* (2001) Acceleration of intestinal polyposis through prostaglandin receptor EP2 in Apc(Delta 716) knockout mice. *Nat Med* **7**: 1048–1051.
36. Y Ikawa, H Fujino, S Otake, T Murayama (2012) Indomethacin antagonizes EP(2) prostanoid receptor activation in LS174T human colon cancer cells. *Eur J Pharmacol* **680**: 16–21.
37. H Fujino, XB Chen, JW Regan, T Murayama (2007) Indomethacin decreases EP2 prostanoid receptor expression in colon cancer cells. *Biochem Biophys Res Commun* **359**: 568–573.
38. TL Edwards, MJ Shrubsole, Q Cai, G Li, Q Dai, DK Rex, *et al.* (2012) A study of prostaglandin pathway genes and interactions with current nonsteroidal anti-inflammatory drug use in colorectal adenoma. *Cancer Prev Res (Phila)* **5**: 855–863.
39. Y Shoji, M Takahashi, T Kitamura, K Watanabe, T Kawamori, T Maruyama, *et al.* (2004) Downregulation of prostaglandin E receptor subtype EP3 during colon cancer development. *Gut* **53**: 1151–1158.
40. JL Goulet, AJ Pace, ML Key, RS Byrum, M Nguyen, SL Tilley, *et al.* (2004) E-prostanoid-3 receptors mediate the proinflammatory actions of prostaglandin E2 in acute cutaneous inflammation. *J Immunol* **173**: 1321–1326.

41. Y Shoji, M Takahashi, N Takasuka, N Niho, T Kitamura, H Sato, *et al.* (2005) Prostaglandin E receptor EP3 deficiency modifies tumor outcome in mouse two-stage skin carcinogenesis. *Carcinogenesis* **26**: 2116–2122.
42. H Fujino (2016) The roles of EP4 prostanoid receptors in cancer malignancy signaling. *Biol Pharm Bull* **39**: 149–155.
43. D Wang, L Fu, H Sun, L Guo, RN DuBois (2015) Prostaglandin E2 promotes colorectal cancer stem cell expansion and metastasis in mice. *Gastroenterology* **149**: 1884–1895.
44. S Otake, K Yoshida, N Seira, CM Sanchez, JW Regan, H Fujino, *et al.* (2015) Cellular density-dependent down-regulation of EP4 prostanoid receptors via the up-regulation of hypoxia-inducible factor-1alpha in HCA-7 human colon cancer cells. *Pharmacol Res Perspect* **3**: e00083.
45. M Dufour, S Faes, A Dormond-Meuwly, N Demartines, O Dormond (2014) PGE2-induced colon cancer growth is mediated by mTORC1. *Biochem Biophys Res Commun* **451**: 587–591.
46. J Chang, J Vacher, B Yao, X Fan, B Zhang, RC Harris, *et al.* (2015) Prostaglandin E receptor 4 (EP4) promotes colonic tumorigenesis. *Oncotarget* **6**: 33500–33511.
47. IG Chae, DH Kim, J Kundu, CH Jeong, JK Kundu, KS Chun (2014) Generation of ROS by CAY10598 leads to inactivation of STAT3 signaling and induction of apoptosis in human colon cancer HCT116 cells. *Free Radic Res* **48**: 1311–1321.
48. H Oshima, BK Popivanova, K Oguma, D Kong, TO Ishikawa, M Oshima (2011) Activation of epidermal growth factor receptor signaling by the prostaglandin E(2) receptor EP4 pathway during gastric tumorigenesis. *Cancer Sci* **102**: 713–719.

Section IV
Autophagy and microRNAs as the Therapeutic Targets in Gastrointestinal Cancers

Chapter 15

Modulation of Autophagy as a Potential Therapeutic Target for Gastrointestinal Cancers: Promises and Uncertainties

Li Ma

Abstract

Autophagy plays a crucial role in the maintenance of cellular homeostasis and genomic integrity. It is upregulated in response to various adverse conditions including hypoxia and anticancer treatment for cell to survive. Autophagy inhibits tumorigenesis; however, it promotes the progression of established tumors. The role of autophagy in cancer is further compounded by the diversity of anti-cancer agents and tumor types. In most cases, anti-cancer treatments induce prosurvival autophagy, whereas in some other cases, autophagy mediates cytotoxic actions of anti-cancer agents. In this chapter, we will discuss the current knowledge of the molecular mechanism and regulation of autophagy, the role of autophagy in cancer and cancer therapy, as well as targeting this process as a potential therapeutic modality in gastrointestinal cancers.

Introduction

Autophagy is a cellular degradation mechanism for the clearance of excessive or dysfunctional proteins or organelles. In normal cells, basal autophagy plays a critical role in maintenance of cellular homeostasis and genomic integrity. The process can also be induced in response to various adverse conditions, including nutrient deprivation, metabolic stress, and hypoxia, for cells to adapt to the stress condition and survive. Dysregulation of autophagy has been shown to be associated with a number of pathological conditions, including cancer, infectious diseases, aging, myopathies, cardiac diseases, and neurodegenerative disorders. With respect to cancer, autophagy can play double roles, each with opposite effects depending on the tumor type, stage, and genetic context. It is generally believed that autophagy inhibits tumorigenesis. However, it also promotes the progression of established tumors. The early stages of tumorigenesis are associated with the downregulation of autophagy-related genes (ATG). Conversely, in advanced stages of tumorigenesis or during anti-cancer therapy, including most of chemotherapy and radiotherapy, autophagy promotes survival of tumor cells leading to therapeutic resistance. Nevertheless, the antitumor effects of some pharmaceutical agents are mediated by autophagy cell death. Therefore, a thorough understanding of the crosstalk between autophagy and cell death and the role of autophagy in different cancer contexts including cancer types and stages in response to anti-cancer therapy is a prerequisite to determine an autophagy-activating or autophagy-inhibiting treatment strategy. In this chapter, we will discuss the current knowledge of the role, molecular mechanism and regulation of autophagy, as well as targeting this process as a potential therapeutic strategy in gastrointestinal (GI) cancers. In addition, the limitations and obstacles currently encountered in the field will be also addressed.

Autophagy

Definition of autophagy

The term "autophagy", derived from the Greek meaning "self-eating", was coined by Christian de Duve in 1960s, based on the observation of degradation of mitochondria and other intracellular structures within lysosomes of rat liver perfused with glucagon.[1] Autophagy involves several intracellular pathways converging on a common phase of lysosomal degradation. There are three main types of autophagy: macroautophagy, microautophagy, and chaperone-mediated autophagy. Macroautophagy is initiated by the formation of a double-membrane structure called phagophore which extends and closes to form an autophagosome. Autophagosomes sequester cytoplasmic components such as damaged proteins and dysfunctional organelles including mitochondria (mitophagy), peroxisomes (pexophagy), endoplasmic reticulum (ER, endophagy), as well as intracellular bacteria and viruses (xenophagy). Autophagosomes ultimately fuse with lysosomes where their contents are degraded and recycled. Microautophagy is characterized by direct lysosomal engulfment of damaged proteins. Chaperone-mediated autophagy involves the association of targeted substrates with chaperone proteins such as hsc70 and hsc90 which facilitate translocation of tagged substrates across the lysosome membrane (Figure 1).[2] Among these three, macroautophagy

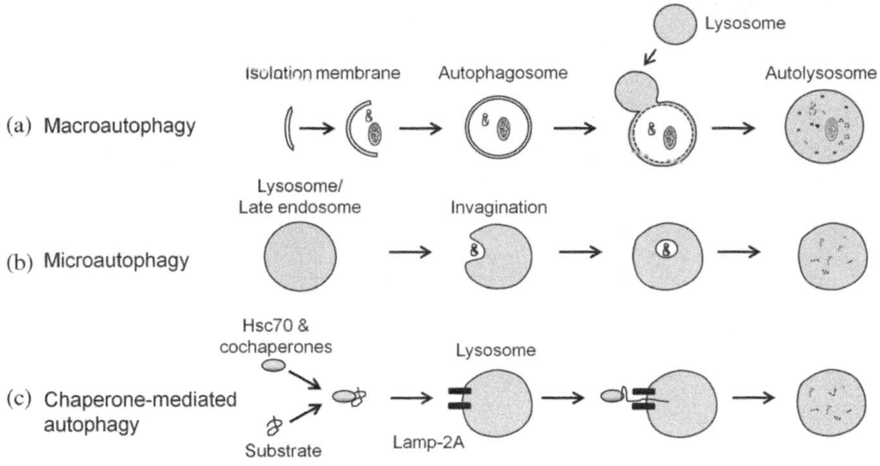

Figure 1. Three main distinct types of autophagy. (a) Macroautophagy: a portion of cytoplasm, including misfolded proteins and damaged organelles, is enclosed by an isolation membrane (also called phagophore) to form an autophagosome. The autophagosome fuses with the lysosome to form autolysosome where the enclosed contents are degraded. (b) Microautophagy: small pieces of the cytoplasm, mainly soluble cytosolic components, are directly engulfed by invagination of the lysosomal or late endosomal membrane. (c) Chaperone-mediated autophagy: substrate proteins are first recognized by cytosolic Hsc70 and cochaperones. They are then translocated into the lysosomal lumen via binding with lysosomal Lamp-2A. Through all three types of autophagy, the resultant degradation products can be reused as building blocks to synthesize large molecules such as proteins and DNAs and to generate energy.

(hereafter referred to as autophagy) is the predominant form, and dysregulation of autophagy has been shown to be associated with various diseases including cancers.

Molecular Basis of Autophagy

The process of autophagy consists of several steps including initiation and nucleation of a double-membrane structure, elongation of the isolation membrane, formation and maturation of the autophagosome, autophagosome–lysosome fusion, and lysosomal degradation (Figure 2(a)).[3] Induction of autophagy is highly controlled by a series of complex regulatory mechanisms; it is regulated by numerous stresses such as nutrient starvation, hypoxia, a reduced ATP/AMP ratio, increased intracellular reactive oxygen species (ROS) levels, bacteria and virus infection or chemical reagents. Its initiation steps are not fully elucidated yet; nevertheless, many signals converge at the inhibition of mammalian target of rapamycin (mTOR), which in turn releases the suppression of the protein complex containing unc-51-like kinase1/2 (ULK1/2), ATG13, ATG101, and focal adhesion kinase family kinase-interacting protein (FIP) 200. The ULK1/2 complex then activates the class III PI3K (PI3K-III or Vps34–Vps15 heterodimer)/Beclin 1 complex composed of proteins such as activating molecule in Beclin-1-regulated autophagy protein 1 (AMBRA 1), ATG14L, UV radiation resistance-associated gene (UVRAG), and Bax-binding protein-1 (Bif-1). Bcl-2 and Bcl-XL prevent activation of this complex by binding to and inhibiting Beclin 1 and AMBRA 1 thereby inhibiting autophagy induction. The activated PI3K-III/Beclin 1 complex is then translocated to ER, the major site of phagophore formation, where it initiates nucleation (Figure 2(b))[4]. During autophagosome nucleation, the PI3K-III complex generates PI3P, which recruits other ATG proteins involved in membrane elongation. Elongation of the membrane involves two ubiquitin-like conjugation systems, ATG12-ATG5 and ATG8/LC3 (microtubule-associated protein 1 light chain 3, Figure 2(c)). ATG12 is initially conjugated to ATG7 (an E1-activating enzyme) and then transferred to ATG10 (an E2-like conjugating enzyme). The ATG12–ATG10 intermediate enables ATG12 to conjugate with ATG5 followed by further conjugation with ATG16. The ATG12–ATG5–ATG16 conjugates form tetramers on the outside of the expanding membrane and enhance LC3 carboxy-terminal lipidation through

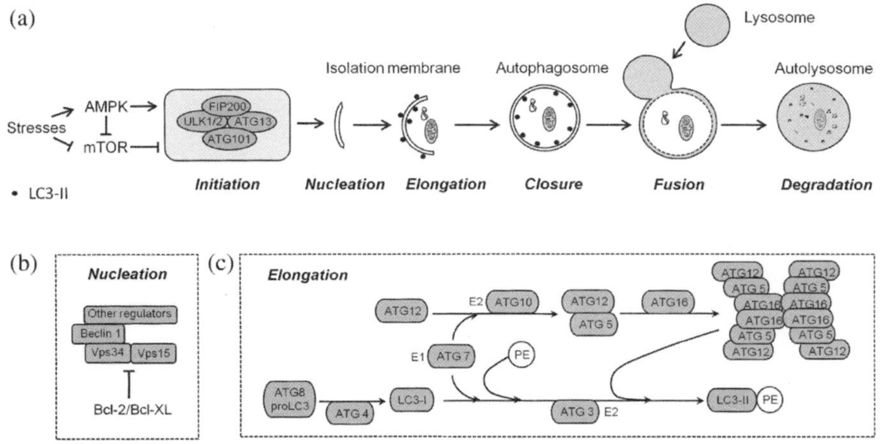

Figure 2. Stages of autophagy. (a) The process of macroautophagy consists of six main stages: initiation and formation of the isolation membrane/phagophore (nucleation), elongation, and completion of the mature autophagosome, fusion of the autophagosome with the lysosome to form an autolysosome, and degradation of the enclosed contents. The initiation is sustained by activation of ULK1 and ULK2 complexes, which are enhanced by AMPK but inhibited by mTOR. (b) The nucleation depends on Vps34-Vps15/Beclin 1 core complex and other proteins, which are inhibited by Bcl-2/Bcl-XL. (c) The elongation of the phagophore is mediated by two ubiquitin-like conjugation systems that together promote the assembly of the ATG12–ATG5–ATG16 complex and the interaction of LC3 with phosphatidylethanolamine (PE), forming autophagosomal membrane bound LC3-II. The resulting mature LC3-II interacts with specific adapter proteins or receptors that are present on the cargo to be engulfed and degraded to accomplish the cargo selection.

the LC3 conjugation system. LC3 is synthesized initially as proLC3, which is cleaved by ATG4 to produce an active cytosolic form, LC3-I. Then, with the catalysis of ATG7 and a conjugating E2 enzyme ATG3, LC3-I interacts with phosphatidylethanolamine, an abundant membrane phospholipid, yielding LC3-II. The resulting mature LC3-II resides on the autophagosome membrane and interacts with specific adapter proteins or receptors that are present on the cargo to be engulfed and degraded.[5] The phagophore expands and closes to form an autophagosome. Upon the formation of autophagosome, ATG5–ATG12–ATG16 and LC3-I (delipidated from LC3-II by ATG4) are recycled. LC3-II associated with the lumenal membrane remains trapped in the autophagosome and is degraded during maturation into the autolysosome, formed by fusion of autophagosome with lysosome.[6] The list of proteins mediating fusion of autophagosomes and lysosomes is not yet complete. Nevertheless, an essential role of the small GTP-binding protein Rab7 as well as the lysosomal membrane proteins LAMP1 and LAMP2 has been identified in this process.[7,8]

Functions of Autophagy

Under normal conditions, autophagy occurs constitutively by breaking down macromolecules in the surrounding environment for producing cellular building blocks and providing energy to maintain homeostasis.[9] Basal autophagy, as part of the cellular surveillance machinery, is also responsible for recognition and removal of misfolded proteins and dysfunctional organelles. In addition, autophagy is involved in normal development and immune response. Dysregulation of autophagy has been implicated in pathologies, including cancer, infectious diseases, aging, myopathies, cardiac diseases, and neurodegenerative disorders. The protective role of autophagy in aging, cardiac diseases, and neurodegenerative diseases is well accepted. However, the effect of autophagy in cancer is far more complex and paradoxical.[9]

Autophagy and Cancer

Autophagy and tumorigenesis

The role of autophagy as a tumor suppressor was initially suggested from genetic studies of Beclin 1. Monoallelic deletion of Beclin 1 is frequently observed in human breast, ovarian, and prostate cancers.[10] In addition, Beclin 1 expression is commonly decreased in breast carcinoma compared with normal breast tissues. Overexpression of Beclin1 in human breast cancer cells inhibits proliferation *in vitro* and reduces tumorigenesis *in vivo* in a mouse xenograft mode.[11] Consistently, genetic deletion of one copy of Beclin 1 gene in mice decreases autophagy and increases the frequency of spontaneous malignancies, including lung adenocarcinoma, hepatocellular carcinoma, and B-cell lymphoma.[10,12] These findings have provided the initial genetic evidence that Beclin 1 functions as a tumor suppressor and suggested that autophagy plays an important role in human tumor suppression.

In addition to Beclin 1, genetic alteration of other autophagy-related genes has been found in various types of cancer. A growing body of evidence suggests that alterations of autophagy-related proteins including mutations and protein expression levels are cancer-type dependent. In GI cancers, upregulation of Beclin 1 is commonly seen in human gastric and colorectal carcinomas,[13–15] which is in contrast to the downregulation of Beclin 1 observed in human breast and ovarian cancers. However, mutations in UVRAG, a Beclin-1-binding protein that positively regulates autophagy, have been frequently observed in gastric carcinomas[16] and colon cancer cells.[17–19] Furthermore, human HCT116 colon cancer cells, which have very low baseline levels of autophagy, contain a monoallelic frameshift mutation in the UVRAG gene which generates a premature stop codon.[18] The ectopic expression of wild-type UVRAG ($UVRAG^{WT}$) in these cells promotes autophagy and suppresses cancer cell proliferation *in vitro* and tumorigenesis *in vivo.*[19] A cancer-related UVRAG frameshift mutation also results in a truncated $UVRAG^{FS}$ which not only loses its proautophagic functions but also antagonizes the effects of $UVRAG^{WT}$ in a dominant-negative manner.[20] The truncated $UVRAG^{FS}$ found in colorectal cancer (CRC) with microsatellite instability (MSI) contributes to tumorigenesis and metastasis.[20] The MSI phenotype is usually caused by deficiency in DNA mismatch repair that progresses with high rates of insertions/deletions to repetitive DNA sequences; approximately, 15% of sporadic CRCs exhibit this phenotype. Immunohistochemical studies in human and animal gastric cancer samples demonstrated a consistent decreased expression of key autophagy-related proteins such as ATG5 and ATG16[21]. Other studies also showed that the mutation of ATG5 was rare in human gastric and colorectal carcinoma[22,23]; however, the expression of ATG5 was lost in 21% of gastric and 23% of colon cancers, respectively.[23] In addition, the downregulation of Bif-1, another positive regulator of autophagy, has been reported in human gastric and colon adenocarcinomas compared to normal tissues.[24,25] Taken together, these findings support the idea that disruption of autophagy is associated with tumorigenesis and that the change is not gene phenotype specific. Rather, different components of the autophagy pathway are affected depending on the context of the cancer.

Mechanisms of tumor suppression by autophagy

Several mechanisms can explain, at least in part, the tumor suppressing role of autophagy. First, autophagy protects cells from genotoxic stress and maintains genome integrity. Defects in autophagy, conferred by either allelic loss of Beclin 1 or a deficiency in ATG5, lead to elevated ROS production and enhanced DNA damage in response to metabolic stress.[26] Furthermore, reduced autophagy promotes gene amplification and chromosomal instability, resulting in aneuploidy. All of these are hallmarks of cancer and suggest that autophagy plays an important role in the maintenance of genomic integrity.[27] The expression of $UVRAG^{FS}$ in colon cancer cells inhibits autophagy and results in extensive centrosome amplification and concomitant aneuploidy.[20] Human MSI gastric cancers that express $UVRAG^{FS}$ demonstrate enhanced chromosome rearrangements compared with $UVRAG^{WT}$ expressing MSI gastric cancers.[20] Another potential mechanism of autophagy-mediated tumor suppression relates to inflammation. Chronic inflammatory conditions promote tumorigenesis partly by elevating ROS accumulation leading to mutations. Autophagy controls inflammation by direct elimination of microorganisms as well as endogenous irritants to prevent excessive inflammation. In many cancers, there are exogenous causes of chronic inflammation such as persistent infection with a pathogen (for example, *H. pylori*-associated gastric cancer) or exposure to toxins (for example, smoking-associated lung cancer).[28] In some other cases, defective autophagy is able to recreate an inflammatory state even without an extrinsic damaging stimulus, because failure to remove misfolded proteins and damage organelles causes cellular dysfunction and necrotic cell death, leading to an inflammatory response.[28] For example, accumulation of p62 due to impaired autophagy activates the pro-inflammatory transcription factor NF-κB and the stress-responsive transcription factor NRF2, thus favoring inflammation and tissue injury.[29]

Autophagy and tumor progression

Although autophagy can suppress tumorigenesis as described above, it may support the survival of rapidly growing cancer cells that have outgrown vascular supply. These cells are constantly under metabolic stress due to inadequate nutrition/oxygen. As nutrient sensors, mTOR, AMPK, and Sirtuins regulate autophagy. Low levels of amino acids and a reduced ATP/AMP ratio activate AMPK and inhibit mTOR leading to the activation of autophagy. Hypoxia-inducible factor-1α (HIF-1α), a key transcription factor induced under hypoxic conditions, can be used by tumor cells to alter metabolism, stimulate angiogenesis, and promote invasion and metastasis.[30] HIF-1α is also responsible for therapy resistance in hypoxic tumors.[30] HIF-1α positively regulates autophagy by upregulating Bcl-2/adenovirus E1B 19 kDa-interacting protein (BNIP3), a BH3-only protein. The induction of BNIP3 and BNIP3L in hypoxic cells disrupts the Beclin 1–Bcl-2 interaction, thereby releasing Beclin 1 to induce autophagy.[30]

Mechanisms of tumor survival by autophagy

Warburg effect and reverse Warburg effect

Altered metabolism is one of the hallmarks of cancer cells. The best-known metabolic abnormality in cancer cells is the Warburg effect, in which there is increased glycolysis even in the presence of oxygen. It had been thought that the Warburg effect was a unique feature of cancer cells arising from mitochondrial dysfunction. Recently, however, human skin keloid fibroblasts were found to generate ATP primarily from anaerobic glycolysis.[31,32] This observation has led to a new hypothesis that epithelial cancer cells are able to induce glycolysis in the adjacent stromal fibroblasts and hijack the energy-rich metabolites from the fibroblasts.[33] The hypothesis considers the tumor microenvironment which consists of connective tissues, blood vessels, immune cells, as well as stromal cells (including myofibroblasts). This tumor stroma accounts for nearly 50% of a tumor's mass. The myofibroblasts and/or cancer-associated fibroblasts may arise from mesenchymal stem cells derived from the bone marrow or from other differentiated cells, such as smooth muscle cells, preexisting fibroblasts, and preadipocytes.[33] Excessive ROS generated by cancer cells due to hypoxia and oxidative stress diffuse into adjacent tumor stromal fibroblasts where they trigger autophagy. The recycled high-energy nutrients, such as ketone bodies, L-lactate, and glutamine, produced by autophagic activity in fibroblasts are released into the intracellular space and reabsorbed by tumor cells to help fuel the tumor cells. This phenomenon, termed the "reverse Warburg effect,"[33] suggests a mechanism of cancer cell survival under stress.

Autophagy and chemoresistance

Autophagy has been suggested as a potential mechanism for resistance to anti-cancer agents. Autophagy could promote cancer cell survival under the stress induced by chemotherapeutics by removing damaged mitochondria and breaking down cellular components to generate alternative sources of energy. One of the most critical clinical problems is the frequent recurrence of the tumors following treatment, often after prolonged dormancy.[34] The survival of tumor cells through autophagy may be a key mechanism to enable long-term tumor cell survival and eventual relapse. Autophagy may allow residual tumor cells to tolerate metabolic stress with the ability to recover once growth conditions are favorable. The induction of autophagy in hypoxic regions may also interfere with therapy, as the tumor cells in these regions are notoriously resistant to the treatments.[35] In addition to chemoresistance, autophagy also contributes to the reduction of radiosensitivity. In human colon cancer cell lines SW480 and SW620, hypoxia-activated autophagy attenuates radiation-induced cell death. The upregulation of HIF-1α as well as miR-210 is associated with activation of autophagy under hypoxic conditions. The inhibition of HIF-1α abolishes both hypoxia-mediated increase in miR-210 and activation of autophagy. Moreover, the silencing of miR-210 attenuates colon cancer cell survival after radiation treatment. The results indicate that the activation of autophagy via HIF-1α/miR-210 contributes to the radioresistance in hypoxic environment.[36] All these suggest that activation of autophagy may be one of the underlying mechanisms of cancer resistance.

Autophagy and cancer stem cells (CSCs)

CSCs are a subpopulation of cancer cells that possess some characteristics of stem cells, specifically self-renewal and differentiation. CSCs are responsible for tumor heterogeneity.[37] Although CSCs have been identified in both solid and non-solid tumors, our current knowledge about the origin and formation of these cells is limited. Given the stem cell-like characteristics of CSCs, it has been proposed that CSCs originate from adult stem cells, progenitor cells or differentiated cells that have acquired "stemness" properties due to genetic and epigenetic alterations.[38] CSCs appear to depend on their own microenvironment for sustenance of the population. The resistance of CSCs to chemotherapy and their relative resistance to radiotherapy help to explain why the macroscopic tumor response to anti-cancer treatments is not always a good predictor of clinical outcome. Recently, autophagy has been shown to be a major factor for the ability of CSCs to survive under stress and to develop therapy resistance.[37] For example, curcumin (an active ingredient in turmeric powder) has been shown to induce apoptosis in colon cancer cells by various mechanisms. However, it promotes the survival of DCLK1-positive colon CSCs via activation of autophagy.[39] These data suggest that targeting autophagy in CSCs may present new opportunities for cancer treatment.

Crosstalk between autophagy and apoptosis in cancer cells

Most forms of cancer treatment activate both apoptosis and autophagy. Crosstalk between the two processes is complex and sometimes contradictory but is certainly important for the overall outcome of anti-cancer therapy.[40] The opposing effects of autophagy can be seen in the survival of BJAB B lymphoma cells upon activation of death ligand receptor. Death receptor agonists Fas Ligand (FasL) and tumor necrosis factor-related apoptosis-inducing ligand (TRAIL) are canonical apoptosis inducers and are both relevant to cancer therapy. High levels of autophagy increase FasL-induced apoptosis, but decrease TRAIL-induced apoptosis in BJAB cells. In contrast, high levels of autophagy inhibit FasL-induced apoptosis in Jurkat A3 T leukemia cells.[41] This may be explained by selective autophagic degradation of Fas-associated phosphatase 1 (Fap-1), a negative regulator of FasL-mediate apoptosis.[41] In Fap-1 expressing BJAB cells, the activation of autophagy increases degradation of Fap-1, therefore enhances FasL-mediated apoptotic cell death. However, in Jurkat cells that rarely express any Fap-1, activation of autophagy promotes cell survival via removing damaged protein and organelles, recycling cellular building blocks and providing energy.[41] Fap-1 specifically modulates FasL but not TRAIL signaling; thus, autophagy increases FasL-induced apoptosis but decreases TRAIL-induced apoptosis in BJAB cells through autophagic prosurvival mechanisms. These results demonstrate a critical role of the crosstalk between autophagy and apoptosis in determining cell fate.

Modes of crosstalk between autophagy and apoptosis in response to stress

Autophagy (self-eating) and apoptosis (self-killing) are two distinct self-destructive processes. In response to stressors, such as DNA damage, deprivation of nutrients, and ischemia/reperfusion, autophagy and apoptosis can occur in the same cells often in a sequence that autophagy precedes apoptosis.[42] Induction of autophagy is usually the initial response, especially when the stress is not lethal. Autophagy suppresses apoptosis and supports cell survival by removing misfolded proteins and damaged organelles and recycling cellular building blocks (Figure 3(a-1)). However, if the stress is too severe and sustained, autophagy can promote apoptosis. In such a case,

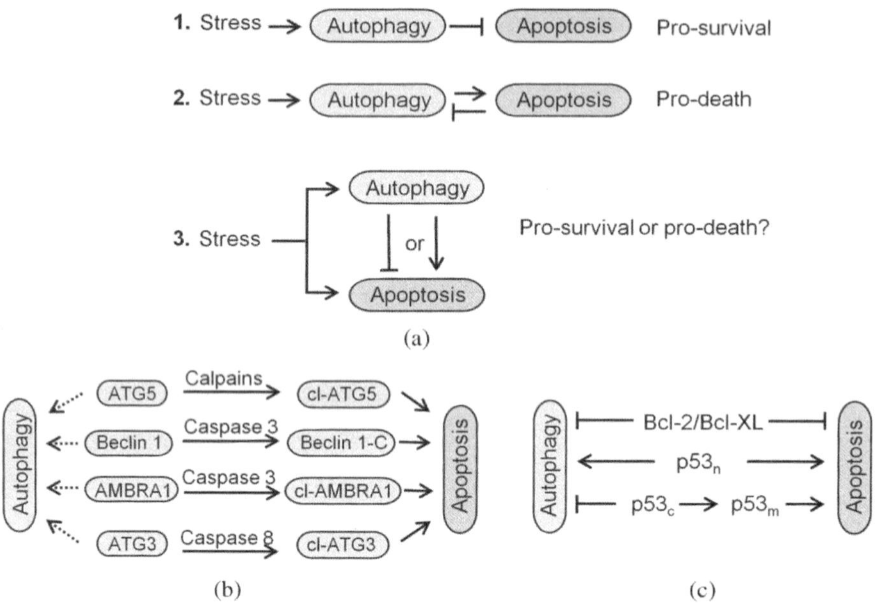

Figure 3. Crosstalk between apoptosis and autophagy. (a) In a cell, (1) a stress induces autophagy, which then inhibits apoptosis to help cell survive, or (2) a stress induces autophagy, which then triggers apoptosis leading to cell death. (3) The same stress induces both autophagy and apoptosis as independent processes. Whether the induced autophagy in this case is prosurvival or prodeath is stressor and cell-type specific. (b) Signals mediating inhibition of autophagy by apoptosis: during sustained exposure to apoptotic stimuli, proautophagic proteins Beclin 1, ATG3, ATG5 as well as AMBRA1 are cleaved by caspases and/or calpains. The cleaved (cl) proautophagic proteins not only lose their ability to induce autophagy but also become proapoptotic to promote apoptosis. (c) Both autophagy and apoptosis are negatively regulated by Bcl-2/Bcl-XL, but positive modulated by nuclear p53 ($p53_n$). Cytosolic p53 ($p53_c$) inhibits autophagy, but increases apoptosis upon translocation to mitochondria ($p53_m$).

apoptosis in turn suppresses prosurvival autophagy and cell death ensues[42] (Figure 3(a-2)). Some stresses, including majority of chemotherapy and radiotherapy, can activate both autophagy and apoptosis simultaneously. Whether the induced autophagy is prosurvival or prodeath is stimulus- and cell-type dependent (Figure 3(a-3)).

Inhibition of apoptosis by autophagy

Mitophagy (mitochondrial autophagy) is one of the principal mechanisms by which autophagy inhibits apoptosis. Impaired mitochondria release several proapoptotic factors upon induction of apoptosis, including cytochrome c. These factors either directly trigger apoptosis or associate with cytosolic factors to form apoptosome. Thus, removal of damaged mitochondria increases the threshold for induction of apoptosis. In addition, autophagy can attenuate apoptosis by selectively reducing the abundance of proapoptotic proteins, such as caspase 8, in the cytosol as well as facilitating the clearance of sequestosome 1 (SQSTM1/p62), a protein that, if overexpressed, can stimulate the production of ROS and cell death.[42]

Activation of apoptosis by autophagy

Autophagy can mediate cell death in a process known as autophagic cell death, especially in cells with attenuated apoptotic activities. In some cases, stress-induced autophagy can also lead to necrotic cell death. There are several mechanisms by which autophagy can facilitate apoptosis. First, the formation of autophagosome at an early stage of autophagy provides a platform for the activation of caspase 8. Second, autophagy can eliminate some endogenous inhibitors of apoptosis by degradation, which promotes apoptosis. Third, proautophagic proteins can serve as precursors of proapoptotic proteins and stimulate apoptosis upon cleavage by caspases or calpains.[42]

Inhibition of autophagy by apoptosis

Caspases, the primary drivers of apoptotic cell death, play a critical role in mediating the inhibition of autophagy by proteolytic processing of autophagy-related proteins (Figure 3(b)). The truncated form of ATG5 generated by calpain-dependent cleavage is a proapoptotic molecule that translocates to mitochondria and inactivates antiapoptotic protein Bcl-XL.[43] Upon cleavage by caspase 3, autophagy-related proteins Beclin 1, AMBRA 1, and ATG3 also lose their proautophagic activity and become proapoptotic facilitating apoptosis.[42]

Signals regulating both autophagy and apoptosis

Many signaling pathways involved in the regulation of autophagy also regulate apoptosis. For example, the binding and subcellular localization of the Bcl-2 family proteins and the transcription factor p53 are very important in the crosstalk between the two systems. The Bcl-2 family is a group of proteins that contain at least one of the four conserved α-helical motifs known as Bcl-2 homology (BH) domains (BH1–BH4). The family is further classified into two groups according to their functions: the antiapoptotic Bcl-2 family proteins (Bcl-2, Bcl-XL, Bcl-w, Mcl-1, Bcl-B, and A1) and the proapoptotic Bcl-2 family proteins (Bax, Bak, Bok, Bad, Bid, Bim, Bmf, Bik, Hrk, Noxa, and PUMA). Bcl-2 and Bcl-XL inhibit both autophagy and apoptosis. They can interact with Beclin 1 and prevent activation of the Vps34–Vps15/Beclin 1 complex, leading to the inhibition of autophagic induction. On the other hand, Bcl-2 and Bcl-XL can also bind and sequester proapoptotic Bax/Bak and prevent their translocation to mitochondria and subsequent cytochrome c release, therefore inhibiting apoptosis[43] (Figure 3(c)). p53, the tumor suppressor, exerts both pro- and antiautophagic activities depending on its subcellular localization and activation status. When present in the cytoplasm, p53 inhibits autophagy by interacting with FIP200 and thus interfering with the ULK1/2 complex.[42] Cytosolic p53 also sequesters Parkin, which prevents Parkin from translocating to the damaged mitochondria and inhibits mitochondrial autophagy.[44] In response to stress, p53 shuttles to the nucleus and promotes transcription of multiple proautophagic genes, including the β1, β2, and γ-subunits of AMPK, damage-regulated autophagy modulator 1 (DRAM1), sestrin 1, sestrin 2, and phosphatase and tensin homolog (PTEN).[42] At the transcriptional level, p53 also upregulates Bax, PUMA, and Bid or reduces the expression of Bcl-2 to induce apoptosis[45] (Figure 3(c)). Under certain circumstances, cytosolic p53 translocates to mitochondria, where it triggers mitochondrial outer membrane permeabilization, and thus induces both mitophagy, at first, and apoptosis, if the proapoptotic stimuli are intense and long enough to overwhelm the protective abilities of mitophagy.[42]

Taken together, most stressors activate both autophagy and apoptosis, either sequentially or concurrently. Whether the induced autophagy is prosurvival or prodeath is dependent on the type of stressors and cells, as well as the severity and duration of the stress.

Targeting Autophagy in GI Cancer

Preclinical studies

Most anti-cancer drugs and ionizing radiation affect autophagy, which in turn influences the outcome of cancer therapies. These effects are not always the same but depend on the nature of the medicine and the context of the cancer. There are diverse classes of anti-cancer drugs including DNA damaging agents, microtubule-targeted drugs, antimetabolites, death receptor agonists, hormonal agents, antiangiogenic agents, proteasome inhibitors, histone deacetylase inhibitors, and kinase inhibitors. Most of them induce autophagy, but a few of them inhibit it. Sometimes autophagy protects tumor cells against treatment, while other times autophagy is a requirement for the therapy to kill the cancer cells. Among all the GI cancers, CRC has received the most extensive attention with respect to the regulation of autophagy in cancer therapy. The majority of the preclinical studies were performed using human cancer cell lines and xenograft models.

Cancer treatments that induce prosurvival autophagy

Fluorouracil (5-FU) is the most common component of front line chemotherapeutics used in GI cancers. 5-FU induces both apoptosis and autophagy in colon cancer cells *in vitro* and xenograft tumor models *in vivo*. The inhibition of autophagy by pharmacological inhibitors or siRNA targeting key autophagy proteins significantly potentiates 5-FU antitumor effects. A study using a mouse colon cancer cell line, colon26, and its xenograft model, discovered that combination of 5-FU with chloroquine (CQ), an autophagy inhibitor, significantly promoted proapoptotic protein expression and apoptosis leading to the enhanced inhibition of tumor growth both *in vivo* and *in vitro.*[46] 5-FU also activated autophagy in HCT116, DLD-1, and DLD-1/5-FU, a specific 5-FU-resistant sub-line of human colon cancer cells. The inhibition of autophagy by 3-methyladenine (3-MA) or small interference RNA targeting ATG7 (ATG7 siRNA) not only significantly augmented 5-FU-induced apoptosis in HCT116 and DLD-1 cells but also resensitized DLD-1/5-FU to the chemotherapeutic. The synergistic effect of 5-FU and 3-MA was further demonstrated in the DLD-1 xenograft tumor model *in vivo.*[47] Interestingly, studies in human colon cancer cells with different p53 statuses showed that cells with wild-type p53 such as HCT116 p53 WT and RKO were hypersensitive to 5-FU treatment. However, p53 deficient (HCT116 $p53^{-/-}$) and mutant (HT-29) cells were resistant to 5-FU.[48] Moreover, 5-FU-induced autophagy was significantly higher in p53 deficient and mutant human colon cells compared with p53 WT cells. The higher levels of autophagy promoted resistance against 5-FU-mediated cytotoxicity in these cells. The suppression of autophagy by 3-MA, CQ, or siRNA targeting ATG5 or Beclin 1, two key autophagy regulators, resensitized these resistant cells to 5-FU.[48] In contrast, in Bax- or PUMA-deficient HCT116 colon cancer cells that were defective in apoptosis, the induction of autophagy via inhibition of mTOR by 5-FU led to cell death. Suppression of autophagy by 3-MA in this case, decreased 5-FU-induced cell death.[49] Thus, whether the activation of autophagy by chemotherapeutics is prosurvival or prodeath depends on many factors including tumor genetic backgrounds.

Oxaliplatin, a third generation platinum-based antineoplastic agent, is commonly used in combination with other anti-cancer drugs (such as 5-FU and leucovorin) to treat advanced colon cancer. However, oxaliplatin also induces autophagy which helps cancer cells survive and develop chemoresistance. Studies have shown that both hypoxia and oxaliplatin are able to induce autophagy in HT29 colon cancer cells *in vitro*. The inhibition of autophagy by CQ or siRNA targeting Beclin 1 or ATG5 sensitizes colon cancer cells to oxaliplatin under hypoxic conditions.[50]

Bevacizumab is an angiogenesis inhibitor which targets vascular endothelial growth factor A (VEGF-A). It inhibits tumor-associated angiogenesis and induces a hypoxic microenvironment in colon cancer xenografts.[50] However, tumor shrinkage as a result of the treatment is variable depending on susceptibility to hypoxia-induced cell death.[51] In addition, both hypoxia and nutrient deprivation are known to induce autophagy, which can counteract the antitumor effect of bevacizumab by enhancing cancer cell survival. Indeed, treatment with oxaliplatin and bevacizumab either alone or in combination upregulates autophagy *in vivo*. The inhibition of autophagy by CQ significantly reduces the growth of HT29-derived xenograft tumor in bevacizumab- and oxaliplatin-treated mice.[50]

Despite increased oncogenic transformation due to disruption of autophagy by UVRAG^{FS}, the truncated form of UVRAG (see section Autophagy and tumorigenesis), UVRAG^{FS}-expressing colon cancer appears to be more responsive to those chemotherapeutics that induce DNA damage and interfere with replication, such as 5-FU, oxaliplatin, and irinotecan, routinely prescribed as adjuvant therapies for CRC patients.[20]

In addition to DNA damaging reagents, histone deacetylase inhibitor vorinostat (VOR), proteasome inhibitor bortezomib, and receptor kinase inhibitor imatinib have all been shown to induce prosurvival autophagy in GI cancer *in vitro* and *in vivo*. Histone deacetylases (HDACs) play an important role in the epigenetic regulation of gene expression. Overexpression and/or hyperactivation of multiple HDACs are associated with epigenetic dysregulation in cancer cells, which leads to malignant progression and anti-cancer drug resistance. Thus, targeting HDAC activity is an appealing therapeutic strategy for many cancers. VOR was the first HDAC inhibitor approved by FDA for cancer therapy. VOR-induced autophagy markedly blunts its anti-cancer activity. The inhibition of autophagy by CQ, 3-MA, or ATG7 siRNA significantly enhances VOR-induced apoptosis in human HCT8 and HT29 colon cancer cells. Furthermore, combination treatment of CQ with VOR in an *in vivo* mouse HCT8 xenograft tumor model also significantly increases tumor cell apoptosis as well as reduces tumor burden when compared to therapy with either agent alone.[52]

Gastrointestinal stromal tumor (GIST) is the most common mesenchymal neoplasm of the GI tract. GISTs express mutant KIT and platelet-derived growth factor receptor A (PDGFRA) that are constitutively activated. This characteristic makes GIST an ideal candidate for KIT/PDGFRA targeting anti-cancer therapy using small molecule-tyrosine kinase inhibitors such as imatinib mesylate. However, clinical studies have shown that these treatments are rarely curative. Often, a sizeable tumor cell subpopulation survives and remains quiescent for years. Eventually, the tumor becomes resistant and treatment fails. In preclinical studies, imatinib induces autophagy as a survival pathway in quiescent GIST cells. The inhibition of autophagy by pharmacological agents or RNAi targeting ATG7 or ATG12 promotes imatinib-induced GIST cell death both *in vitro* and *in vivo*. Thus, combining imatinib with drugs that inhibit autophagy represents a potentially valuable strategy to promote cytotoxicity and to diminish both cellular quiescence and acquired resistance in GIST patients.[53] Indeed, surgically resected samples taken from imatinib-treated GIST patients show evidence of an increase in autophagy. Biochemical and immunohistochemical evidence from these tissues have demonstrated high levels of proautophagic Beclin 1/PI3K-III and low levels of antiautophagic Beclin 1/Bcl-2 complexes.[54]

While autophagy degrades mainly long-lived proteins and subcellular organelles, the ubiquitin–proteasome system (UPS) is a major degradation system for short-lived proteins. The inhibition of UPS enhances autophagy as a compensatory response; however, the reverse is not the case.[55] Cancer cells are usually associated with higher levels of basal proteasomal activity, which renders the proteasome an attractive target for anti-cancer therapy.[55] The proteasome inhibitor bortezomib has been approved for clinical use to treat refractory or relapsed multiple myeloma. However, its effects on other tumors have not been fully defined yet. Recent studies in human colon cancer cells and their mouse xenograft models have shown that the combination of bortezomib with autophagy inhibitors potentiates cell death both *in vitro* and *in vivo*.[56] Interestingly, KRAS mutant colon cancer cells HT-29-$KRas^{V12}$ and T80-$KRas^{v12}$ demonstrate an enhanced ability to activate autophagy in response to bortezomib treatment. Thus, autophagy suppression has more profound effects on potentiating bortezomib-induced apoptosis in these KRAS mutant transformed cells than their parent cells, reflecting a stronger dependence of KRAS mutant cells on autophagy for survival under stress.[56]

Radiotherapy is one of the most commonly used strategies for treating solid tumors. Radiation induces autophagy in human esophageal squamous carcinoma cells and inhibition of autophagy with 3-MA enhances cytotoxicity of radiotherapy.[57] Furthermore, in human colon cancer SW480 and SW620 cells, hypoxia-activated autophagy compromises radiation-induced cell death.[36]

Cancer treatments that induce prodeath autophagy

Most studies show that autophagy is primarily protective and induction of autophagy during anti-cancer treatment leads to chemoresistance. However, in some cases, autophagy is not protective but is actually necessary for the antitumor effect of the drug. In these cases, the inhibition of autophagy reduces tumor cell death and increases tumor growth.[58] Resveratrol (3,4′,5-tri-hydroxy-trans-stilbene), a polyphenol found in grapes, can inhibit cell proliferation and induce growth arrest and/or cell death in several types of cancer cells, including colon cancer cells. Resveratrol blocks both anchorage-dependent and anchorage-independent growth of HT-29 and COLO 201 human colon cancer cells in a dose- and time-dependent manner. It activates both apoptosis and autophagy. The inhibition of autophagy by 3-MA diminishes resveratrol-induced apoptosis, suggesting that autophagy induced by resveratrol promotes apoptosis.[59]

Cancer treatments that inhibit autophagy

Most cancer therapeutics induce autophagy, prosurvival, or prodeath. However, microtubule inhibitors such as vinblastine, block autophagy[60] via disruption of microtubule dynamics to prevent fusion of autophagosomes with lysosomes.[61] Therefore, vinblastine has been shown particularly beneficial when used in combination with prosurvival autophagy inducing anti-cancer therapeutics. Ceramide is a sphingolipid metabolite that induces cancer cell death. Ceramide can be generated by exposure to chemotherapy or ionizing radiation, or it can be administered in the form of short-chain analogs. Ceramide has been shown to inhibit colon cancer cell proliferation and induce apoptosis, but it is also a strong autophagy inducer. Interestingly, the combination of ceramide, an autophagy inducer with vinblastine, and an autophagy inhibitor synergistically enhances apoptotic cell death in LS174T human colon cancer cells.[62]

Clinical trials targeting autophagy in GI cancer

Both *in vitro* and *in vivo* studies in preclinical models suggest that modulation of autophagy can be used as a therapeutic modality to enhance the efficacy of conventional therapies, including chemotherapy and radiotherapy. Currently, more than 30 clinical trials are investigating the effects of autophagy inhibition in combination with cytotoxic chemotherapies and targeted agents in various cancers, including CRC. CQ and HCQ are FDA approved agents with autophagy inhibiting properties in clinical use. Based on the preclinical finding that the inhibition of autophagy significantly augmented the anti-cancer activity of HDAC inhibitor VOR,[52] a phase I clinical trial (NCT01023737) was performed to investigate the safety, preliminary efficacy, pharmacokinetics, and pharmacodynamics of the combination of HCQ and VOR in patients with advanced solid tumors, among which 12 had CRCs.[63] These CRC patients were assigned as follows: 1 in Cohort 1, 2 in Cohort 2, 6 in Cohort 3, and 3 in Cohort 4, with escalating daily oral doses of HCQ (400–800 mg) in combination with VOR (300–400 mg). The patients enrolled in Cohort 4 (HCQ 800 mg + VOR 400 mg) experienced dose limiting toxicities and were withdrawn from the study. The dosing utilized in Cohort 3 (HCQ 600 mg + VOR 400 mg daily) was defined as the maximum tolerated dose and was further recommended as a phase II regimen. Tumor responses were observed in four out of six CRC patients enrolled in Cohort 3, among which two patients achieved prolonged stable disease. Interestingly, both of these patients had tumors with activating mutations in KRAS.[63] This observation may be significant because of the preclinical finding that mutations in RAS confer higher levels of basal autophagy. The phase I clinical trial has demonstrated that the inhibition of autophagy with HCQ is a novel and safe strategy that may enhance the efficacy of VOR. Based on these data, there is now an ongoing phase II clinical study of "Vorinostat Plus Hydroxychloroquine versus Regorafenib in Refractory Metastatic Colorectal Cancer (mCRC) Patients" (NCT02316340). There are also several other ongoing clinical trials testing the combination of autophagy inhibition with chemotherapy in treatment of CRCs (Table 1).

Overall, preclinical studies and clinical trials suggest that autophagy inhibition may enhance the efficacy of the majority of conventional therapies in GI cancers. However, larger clinical trials and a comprehensive analysis of the data will eventually provide more definitive answers regarding the effects of manipulation of autophagy in these patients.

Table 1. Clinical trials on targeting autophagy in GI cancers.

Tumor type	Clinical study status	Therapeutic combination	Trial ID
Advanced solid tumor (including 12 colorectal cancers)	Phase I	HCQ + vorinostat	NCT01023737
Refractory metastatic colorectal cancer	Phase II	HCQ + vorinostat	NCT02316340
Advanced or metastatic colorectal cancer	Phase I/II	HCQ + FOLFOX/ bevacizumab	NCT01206530
Metastatic colorectal cancer	Phase II	HCQ + bevacizumab	NCT01006369

Limitations and Uncertainties of Autophagy Modulation in Cancer Therapy

Despite the rapid progresses made in the field of modulation of autophagy in cancer therapy, there are still many limitations and uncertainties awaiting us.

Variation of autophagic response in different cancer context

The induction or inhibition of autophagy in response to a cancer therapy is agent-type dependent. In most cases, treatment increases autophagy. For example, in a screen of 80 cytotoxic anti-cancer agents that caused high levels of autophagosome accumulation in human osteosarcoma U2OS cells and cervical carcinoma HeLa cells, 59 induced both autophagosome formation and autophagic flux and, thus, truly increased autophagy. The remaining 21 compounds induced higher numbers of autophagosomes yet failed to stimulate an autophagic flux (for example, microtubule inhibitors block autophagy by inhibiting fusion of autophagosomes with the lysosomes).[60] The situation is even more complex because some agents can both increase the formation of autophagosomes and block their fusion with lysosomes.[58] In addition to the agent-dependent variation of autophagic response in cancer cells, the result of induced autophagy can either be cytoprotective or cytotoxic depending on the type of cancer. As mentioned previously, FasL-stimulated autophagy promotes apoptosis in BJAB B lymphoma cells but inhibits apoptosis in Jurkat A3 T leukemia cells.[41] Furthermore, results obtained with the same chemotherapeutic in the same cell line were variable. In tamoxifen-treated MCF7 breast cancer cells, there seems general agreement that tamoxifen increases autophagy. However, in some studies tamoxifen resistance in MCF7 cells was caused by the induction of autophagy and in others it was overcome by the activation of autophagy.[58] It is not clear as to what caused the discrepancies in these studies, yet the incompatible conclusions obviously add little to help determine whether autophagy inhibitors or autophagy enhancers should be investigated in breast cancer patients when treated with tamoxifen. Taken together, based on the complexity of the relationship between autophagy and cancer therapy, a more thorough understanding of the molecular mechanisms of how an antitumor intervention affects autophagy and whether it is cytoprotective or cytotoxic is essential before development of rational approaches to manipulate autophagy for clinical benefit. We also need to identify which tumors are most effectively treated by autophagy manipulation.

Off-target effects of autophagy inhibition

Overall, *in vivo* preclinical studies and clinical trials suggest that the inhibition of autophagy may enhance the efficacy of the majority of conventional therapies in cancer. However, the suppression of autophagy may exacerbate preexisting problems in organs such as brain and heart in which basal autophagy is critical to maintain cellular homeostasis. Furthermore, the inhibition of autophagy may also worsen chemotherapy-related organ injuries and decrease organ function. For example, most of the chemotherapeutics often cause bone marrow depression, and the inhibition of autophagy may worsen this condition. Anthracycline antibiotics, such as doxorubicin and daunorubicin, cause cardiotoxicity in a dose-dependent manner, presumably through DNA damage, and the addition of autophagy inhibitor to the therapeutic regimen could worsen the cardiotoxicity. Therefore, caution is needed when considering the addition of autophagy inhibitors to chemotherapy.[64]

Targeting autophagy in CSCs appears to be an attractive strategy to treat cancer. However, the similarity between normal tissue stem cells and

CSCs with respect to autophagy might lead to possible off-target effects of autophagy-based anti-CSC therapies. Determining the specific autophagy requirements for normal stem cells and CSCs may be an essential requisite to designing strategies targeting autophagy in CSCs that spare normal stem cells.[65]

Autophagy also affects antitumor immune responses, including antigen presentation and stimulation of immune reaction from released immunogenic molecules. Thus, adverse effects on antitumor immune functions may override any benefit from causing more direct tumor cell death by suppression of autophagy. Indeed, a recent study demonstrated that autophagy inhibition could enhance radiosensitivity *in vitro*, as well as *in vivo* in immune deficient mice but caused radioresistance in immune competent mice,[66] suggesting a negative impact of autophagy suppression on antitumor immune response.

Challenges of monitoring autophagic activity *in vivo* in patients

Another challenge we are facing when considering the possibilities of treating patients with autophagy regulators is how to determine autophagic response to a treatment in patients *in vivo*. There are methods to measure this dynamic process *in vitro*, for example, to compare the levels of autophagic intermediates such as autophagosomes in the presence and absence of an autophagosome–lysosome fusion inhibitor and determine whether autophagic flux is increased or decreased. However, we have not found a good way to assess this dynamism in humans. This makes it inherently difficult to determine whether an intervention affects autophagy or not in a patient. We need to develop ways to monitor the amount of autophagy and autophagic flux *in vivo* especially in humans so that we can develop useful pharmacodynamic markers for clinical assessment of autophagy manipulation.

Uncertainty: The role of CQ in cancer treatment

Although CQ and HCQ have been evaluated and used in clinical trials as autophagy blockers for cancer treatment, these drugs are known to have additional effects. It is not fully elucidated yet whether their anti-cancer action is solely dependent on its direct inhibition in autophagy as we originally intended. A preclinical study suggests that the antiproliferative effect of CQ in some cancer cells is independent of its suppressive actions on autophagy.[67] In this study, the deletion of ATG7 completely blocked autophagy in several tumor lines but did not inhibit cell proliferation *in vitro* or tumorigenesis *in vivo*. Furthermore, CQ but not knockout of ATG7 sensitized cells to irradiation and to several anti-cancer agents tested. The degree of synergy by CQ was similar in both wild-type and ATG7-deficient cells. All these suggest that the mechanisms underlying CQ-induced inhibition of proliferation may be multifactorial and could include defects in DNA synthesis and repair, inhibition of topoisomerases, as well as mitochondrial membrane permeabilization, all of which may occur independently or as a consequence of lysosomal inhibition.[67] Moreover, another recent study that focused on the role of CQ in tumor angiogenesis has also revealed an autophagosome–lysosome fusion inhibiting independent role of CQ in tumor growth.[68] Both CQ and knockdown of ATG5 induced melanoma cancer cell death, and reduced tumor growth and metastasis. However, ATG5 knockdown overall did not phenocopy the effects of CQ on the tumor stroma. CQ but not knockdown of ATG5 improved tumor oxygenation by normalizing tumor vessel structure and function and increasing perfusion. By reducing hypoxia in tumor stroma, CQ may indirectly inhibit the reverse Warburg effect and improve chemotherapy delivery and response, thus enhancing the anti-cancer therapy.[68] These findings shed additional light on the mechanisms of how CQ functions as an adjuvant therapy in cancer treatment. It indeed improves our current understanding and continues to support the ongoing clinical trials of CQ in combination treatment in cancer, although it challenges our original intention using CQ solely as an autophagy inhibitor.

Concluding Remarks

Given the diversity of tumor types and antitumor therapeutics, as well as the numerous oncogenic drivers involved in cancer, the role of autophagy during cancer progression and treatment will likely continue to remain complex. The controversial and context-dependent role of autophagy during initiation and advanced progression of tumors as well as cancer treatment emphasize the need for a comprehensive understanding of the cell biological mechanisms regulating autophagy during these processes. Thus, when seeking to modulate autophagy in order to enhance treatment efficacy, we should first evaluate whether the potentially cotreated anti-cancer drug increases or inhibits autophagy in the target cancers, and whether the induced autophagy is cytoprotective or cytotoxic. Second, we should identify which cancers respond well to autophagy targeting therapy. For GI cancer, preclinical studies have demonstrated that the majority of the cytotoxic antitumor drugs induce autophagy which antagonizes the cytotoxic effect of the chemotherapeutics. The inhibition of autophagy enhances the efficacy of the conventional chemotherapy. These findings have warranted a few ongoing clinical trials on autophagy targeting therapy in GI cancer, primarily in CRC. The results of these studies will no doubt provide further insight into autophagy targeting adjuvant therapy and help to develop better therapeutic strategies. Even with rapid progress made thus far in this field, in order to identify new strategies that selectively target autophagy in cancer cells and CSCs without harming normal tissue and normal stem cells, we must continue to discern the cellular and metabolic functions of autophagy in both normal and tumor cells. With such knowledge, we may be able to develop cancer specific autophagy targeting agent alternatives to HCQ, the major current clinical option for inhibiting autophagy in patients, which has been shown to have off-target effects. In addition, we also need to develop a better way to monitor autophagic activity in response to therapeutic intervention in patients *in vivo*. Ultimately, we may be able to develop very effective anti-cancer treatment modalities by combining a certain class of autophagy modulators with molecular-targeted drugs directed against specific cellular targets in each different type of cancer and CSCs.

Acknowledgment

The author thanks Dr. James Dilger for his critical reading and editing of the manuscript.

References

1. RL Deter, C De Duve (1967) Influence of glucagon, an inducer of cellular autophagy, on some physical properties of rat liver lysosomes. *J Cell Biol* **33**: 437–449.

2. N Mizushima, M Komatsu (2011) Autophagy: Renovation of cells and tissues. *Cell* **147**: 728–741.
3. I Tanida (2011) Autophagy basics. *Microbiol Immunol* **55**: 1–11.
4. R Kang, HJ Zeh, MT Lotze, D Tang (2011) The Beclin 1 network regulates autophagy and apoptosis. *Cell Death Differ* **18**: 571–580.
5. T Johansen, T Lamark (2011) Selective autophagy mediated by autophagic adapter proteins. *Autophagy* **7**: 279–296.
6. J Van Limbergen, C Stevens, E Nimmo, D Wilson, J Satsangi (2009) Autophagy: From basic science to clinical application. *Mucosal Immunol* **2**: 315–330.
7. S Jager, C Bucci, I Tanida, T Ueno, E Kominami, P Saftig, EL Eskelinen (2004) Role for Rab7 in maturation of late autophagic vacuoles. *J Cell Sci* **117**: 4837–4848.
8. EL Eskelinen (2006) Roles of LAMP-1 and LAMP-2 in lysosome biogenesis and autophagy. *Mol Aspects Med* **27**: 495–502.
9. AM Choi, SW Ryter, B Levine (2013) Autophagy in human health and disease. *N Engl J Med* **368**: 651–662.
10. X Qu, J Yu, G Bhagat, N Furuya, H Hibshoosh, A Troxel, J Rosen, E-L Eskelinen, N Mizushima, Y Ohsumi (2003) Promotion of tumorigenesis by heterozygous disruption of the beclin 1 autophagy gene. *J Clinical Invest* **112**: 1809.
11. XH Liang, S Jackson, M Seaman, K Brown, B Kempkes, H Hibshoosh, B Levine (1999) Induction of autophagy and inhibition of tumorigenesis by beclin 1. *Nature* **402**: 672–676.
12. Z Yue, S Jin, C Yang, AJ Levine, N Heintz (2003) Beclin 1, an autophagy gene essential for early embryonic development, is a haploinsufficient tumor suppressor. *Proc Natl Acad Sci USA* **100**: 15077–15082.
13. CH Ahn, EG Jeong, JW Lee, MS Kim, SH Kim, SS Kim, NJ Yoo, SH Lee (2007) Expression of beclin-1, an autophagy-related protein, in gastric and colorectal cancers. *Apmis* **115**: 1344–1349.
14. JM Park, S Huang, TT Wu, NR Foster, FA Sinicrope (2013) Prognostic impact of Beclin 1, p62/sequestosome 1 and LC3 protein expression in colon carcinomas from patients receiving 5-fluorouracil as adjuvant chemotherapy. *Cancer Biol Ther* **14**: 100–107.
15. SH Wei, W Li, Y Liu, DK Gao, J Pan, CW Gu, HR Wu (2014) Disturbance of autophagy-lysosome signaling molecule expression in human gastric adenocarcinoma. *Oncol Lett* **7**: 635–640.
16. MS Kim, EG Jeong, CH Ahn, SS Kim, SH Lee, NJ Yoo (2008) Frameshift mutation of UVRAG, an autophagy-related gene, in gastric carcinomas with microsatellite instability. *Hum Pathol* **39**: 1059–1063.

17. T Goi, M Kawasaki, T Yamazaki, K Koneri, K Katayama, K Hirose, A Yamaguchi (2003) Ascending colon cancer with hepatic metastasis and cholecystolithiasis in a patient with situs inversus totalis without any expression of UVRAG mRNA: Report of a case. *Surg Today* **33**: 702–706.
18. Y Ionov, N Nowak, M Perucho, S Markowitz, JK Cowell (2004) Manipulation of nonsense mediated decay identifies gene mutations in colon cancer cells with microsatellite instability. *Oncogene* **23**: 639–645.
19. C Liang, P Feng, B Ku, I Dotan, D Canaani, BH Oh, JU Jung (2006) Autophagic and tumour suppressor activity of a novel Beclin1-binding protein UVRAG. *Nat Cell Biol* **8**: 688–699.
20. S He, Z Zhao, Y Yang, D O'Connell, X Zhang, S Oh, B Ma, J-H Lee, T Zhang, B Varghese (2015) Truncating mutation in the autophagy gene UVRAG confers oncogenic properties and chemosensitivity in colorectal cancers. *Nat Commun* **6**.
21. RA Vigen, Y Kodama, T Viset, R Fossmark, H Waldum, M Kidd, TC Wang, IM Modlin, D Chen, CM Zhao (2013) Immunohistochemical evidence for an impairment of autophagy in tumorigenesis of gastric carcinoids and adenocarcinomas in rodent models and patients. *Histol Histopathol* **28**: 531–542.
22. MR Kang, MS Kim, JE Oh, YR Kim, SY Song, SS Kim, CH Ahn, NJ Yoo, SH Lee (2009) Frameshift mutations of autophagy-related genes ATG2B, ATG5, ATG9B and ATG12 in gastric and colorectal cancers with microsatellite instability. *J Pathol* **217**: 702–706.
23. CH An, MS Kim, NJ Yoo, SW Park, SH Lee (2011) Mutational and expressional analyses of ATG5, an autophagy-related gene, in gastrointestinal cancers. *Pathol Res Pract* **207**: 433–437.
24. JW Lee, EG Jeong, YH Soung, SW Nam, JY Lee, NJ Yoo, SH Lee (2006) Decreased expression of tumour suppressor Bax-interacting factor-1 (Bif-1), a Bax activator, in gastric carcinomas. *Pathology* **38**: 312–315.
25. D Coppola, F Khalil, SA Eschrich, D Boulware, T Yeatman, HG Wang (2008) Down-regulation of Bax-interacting factor-1 in colorectal adenocarcinoma. *Cancer* **113**: 2665–2670.
26. R Mathew, CM Karp, B Beaudoin, N Vuong, G Chen, HY Chen, K Bray, A Reddy, G Bhanot, C Gelinas, RS Dipaola, V Karantza-Wadsworth, E White (2009) Autophagy suppresses tumorigenesis through elimination of p62. *Cell* **137**: 1062–1075.
27. R Mathew, S Kongara, B Beaudoin, CM Karp, K Bray, K Degenhardt, G Chen, S Jin, E White (2007) Autophagy suppresses tumor progression by limiting chromosomal instability. *Genes Dev* **21**: 1367–1381.
28. E White, C Karp, AM Strohecker, Y Guo, R Mathew (2010) Role of autophagy in suppression of inflammation and cancer. *Curr Opinion Cell Biol* **22**: 212–217.

29. B Levine, N Mizushima, HW Virgin (2011) Autophagy in immunity and inflammation. *Nature* **469**: 323–335.
30. S Roy, J Debnath (2010) Autophagy and tumorigenesis. In: *Seminars in Immunopathology*. Berlin: Springer.
31. AS Vincent, TT Phan, A Mukhopadhyay, HY Lim, B Halliwell, KP Wong (2008) Human skin keloid fibroblasts display bioenergetics of cancer cells. *J Invest Dermatol* **128**: 702–709.
32. S Pavlides, D Whitaker-Menezes, R Castello-Cros, N Flomenberg, AK Witkiewicz, PG Frank, MC Casimiro, C Wang, P Fortina, S Addya, RG Pestell, UE Martinez-Outschoorn, F Sotgia, MP Lisanti (2009) The reverse Warburg effect: Aerobic glycolysis in cancer associated fibroblasts and the tumor stroma. *Cell Cycle* **8**: 3984–4001.
33. CD Gonzalez, S Alvarez, A Ropolo, C Rosenzvit, MF Gonzalez Bagnes, MI Vaccaro (2014) Autophagy, Warburg, and Warburg reverse effects in human cancer. *BioMed Res Int* **2014**.
34. JA Aguirre-Ghiso (2006) The problem of cancer dormancy: understanding the basic mechanisms and identifying therapeutic opportunities. *Cell Cycle* **5:** 1740–1743.
35. R Mathew, V Karantza-Wadsworth, E White (2007) Role of autophagy in cancer. *Nat Rev Cancer* 7: 961–967.
36. Y Sun, X Xing, Q Liu, Z Wang, Y Xin, P Zhang, C Hu, Y Liu (2015) Hypoxia-induced autophagy reduces radiosensitivity by the HIF-1alpha/miR-210/Bcl-2 pathway in colon cancer cells. *Int J Oncol* **46**: 750–756.
37. R Ojha, S Bhattacharyya, SK Singh (2015) Autophagy in cancer stem cells: A potential link between chemoresistance, recurrence, and metastasis. *Biores Open Access* **4**: 97–108.
38. SS Franco, H Raveh-Amit, J Kobolák, MH Alqahtani, A Mobasheri, A Dinnyes (2015) The crossroads between cancer stem cells and aging. *BMC Cancer* **15**: S1.
39. C Kantara, M O'Connell, S Sarkar, S Moya, R Ullrich, P Singh (2014) Curcumin promotes autophagic survival of a subset of colon cancer stem cells, which are ablated by DCLK1-siRNA. *Cancer Res* **74**: 2487–2498.
40. MP Tschan, HU Simon (2010) The role of autophagy in anticancer therapy: Promises and uncertainties. *J Intern Med* **268**: 410–418.
41. JM Gump, L Staskiewicz, MJ Morgan, A Bamberg, DW Riches, A Thorburn (2014) Autophagy variation within a cell population determines cell fate through selective degradation of Fap-1. *Nat Cell Biol* **16**: 47–54.
42. G Mariño, M Niso-Santano, EH Baehrecke, G Kroemer (2014) Self-consumption: The interplay of autophagy and apoptosis. *Nat Rev Mol Cell Biol* **15**: 81–94.

43. F Zhou, Y Yang, D Xing (2011) Bcl-2 and Bcl-xL play important roles in the crosstalk between autophagy and apoptosis. *FEBS J* **278**: 403–413.
44. A Hoshino, Y Mita, Y Okawa, M Ariyoshi, E Iwai-Kanai, T Ueyama, K Ikeda, T Ogata, S Matoba (2013) Cytosolic p53 inhibits Parkin-mediated mitophagy and promotes mitochondrial dysfunction in the mouse heart. *Nat Commun* **4**: 2308.
45. V Nikoletopoulou, M Markaki, K Palikaras, N Tavernarakis (2013) Crosstalk between apoptosis, necrosis and autophagy. *Biochim Biophys Acta* **1833**: 3448–3459.
46. K Sasaki, NH Tsuno, E Sunami, K Kawai, K Hongo, M Hiyoshi, M Kaneko, K Murono, N Tada, T Nirei, K Takahashi, J Kitayama (2012) Resistance of colon cancer to 5-fluorouracil may be overcome by combination with chloroquine, an *in vivo study. Anticancer Drugs* **23**: 675–682.
47. J Li, N Hou, A Faried, S Tsutsumi, H Kuwano (2010) Inhibition of autophagy augments 5-fluorouracil chemotherapy in human colon cancer *in vitro* and *in vivo* model. *Eur J Cancer* **46**: 1900–1909.
48. X Sui, N Kong, X Wang, Y Fang, X Hu, Y Xu, W Chen, K Wang, D Li, W Jin, F Lou, Y Zheng, H Hu, L Gong, X Zhou, H Pan, W Han (2014) JNK confers 5-fluorouracil resistance in p53-deficient and mutant p53-expressing colon cancer cells by inducing survival autophagy. *Sci Rep* **4**: 4694.
49. HY Xiong, XL Guo, XX Bu, SS Zhang, NN Ma, JR Song, F Hu, SF Tao, K Sun, R Li, MC Wu, LX Wei (2010) Autophagic cell death induced by 5-FU in Bax or PUMA deficient human colon cancer cell. *Cancer Lett* **288**: 68–74.
50. M Selvakumaran, RK Amaravadi, IA Vasilevskaya, PJ O'Dwyer (2013) Autophagy inhibition sensitizes colon cancer cells to antiangiogenic and cytotoxic therapy. *Clin Cancer Res* **19**: 2995–3007.
51. M Selvakumaran, KS Yao, MD Feldman, PJ O'Dwyer (2008) Antitumor effect of the angiogenesis inhibitor bevacizumab is dependent on susceptibility of tumors to hypoxia-induced apoptosis. *Biochem Pharmacol* **75**: 627–638.
52. JS Carew, EC Medina, JA Esquivel, 2nd, D Mahalingam, R Swords, K Kelly, H Zhang, P Huang, AC Mita, MM Mita, FJ Giles, ST Nawrocki (2010) Autophagy inhibition enhances vorinostat-induced apoptosis via ubiquitinated protein accumulation. *J Cell Mol Med* **14**: 2448–2459.
53. A Gupta, S Roy, AJ Lazar, WL Wang, JC McAuliffe, D Reynoso, J McMahon, T Taguchi, G Floris, M Debiec-Rychter, P Schoffski, JA Trent, J Debnath, BP Rubin (2010) Autophagy inhibition and antimalarials promote cell death in gastrointestinal stromal tumor (GIST). *Proc Natl Acad Sci USA* **107**: 14333–14338.
54. F Miselli, T Negri, A Gronchi, M Losa, E Conca, S Brich, E Fumagalli, M Fiore, PG Casali, MA Pierotti, E Tamborini, S Pilotti (2008) Is autophagy

rather than apoptosis the regression driver in imatinib-treated gastrointestinal stromal tumors? *Transl Oncol* **1**: 177–186.

55. A Lilienbaum (2013) Relationship between the proteasomal system and autophagy. *Int J Biochem Mol Biol* **4**: 1.
56. WX Ding, HM Ni, W Gao, X Chen, JH Kang, DB Stolz, J Liu, XM Yin (2009) Oncogenic transformation confers a selective susceptibility to the combined suppression of the proteasome and autophagy. *Mol Cancer Ther* **8**: 2036–2045.
57. YS Chen, HX Song, Y Lu, X Li, T Chen, Y Zhang, JX Xue, H Liu, B Kan, G Yang, T Fu (2011) Autophagy inhibition contributes to radiation sensitization of esophageal squamous carcinoma cells. *Dis Esophagus* **24**: 437–443.
58. A Thorburn, DH Thamm, DL Gustafson (2014) Autophagy and cancer therapy. *Mol Pharmacol* **85**: 830–838.
59. H Miki, N Uehara, A Kimura, T Sasaki, T Yuri, K Yoshizawa, A Tsubura (2012) Resveratrol induces apoptosis via ROS-triggered autophagy in human colon cancer cells. *Int J Oncol* **40**: 1020–1028.
60. S Shen, O Kepp, M Michaud, I Martins, H Minoux, D Metivier, MC Maiuri, RT Kroemer, G Kroemer (2011) Association and dissociation of autophagy, apoptosis and necrosis by systematic chemical study. *Oncogene* **30**: 4544–4556.
61. R Köchl, XW Hu, EY Chan, SA Tooze (2006) Microtubules facilitate autophagosome formation and fusion of autophagosomes with endosomes. *Traffic* **7**: 129–145.
62. PP Adiseshaiah, JD Clogston, CB McLeland, J Rodriguez, TM Potter, BW Neun, SL Skoczen, SS Shanmugavelandy, M Kester, ST Stern, SE McNeil (2013) Synergistic combination therapy with nanoliposomal C6-ceramide and vinblastine is associated with autophagy dysfunction in hepatocarcinoma and colorectal cancer models. *Cancer Lett* **337**: 254–265.
63. D Mahalingam, M Mita, J Sarantopoulos, L Wood, RK Amaravadi, LE Davis, AC Mita, TJ Curiel, CM Espitia, ST Nawrocki, FJ Giles, JS Carew (2014) Combined autophagy and HDAC inhibition: A phase I safety, tolerability, pharmacokinetic, and pharmacodynamic analysis of hydroxychloroquine in combination with the HDAC inhibitor vorinostat in patients with advanced solid tumors. *Autophagy* **10**: 1403–1414.
64. T Kimura, Y Takabatake, A Takahashi, Y Isaka (2013) Chloroquine in cancer therapy: A double-edged sword of autophagy. *Cancer Res* **73**: 3–7.
65. JL Guan, AK Simon, M Prescott, JA Menendez, F Liu, F Wang, C Wang, E Wolvetang, A Vazquez-Martin, J Zhang (2013) Autophagy in stem cells. *Autophagy* **9**: 830–849.

66. A Ko, A Kanehisa, I Martins, L Senovilla, C Chargari, D Dugue, G Marino, O Kepp, M Michaud, J Perfettini (2014) Autophagy inhibition radiosensitizes *in vitro*, yet reduces radioresponses in vivo due to deficient immunogenic signalling. *Cell Death Differ* **21**: 92–99.
67. CH Eng, Z Wang, D Tkach, L Toral-Barza, S Ugwonali, S Liu, SL Fitzgerald, E George, E Frias, N Cochran, R De Jesus, G McAllister, GR Hoffman, K Bray, L Lemon, J Lucas, VR Fantin, RT Abraham, LO Murphy, B Nyfeler (2015) Macroautophagy is dispensable for growth of KRAS mutant tumors and chloroquine efficacy. *Proc Natl Acad Sci USA*.
68. H Maes, A Kuchnio, A Peric, S Moens, K Nys, K De Bock, A Quaegebeur, S Schoors, M Georgiadou, J Wouters, S Vinckier, H Vankelecom, M Garmyn, AC Vion, F Radtke, C Boulanger, H Gerhardt, E Dejana, M Dewerchin, B Ghesquiere, W Annaert, P Agostinis, P Carmeliet (2014) Tumor vessel normalization by chloroquine independent of autophagy. *Cancer Cell* **26**: 190–206.

Chapter 16

microRNAs as Therapeutic Targets for Gastric Cancer

Takatsugu Ishimoto and Hideo Baba

Abstract

Gastric cancer (GC) remains a leading cause of cancer-related deaths worldwide. microRNAs (miRNAs) are small non-coding RNAs that function as key post-transcriptional regulators of gene expression. Accumulating evidence suggests that dysregulation of miRNAs is intimately involved in carcinogenesis, cancer invasion, metastases, and drug resistance of GC. This chapter summarizes recent findings on the miRNA-mediated mechanisms underlying aggressive behaviors of GC that will help to support the design of novel therapeutic strategies.

Introduction

Gastric cancer (GC) is one of the most common cancers and the third leading cause of cancer deaths worldwide.[1] Despite recent advances in treatment strategies against GC, the survival rate of patients with advanced GC remains poor because of distant metastases and recurrences. GC is divided into two major histological types, intestinal type, and diffuse-type GCs, based on the Lauren classification.[2] Intestinal-type GCs tend to be associated with liver or lymph node metastases, whereas diffuse-type GCs are more likely to cause peritoneal dissemination. To date, multiple types of conventional chemotherapy agents have been unable to treat these metastases successfully. Thus, elucidation of the precise mechanisms associated with GC progression is required to identify critical molecular targets for the development of novel targeted therapeutic agents for advanced GC.

There is unambiguous evidence that carcinogenic processes involve a series of genetic aberrations including gene amplification,[3] and that epigenetic changes are also crucial factors for multiple steps of tumor progression.[4,5] The epigenetic changes that are regulated by DNA methylases, chromatin modifiers, and non-coding RNAs have received extensive attention during the last decade.[6,7] In particular, microRNAs (miRNAs) induce post-transcriptional repression of their target genes by partial complementary base pairing to sequences in the 3′-untranslated region of the messenger RNA (mRNA). Most miRNAs regulate the expression of multiple target genes and many are implicated in diverse human pathologic conditions.[8–10] Emerging evidence suggests that miRNA aberrations are associated with the development and progression of various types of cancer, including GC, by regulating the expression of oncogenes or tumor suppressor genes.[11–13] In this chapter, we summarize the most recent updates on the functional roles of miRNAs in GCs and also discuss their application as therapeutic targets against GC.

miRNAs Associated with Gastric Carcinogenesis

Gastric carcinogenic processes are composed of diverse steps that predispose normal epithelial cells to neoplastic transformation; these processes are modulated through genetic/epigenetic alterations and affected by infectious agents such as *Helicobacter pylori* or Epstein–Barr virus (EBV).[14–17] Cytotoxin-associated gene A (CagA) derived from *H. pylori* is delivered into gastric epithelial cells via a bacterial conjugation system called the type IV secretion system and can induce malignant transformation by perturbing multiple host signaling pathways.[18,19] Accumulating evidence indicates that constant infection with these agents is implicated in the expression of various miRNAs and their unique target genes, and regulates the properties of gastric epithelial cells. In other words, environmental factors have an effect on the expression of tumor-suppressive-miRNAs (TS-miRs) and oncogenic-miRNAs (onco-miRs), and thus promote gastric carcinogenic processes (Table 1).

Helicobacter pylori

Petrocca *et al.* explored global miRNA expression in 20 intestinal type GCs and paired adjacent gastric tissue and in 6 GC cell lines using a custom miRNA microarray. They demonstrated that E2F1 controls the expression of miR-106b, miR-93, and miR-25, a cluster of intronic miRNAs hosted in the *Mcm7* gene, whereas miR-106b and miR-93 regulate E2F1 expression.[20] Following this miRNA microarray analysis, Gao *et al.* shed light on the role of miR-218 in *H. pylori*-associated gastric cancer, showing that the miR-218 expression was reduced significantly in GC tissues and in *H. pylori*-infected gastric mucosa and that the downregulation of miR-218 was associated with nuclear factor-κB (NF-κB) activation.[21] Suzuki *et al.* demonstrated the epigenetic silencing of miR-34b/c in GC and its involvement in the development of an epigenetic field defect during gastric carcinogenesis related to *H. pylori*.[22] Feng *et al.* demonstrated that increased expression of forkhead box M1 and decreased expression of miR-370 are associated with gastric carcinogenesis mediated by *H. pylori* by suppressing P27Kip1 expression.[23] We reported miR-328 downregulation and *de novo* expression of CD44v9 in *H. pylori*-infected gastric mucosa adjacent to GC when compared with the mucosa adjacent to GC not infected with *H. pylori*.[24] It was shown that epigenetic silencing of miR-210 by chronic inflammation promoted the growth of gastric epithelium through upregulation of stathmin 1 and demethyladenosine transferase 1 during persistent *H. pylori* infection.[25] Shen *et al.* also showed that epigenetic silencing of miR-490-3p reactivated the SWI/SNF chromatin remodeling complex subunit and promoted *H. pylori*-induced gastric carcinogenesis.[26] Furthermore, two research groups showed that miR-21 and miR-222 were significantly upregulated in gastric mucosa infected with *H. pylori* and played an important role in gastric carcinogenesis as oncomiRs by suppressing the expression of reversion-inducing cysteine-rich protein with Kazal motifs (RECK).[27,28]

Some researchers have explored the role of miRNA in gastric carcinogenesis using established mouse models. Kong *et al.* demonstrated that the expression level of miR-7, a possible tumor suppressor (TS)-miR,

Table 1. miRNAs involved in the pathogen-related carcinogenesis.

microRNA expression	Targets	Onco/TS-miR	Effects and related pathogen	Reference
miR-218↓	ECOP	TS-miR	Apoptosis and inhibitory effect on cell proliferation, *H. pylori*	(21)
miR-34b/c↓	Not reported	TS-miR	Inhibitory effect on cell proliferation, *H. pylori*	(22)
miR-370↓	FOXM1	TS-miR	Inhibitory effect on cell proliferation, *H. pylori*	(23)
miR-328↓	CD44	TS-miR	*H. pylori*	(24)
miR-210↓	STMN1, DIMT1	TS-miR	Inhibitory effect on cell proliferation, *H. pylori*	(25)
miR-490-3p↓	SMARCD1	TS-miR	Inhibitory effect on growth *in vitro* and *in vivo, H. pylori*	(26)
miR-7↓	LPHN2, BASP1, MAFG	TS-miR	Inhibitory effect on cell proliferation and colony forming ability, *H. pylori*	(29)
let-7↓	Ras	TS-miR	*H. pylori*	(32)
miR-200↓	ZEB1, ZEB2	TS-miR	Cell-to-cell adhesion, EBV	(35)
ebv-miR-BART4-5p↑	Bid	OncomiR	Anti-apoptosis, EBV	(36)
miR-21↑	RECK	OncomiR	Anti-apoptosis, cell proliferation, migration and invasion, *H. pylori*	(27)
miR-222↑	RECK	OncomiR	Cell proliferation and colony forming ability, *H. pylori*	(28)

was significantly decreased in mouse gastric mucosa with *Helicobacter felis* infection. They further showed that the suppression of the miR-7 expression could maintain the undifferentiated state of gastric epithelial cells and thus promote gastric tumorigenesis in *K19-Wnt1/C2mE* mice.[29] Hatakeyama *et al.* explored the mechanism underlying *H. pylori*-induced carcinogenesis and demonstrated that CagA protein derived from *H. pylori*-induced gastric carcinogenesis through the microbial–host cell interaction.[30,31] It was further showed that CagA decreased let-7 expression and increased Ras oncoprotein expression in the stomach of CagA transgenic mice, indicating that let-7 plays an important role in gastric carcinogenesis mediated by CagA.[32]

Epstein–Barr virus

EBV-related GC accounts for almost 10% of all cases of GC and is one of four molecular subtypes of GCs according to a recent report from The Cancer Genome Atlas.[33] Multiple EBV latent genes are considered to contribute to malignant transformation by disrupting diverse intracellular signaling, including alterations in miRNAs.[34] Shinozaki *et al.* demonstrated that the expression of the miR-200 family was downregulated in EBV-related GCs compared with that in EBV-negative GCs. Downregulation of the miR-200 family and the subsequent upregulation of ZEB1/ZEB2 by transfection with EBV latent genes led to a loss of E-cadherin expression, which plays an important role in EBV-related carcinogenesis.[35] More recently, these researchers also showed that EBV-miR-BART4-5p, an EBV encoded miRNA, plays a partial role in suppressing the proapoptotic protein Bid, leading to reduced apoptosis and EBV-associated carcinogenesis.[36]

miRNAs Associated with Refractory GC

5-Fluorouracil (5-FU) and its prodrugs have been mainly used for the treatment of advanced GC in clinical practice. Although several molecular-targeted drugs have been assessed in diverse combinations with conventional chemotherapy agents against advanced GCs, the prognosis of these patients remains poor. Elucidation of the molecular mechanisms underlying treatment resistance is needed in order to identify novel therapeutic targets in patients with advanced GC. Xia *et al.* previously showed that the expression of miR-15b and miR-16 was decreased in SGC7901/VCR cells, which are the multidrug-resistant (MDR) GC cells, concurrent with the upregulation of Bcl-2 protein. The overexpression of these miRNAs could sensitize cells to anti-cancer drugs by targeting BCL2.[37] Li *et al.* also showed that the miR-185 expression was significantly decreased in GC tissues and cell lines, and that the overexpression of miR-185 enhanced the sensitivity of GC cell lines to chemotherapeutic agents by suppressing apoptosis repressor with caspase recruitment domain (ARC). Moreover, they showed that runt-related transcription factor (RUNX3) was implicated in the induction of the miR-185 expression.[38] Recent studies demonstrated that RUNX3 is targeted by several miRNAs. For example, miR-106a was found to be highly expressed in MDR GC cell lines and to enhance the drug resistance of GC cells through RUNX3 suppression.[39] The expression of miR-301a was increased in both GC tissues and cells, and enhanced cell proliferation, soft agar colony formation, migration and invasion, and evasion of cisplatin-induced cell apoptosis through a reduction in the RUNX3 expression.[40] Liu *et al.* reported that the expression of miR-23a was frequently increased and that of interferon regulator factor 1 (IRF1) was decreased in GC tissues, demonstrating that miR-23a suppressed paclitaxel-induced apoptosis in GC cells through suppression of IRF1.[41]

The accumulation of abundant reactive oxidative species (ROS) associated with metabolic disorders and oncogenic stress may cause a redox adaptation response, resulting in the development of oxidative-stress-resistant cancer cells.[42] The redox adaptation mechanism not only confers a survival advantage on cancer cells under excess ROS conditions, but also confers resistance to diverse chemotherapeutic drugs.[43] We have identified a new redox adaptation mechanism through the miRNA–target gene pathway in which macrophages in the tumor stroma cause upregulation of CD44variant9 (v9) through suppression of miR-328 in gastrointestinal cancer. CD44v contributes to ROS defense by enhancing the synthesis of reduced glutathione; thus, upregulation of CD44v induces cell proliferation and resistance to chemotherapeutic agent.[44,45] Knockdown of miR-221 and miR-222 inhibited GC cell proliferation and invasion and increased radiosensitivity through the induction of PTEN expression.[46] Although trastuzumab has recently been used for the treatment of advanced GC in clinical practice, we have demonstrated that particular miRNAs regulate crucial molecules related to the sensitivity of GC cells to trastuzumab. For example, the miR-21–PTEN and miR-223–FBXW7 pathways control sensitivity to trastuzumab via the modulation of apoptosis in human epidermal growth factor receptor 2 (HER2)-positive GC cells.[47,48] The study by Bao *et al.* has shed light on defining the molecular mechanism by which HER2 signaling could cause GC progression, and also reveals that HER2 can interact with CD44 to upregulate CXCR4 by epigenetic silencing of miR-139 in GC cells.[49]

miRNAs Involved in Metastatic Processes

As a result of their invasiveness, GC cells frequently metastasize into the lymph nodes, lung, liver, omentum, and peritoneum.[50,51] Although a number of molecules have been reported to be involved in these metastatic processes, the crucial therapeutic target(s) for prevention of metastasis remain unclear. Accumulating evidence indicates that diverse miRNAs are involved in multiple steps of GC metastasis Table 2.

Migration, invasion, and epithelial–mesenchymal transition

It was demonstrated that the expression of miR-101 was downregulated in GC tissues and that overexpression of miR-101 inhibited not only GC cell growth and invasion *in vitro*, but also tumorigenesis *in vivo*, by targeting EZH2, Cox-2, Mcl-1, and Fos.[52] There are intriguing studies looking into the mechanism underlying miR-101 downregulation in several types of cancers. Indeed, Varambally *et al.* detected genomic loss of miR-101 in 66.7% of metastatic prostate cancers (PCs) and in 37.5% of localized PCs. They proposed that the upregulation of enhancer of zeste homolog 2 (EZH2) resulting from the genomic loss of miR-101 resulted in PC progression.[53] It was subsequently reported that the miR-101 expression was significantly decreased in GC when compared with normal tissue as a result of deletions and/or microdeletions at the miR-101 genomic locus. The loss of miR-101 caused functional deregulation of E-cadherin through EZH2 overexpression in intestinal type GC.[54] Li *et al.* demonstrated that miR-495 and miR-551a expressions were decreased in GC tissues and that these miRNAs suppressed the expression of phosphatase of regenerating liver-3 (PRL-3). Furthermore, the ectopic expression of miR-495 or miR-551a inhibited GC cell migration

Table 2. miRNAs involved in metastatic processes.

microRNA expression	Targets	Onco/TS-miR	Effects	Reference
miR-101↓	EZH2, Cox-2, Mcl-1, Fos	TS-miR	Inhibitory effect on growth *in vitro* and *in vivo* and invasion	(52)(53)(54)
miR-495↓, miR-551a↓	PRL-3	TS-miR	Inhibitory effect on migration and invasion	(55)
miR-610↓	VASP	TS-miR	Inhibitory effect on migration and invasion	(56)
miR-146a↓	WASF2	TS-miR	Inhibitory effect on migration and invasion	(57)
miR-148a↓	MMP7, ROCK1	TS-miR	Inhibitory effect on migration, invasion and metastases *in vivo*	(58)(78)
miR-1207-5p↓, miR-1266↓	hTERT	TS-miR	Inhibitory effect on growth and invasion	(59)
miR-183↓	Bmi-1	TS-miR	Inhibitory effect on growth, colony formation and invasion	(60)
miR-874↓	aquaporin-3, STAT3	TS-miR	Inhibitory effect on growth *in vitro* and *in vivo*, migration, invasion and angiogenesis	(61)(74)
miR-29a/b/c↓	cyclin D2, MMP2	TS-miR	Inhibitory effect on growth *in vitro* and *in vivo* and invasion	(62)
miR-200b↓	ZEB2	TS-miR	Inhibitory effect on growth, migration, invasion and metastases *in vivo*	(68),(86)
miR-204↓	SIRT1	TS-miR	Inhibitory effect on EMT and invasion	(69)
miR-200 family↓	ZEB1, ZEB2	TS-miR	Inhibitory effect on EMT	(70)
miR-125a↓, miR-126↓	VEGF-A	TS-miR	Inhibitory effect on angiogenesis	(72)(73)

miR-409↓	radixin	TS-miR	Inhibitory effect on migration, invasion and metastases *in vivo*	(79)
miR-625↓	ILK	TS-miR	Inhibitory effect on migration, invasion and metastases *in vivo*	(80)
miR-218↓	Robo1	TS-miR	Inhibitory effect on invasion and metastases *in vivo*	(81)
miR-126↓	Crk	TS-miR	Inhibitory effect on growth *in vitro* and *in vivo*, invasion and metastases in vivo	(82)
let-7f↓	MYH9	TS-miR	Inhibitory effect on migration, invasion and metastases *in vivo*	(83)
miR-335↓	Bcl-w, specificity protein 1	TS-miR	Inhibitory effect on invasion and metastases *in vivo*	(84)
miR-7↓	IGF1R	TS-miR	Inhibitory effect on EMT and metastases *in vivo*	(85)
miR-145↓	N-cadherin	TS-miR	Inhibitory effect on migration, invasion and metastases *in vivo*	(87)
miR-516a-3p↓	sulfatase 1	TS-miR	Inhibitory effect on metastases *in vivo*	(88)
miR-192↑, miR-215 ↑	ALCAM	OncomiR	Growth and migration	(63)
miR-423-5p↑	TFF1	OncomiR	Growth, inhibitory effect on migration and invasion	(64)
miR-363↑	MBP-1	OncomiR	Growth, EMT and sphere formation	(67)
miR-130a↑, miR-495↑	RUNX3	OncomiR	Growth and angiogenesis	(75)
miR-223↑	EPB41L3	OncomiR	Migration, invasion and metastases *in vivo*	(89)
miR-370↑	TGF-β-RII	OncomiR	Metastases *in vivo*	(90)
miR-19a/b↑	MXD1	OncomiR	Migration, invasion and metastases *in vivo*	(91)

and invasion through the suppression of PRL-3.[55] Report by Wang *et al.* demonstrated that the expression of miR-610 was downregulated in GC tissues, and that miR-610 significantly inhibited the migration and invasion of GC cells through suppression of vasodilator-stimulated phosphoprotein.[56] It was showed that the miR-146a expression was inversely correlated with the WASP family verprolin homologous protein 2 (WASF2) expression in GC cells and that the ectopic expression of miR-146a inhibited GC cell migration and invasion via suppression of WASF2.[57] Sakamoto *et al.* showed that downregulation of miR-148a was significantly correlated with advanced clinical stage, lymph node metastasis, and poor clinical outcome. Furthermore, the ectopic expression of miR-148a suppressed GC cell invasion by regulating the expression of matrix metalloproteinase 7 (MMP7).[58] Also, Chen *et al.* showed that the expression of miR-1207-5p and miR-1266 was significantly decreased in GC tissues, and that these miRNAs inhibited GC proliferation and invasion by targeting telomerase reverse transcriptase.[59] Similarly, it was reported that the expression of miR-183 was significantly reduced in GC tissues compared with corresponding normal tissues, and that miR-183 suppressed GC cell growth, colony formation, and invasion through suppression of Bmi-1.[60] Report by Jiang *et al.* showed that miR-874 expression was significantly decreased in GC tissues and that the ectopic expression of miR-874 inhibited GC cell proliferation, migration, invasion, and tumorigenicity via suppression of aquaporin-3.[61] Also Gong *et al.* demonstrated that the expression of miR-29 family members (miR-29a/b/c) was downregulated in GC tissues when compared with adjacent controls. They further proved that the ectopic expression of the miR-29 family inhibited not only GC cell growth and invasion *in vitro*, but also tumorigenesis *in vivo*, by suppressing cyclin D2 (CCND2) and MMP2.[62] These miRNAs play crucial roles in the invasive behavior of GC cells as TS-miRs; however, oncogenic (onco)-miRs have also been reported. Furthermore, Jin *et al.* reported that the miR-192 and miR-215 expressions were significantly increased in GC tissues and promoted GC cell proliferation and migration via the suppression of activated leukocyte cell adhesion molecule.[63] Similarly, Liu *et al.* showed that the miR-423-5p expression was significantly increased in GC tissues and suppressed the expression of trefoil factor family1 (TFF1). The ectopic expression of miRNA-423-5p enhanced GC cell proliferation and decreased GC cell migration and invasion.[64]

Epithelial–mesenchymal transition (EMT) in solid cancer cells is intimately involved in cancer progression and metastasis.[65] Several miRNAs have been directly or indirectly associated with the EMT in diverse types of tumor, including GC.[66] Hsu *et al.* showed that the ectopic expression of miR-363 enhanced GC cell proliferation, viability, EMT, and sphere formation ability through downregulation of c-myc promoter binding protein 1 (MBP-1).[67] Likewise, we previously reported that the downregulation of miR-200b was involved in EMT through upregulation of zinc finger E-Box binding homeobox 2 (ZEB2) and promoted GC cell proliferation, migration, and invasion.[68] Zhang *et al.* demonstrated that miR-204 played a crucial role in regulating metastasis of GC through post-transcriptional repression of SIRT1. Furthermore, they showed that the downregulation of miR-204 enhanced EMT and invasion of GC cells by activating the SIRT1-LKB1 pathway.[69] Although Smad3 is known as a mediator of transforming growth factor-β (TGF-β) signaling, it was showed that Smad3 modulated EMT of GC cells by regulating the expression of miR-200 family members in a TGF-β-independent manner.[70]

Tumor angiogenesis

Tumor angiogenesis is essential for metastatic tumor formation, and various intracellular signaling factors including miRNAs have been shown to regulate angiogenic potential in solid tumors.[71] Vascular endothelial growth factor (VEGF) is well known to play a crucial role in modulating the endothelial cell function during blood vessel formation. Studies have demonstrated that particular miRNAs control tumor angiogenesis through the regulation of VEGF-A expression in GCs. The expression of miR-125a and miR-126 was found to be significantly downregulated in GC tissues compared with normal gastric tissues and was inversely correlated with tumor microvessel density and the VEGF-A expression at the protein level.[72,73] Furthermore, the ectopic expression of miR-126 significantly suppressed VEGF-A expression and inhibited the growth of GC cells both *in vitro* and *in vivo*.[73] Zhang *et al.* showed that the miR-874 expression was downregulated and inversely correlated with signal transducer and activator of transcription factor 3 (STAT3) protein in GC tissues, and that downregulation of miR-874 caused tumor angiogenesis through STAT3 upregulation in GC.[74] Work by Lee *et al.*

showed that the combination of the miR-130a and miR-495 inhibited the RUNX3 expression at the protein level and significantly decreased apoptosis. In contrast, the depletion of these miRNAs significantly reduced angiogenesis *in vivo*. These results suggested that the downregulation of RUNX3 by miR-130a and miR-495 cooperatively increased cell proliferation and tumor angiogenesis in GC.[75]

Metastatic tumor formation using *in vivo* models

Tumor formation at distant organs is required for cancer metastasis, and a number of studies using animal models have been conducted to recapitulate human cancer metastases.[76,77] The effect of miRNA expression on cancer metastasis has been investigated by the alteration of certain miRNAs in animal models of metastatic tumor formation. Zheng *et al.* demonstrated that the ectopic expression of miR-148a inhibited GC cell migration and invasion *in vitro* and lung metastasis formation in an *in vivo* model, and reduced the mRNA and protein levels of Rho-activated protein kinase (ROCK1), whereas miR-148a silencing significantly increased ROCK1 expression.[78] They also showed that the overexpression of miR-409 significantly suppressed GC cell migration and invasion *in vitro* and the capacity to develop distal pulmonary metastases and peritoneal dissemination *in vivo* model by directly targeting radixin.[79] In a separate study, it was demonstrated that the overexpression of miR-625 in GC cells significantly impaired their migration and invasion *in vitro* and lung metastases *in vivo* by directly targeting integrin-linked kinase.[80] Also Tie *et al.* showed that the overexpression of miR-218 suppressed Robo1 expression and GC cell invasion *in vitro*, and lung and liver metastasis *in vivo*.[81] Other investigators demonstrated that the overexpression of miR-126 in GC cells significantly suppressed migratory and invasive cell growth *in vitro* and tumorigenicity and lung metastasis *in vivo* by directly targeting Crk.[82] Liang *et al.* demonstrated that the expression of let-7f was decreased in metastatic GC cell lines and tissues. The overexpression of let-7f in GC cells inhibited invasion and migration *in vitro* and liver metastasis *in vivo* by directly targeting the tumor metastasis-associated gene MYH9.[83] It was found that the overexpression of miR-335 inhibited GC cell invasion *in vitro* and lung metastasis *in vivo* by suppressing Bcl-w and specificity protein 1.[84] A few studies have demonstrated that certain miRNAs regulate the expression of EMT-related genes and metastatic tumor formation in *in vivo* models. A report by Zhao *et al.* demonstrated that the miR-7 expression was significantly decreased in metastatic tissues and highly metastatic GC cells. Furthermore, the downregulation of Snail by miR-7 in GC cells inhibited EMT *in vitro* and liver metastasis *in vivo* by targeting IGF1R.[85] Kurashige *et al.* showed that cancer-associated fibroblasts caused the epigenetic repression of miR-200b, and thus enhanced GC cell invasion *in vitro* and peritoneal dissemination *in vivo* through ZEB2 reactivation.[86] Likewise, Gao *et al.* recently showed that the ectopic expression of miR-145 significantly suppressed GC cell migration and invasion *in vitro* and lung metastasis *in vivo* by directly targeting N-cadherin.[87] Furthermore, Takei *et al.* demonstrated the possible potential of miR-516a-3p for antimetastasis therapy using a peritoneal dissemination model. They showed that the injection of the atelocollagen-containing miR-516a-3p expression vector into orthotopic 44As3 tumors, which possess a high metastatic potential, reduced disseminated metastases, and increased the overall survival period compared with the control.[88] These studies indicate that the above miRNAs function as TS-miRs in suppressing GC cell invasion and metastasis. Conversely, oncomiRs that promote the metastatic potential of GC cells have also been explored. Indeed, the report by Li *et al.* demonstrated that the expression of miR-223 was increased in metastatic GC cells, that ectopic expression of miR-223 promoted GC cell migration and invasion *in vitro* and liver metastasis *in vivo* by suppressing erythrocyte membrane protein band 4.1-like 3 (EPB41L3).[89] Also, it was reported that the overexpression of miR-370 increased abdominal metastases *in vivo* through the downregulation of TGF-β-RII,[90] and miR-19a/b expression was increased in GC tissues and associated with metastasis in GC patients. The overexpression of miR-19a/b promoted GC cell migration and invasion *in vitro,* and liver and lung metastases *in vivo*, through MXD1 suppression.[91]

Future Perspectives

From the review of miRNA dysregulation in GC presented in this chapter, it is apparent that many miRNAs have been identified that regulate GC cell behaviors such as proliferation, apoptosis, drug resistance, motility, invasion, EMT, and angiogenesis, by modulating the expression of target genes.

Therefore, miRNA-targeting therapies might not only attenuate the hallmarks of GC cells, but may also sensitize them to conventional chemotherapies. However, the fact remains that miRNAs interact with various target genes and give rise to a large variety of phenomena. The combination of candidate miRNAs that cause GC progression should be investigated for development of more sophisticated therapeutics targeting miRNAs in GC. Moreover, specific delivery systems of miRNA modulators into GC tissues must be developed for miRNA-targeting therapies.

References

1. LA Torre, F Bray, RL Siegel, J Ferlay, J Lortet-Tieulent, A Jemal (2015) Global cancer statistics, 2012. *CA Cancer J Clin* **65**: 87–108.
2. P Lauren (1965) The two histological main types of gastric carcinoma: Diffuse and so-called intestinal-type carcinoma. An attempt at a histo-clinical classification. *Acta Pathol Microbiol Scand* **64**: 31–49.
3. B Vogelstein, N Papadopoulos, VE Velculescu, S Zhou, LA Diaz, KW Jr., Kinzler (2013) Cancer genome landscapes. *Science* **339**: 1546–1558.
4. SB Baylin, PA Jones (2011) A decade of exploring the cancer epigenome — biological and translational implications. *Nat Rev Cancer* **11**: 726–734.
5. ND Marjanovic, RA Weinberg, CL Chaffer (2013) Cell plasticity and heterogeneity in cancer. *Clin Chem* **59**:168–179.
6. M Ptashne (2007) On the use of the word 'epigenetic'. *Curr Biol* **17**: R233–236.
7. M Esteller (2011) Non-coding RNAs in human disease. *Nat Rev Genet* **12**: 861–874.
8. BP Lewis, CB Burge, DP Bartel (2005) Conserved seed pairing, often flanked by adenosines, indicates that thousands of human genes are microRNA targets. *Cell* **120**: 15–20.
9. I Alvarez-Garcia, EA Miska (2005) MicroRNA functions in animal development and human disease. *Development* **132**: 4653–4662.
10. C Xia, K Rajewsk (2009) MicroRNA control in the immune system: Basic principles. *Cell* **136**: 26–36.
11. B Zhang, X Pan, GP Cobb, TA Anderson (2007) MicroRNAs as oncogenes and tumor suppressors. *Dev Biol* **302**: 1–12.
12. S Song, JA Ajani (2013) The role of microRNAs in cancers of the upper gastrointestinal tract. *Nat Rev Gastroenterol Hepatol* **10**: 109–118.

13. T Ishimoto, H Baba, D Izumi, H Sugihara, J Kurashige, M Iwatsuki, P Tan (2016) Current perspectives toward the identification of key players in gastric cancer microRNA dysregulation. *Int J Cancer* **138**: 1337–1349.
14. P Correa (1988) A human model of gastric carcinogenesis. *Cancer Res* **48**: 3554–3560.
15. N Uemura, S Okamoto, S Yamamoto, N Matsumura, S Yamaguchi, M Yamakido, K Taniyama, N Sasaki, RJ Schlemper (2001) Helicobacter pylori infection and the development of gastric cancer. *N Engl J Med* **345**: 784–789.
16. AM Shanks, EM El-Omar (2009) Helicobacter pylori infection, host genetics and gastric cancer. *J Dig Dis* **10**: 157–164.
17. Y Yoda, H Takeshima, T Niwa, JG Kim, T Ando, R Kushima, T Sugiyama, H Katai, H Noshiro, T Ushijima (2015) Integrated analysis of cancer-related pathways affected by genetic and epigenetic alterations in gastric cancer. *Gastric Cancer* **18**: 65–76.
18. M Hatakeyama (2008) Linking epithelial polarity and carcinogenesis by multi-tasking Helicobacter pylori virulence factor CagA. *Oncogene* **27**: 7047–7054.
19. M Hatakeyama (2014) *Helicobacter pylori* CagA and gastric cancer: A paradigm for hit-and-run carcinogenesis. *Cell Host Microbe* **15**: 306–316.
20. F Petrocca, R Visone, MR Onelli, MH Shah, MS Nicoloso, I de Martino, D Iliopoulos, E Pilozzi, CG Liu, M Negrini, L Cavazzini, S Volinia, H Alder, LP Ruco, G Baldassarre, CM Croce, A Vecchione (2008) E2F1-regulated microRNAs impair TGFbeta-dependent cell-cycle arrest and apoptosis in gastric cancer. *Cancer Cell* **13**: 272–286.
21. C Gao, Z Zhang, W Liu, S Xiao, W Gu, H Lu (2010) Reduced microRNA-218 expression is associated with high nuclear factor kappa B activation in gastric cancer. *Cancer* **116**: 41–49.
22. H Suzuki, E Yamamoto, M Nojima, M Kai, HO Yamano, K Yoshikawa, T Kimura, T Kudo, E Harada, T Sugai, H Takamaru, T Niinuma, R Maruyama, H Yamamoto, T Tokino, K Imai, M Toyota, Y Shinomura (2010) Methylation-associated silencing of microRNA-34b/c in gastric cancer and its involvement in an epigenetic field defect. *Carcinogenesis* **31**: 2066–2073.
23. Y Feng, L Wang, J Zeng, L Shen, X Liang, H Yu, S Liu, Z Liu, Y Sun, W Li, C Chen, J Jia (2013) FoxM1 is overexpressed in Helicobacter pylori-induced gastric carcinogenesis and is negatively regulated by miR-370. *Mol Cancer Res* **11**: 834–844.
24. T Ishimoto, D Izumi, M Watanabe, N Yoshida, K Hidaka, K Miyake, H Sugihara, H Sawayama, Y Imamura, M Iwatsuki, S Iwagami, Y Baba, H Horlad, Y Komohara, M Takeya, H Baba (2015) Chronic inflammation with

Helicobacter pylori infection is implicated in CD44 overexpression through miR-328 suppression in the gastric mucosa. *J Gastroenterol* **50**(7): 751–7.

25. K Kiga, H Mimuro, M Suzuki, A Shinozaki-Ushiku, T Kobayashi, T Sanada, M Kim, M Ogawa, YW Iwasaki, H Kayo, Y Fukuda-Yuzawa, M Yashiro, M Fukayama, T Fukao, C Sasakawa (2014) Epigenetic silencing of miR-210 increases the proliferation of gastric epithelium during chronic Helicobacter pylori infection. *Nat Commun* **5**: 4497.
26. J Shen, Z Xiao, WK Wu, MH Wang, KF To, Y Chen, W Yang, MS Li, VV Shin, JH Tong, W Kang, L Zhang, M Li, L Wang, L Lu, RL Chan, SH Wong, J Yu, MT Chan, FK Chan, JJ Sung, AS Cheng, CH Cho (2015) Epigenetic silencing of miR-490-3p reactivates the chromatin remodeler SMARCD1 to promote Helicobacter pylori-induced gastric carcinogenesis. *Cancer Res* **75**(4): 754–765.
27. Z Zhang, Z Li, C Gao, P Chen, J Chen, W Liu, S Xiao, H Lu (2008) MiR-21 plays a pivotal role in gastric cancer pathogenesis and progression. *Lab Invest* **88**: 1358–1366.
28. N Li, B Tang, ED Zhu, BS Li, Y Zhuang, S Yu, DS Lu, QM Zou, B Xiao, XH Mao (2012) Increased miR-222 in *H. pylori*-associated gastric cancer correlated with tumor progression by promoting cancer cell proliferation and targeting RECK. *FEBS Lett* **586**: 722–728.
29. D Kong, YS Piao, S Yamashita, H Oshima, K Oguma, S Fushida, T Fujimura, T Minamoto, H Seno, Y Yamada, K Satou, T Ushijima, TO Ishikawa, M Oshima (2012) Inflammation-induced repression of tumor suppressor miR-7 in gastric tumor cells. *Oncogene* **31**: 3949–3960.
30. M Hatakeyama (2004) Oncogenic mechanisms of the Helicobacter pylori CagA protein. *Nat Rev Cancer* **4**: 688–694.
31. M Hatakeyama (2006) Helicobacter pylori CagA — a bacterial intruder conspiring gastric carcinogenesis. *Int J Cancer* **119**: 1217–1223.
32. Y Hayashi, M Tsujii, J Wang, J Kondo, T Akasaka, Y Jin, W Li, T Nakamura, T Nishida, H Iijima, S Tsuji, S Kawano, N Hayashi, T Takehara (2013) CagA mediates epigenetic regulation to attenuate let-7 expression in *Helicobacter pylori*-related carcinogenesis. *Gut* **62**: 1536–1546.
33. Cancer Genome Atlas Research N (2014) Comprehensive molecular characterization of gastric adenocarcinoma. *Nature* **513**: 202–209.
34. SW Tsao, CM Tsang, KF To, KW Lo (2015) The role of Epstein–Barr virus in epithelial malignancies. *J Pathol* **235**: 323–333.
35. A Shinozaki, T Sakatani, T Ushiku, R Hino, M Isogai, S Ishikawa, H Uozaki, K Takada, M Fukayama (2010) Downregulation of microRNA-200 in EBV-associated gastric carcinoma. *Cancer Res* **70**: 4719–4727.

36. A Shinozaki-Ushiku, A Kunita, M Isogai, T Hibiya, T Ushiku, K Takada, M Fukayama (2015) Profiling of virus-encoded microRNAs in Epstein-Barr virus-associated gastric carcinoma and their roles in gastric carcinogenesis. *J Virol* **89**: 5581–5591.
37. L Xia, D Zhang, R Du, Y Pan, L Zhao, S Sun, L Hong, J Liu, D Fan (2008) miR-15b and miR-16 modulate multidrug resistance by targeting BCL2 in human gastric cancer cells. *Int J Cancer* **123**: 372–379.
38. Q Li, JX Wang, YQ He, C Feng, XJ Zhang, JQ Sheng, PF Li (2014) MicroRNA-185 regulates chemotherapeutic sensitivity in gastric cancer by targeting apoptosis repressor with caspase recruitment domain. *Cell Death Dis* **5**: e1197.
39. Y Zhang, Q Lu, X Cai (2013) MicroRNA-106a induces multidrug resistance in gastric cancer by targeting RUNX3. *FEBS Lett* **587**: 3069–3075.
40. M Wang, C Li, B Yu, L Su, J Li, J Ju, Y Yu, Q Gu, Z Zhu, B Liu (2013) Overexpressed miR-301a promotes cell proliferation and invasion by targeting RUNX3 in gastric cancer. *J Gastroenterol* **48**: 1023–1033.
41. X Liu, J Ru, J Zhang, LH Zhu , M Liu, X Li, H Tang (2013) miR-23a targets interferon regulatory factor 1 and modulates cellular proliferation and paclitaxel-induced apoptosis in gastric adenocarcinoma cells. *PLoS One* **8**: e64707.
42. S Pervaiz, MV Clement (2004) Tumor intracellular redox status and drug resistance — serendipity or a causal relationship? *Curr Pharm Des* **10**: 1969–1977.
43. D Trachootham, J Alexandre, P Huang (2009) Targeting cancer cells by ROS-mediated mechanisms: A radical therapeutic approach? *Nat Rev Drug Discov* **8**: 579–591.
44. T Ishimoto, O Nagano, T Yae, M Tamada, T Motohara, H Oshima, M Oshima, T Ikeda, R Asaba, H Yagi, T Masuko, T Shimizu, T Ishikawa, K Kai, E Takahashi, Y Imamura, Y Baba, M Ohmura, M Suematsu, H Baba, H Saya (2011) CD44 variant regulates redox status in cancer cells by stabilizing the xCT subunit of system xc(-) and thereby promotes tumor growth. *Cancer Cell* **19**: 387–400.
45. T Ishimoto, H Sugihara, M Watanabe, H Sawayama, M Iwatsuki, Y Baba, H Okabe, K Hidaka, N Yokoyama, K Miyake, M Yoshikawa, O Nagano, Y Komohara, M Takeya, H Saya, H Baba (2014) Macrophage-derived reactive oxygen species suppress miR-328 targeting CD44 in cancer cells and promote redox adaptation. *Carcinogenesis* **35**: 1003–1011.
46. Z Chun-Zhi, H Lei, Z An-Ling, F Yan-Chao, Y Xiao, W Guang-Xiu, J Zhi-Fan, P Pei-Yu, Z Qing-Yu, K Chun-Sheng (2010) MicroRNA-221 and microRNA-222 regulate gastric carcinoma cell proliferation and radioresistance by targeting PTEN. *BMC Cancer* **10**: 367.

47. K Eto, M Iwatsuki, M Watanabe, S Ida, T Ishimoto, S Iwagami, Y Baba, Y Sakamoto, Y Miyamoto, N Yoshida, H Baba (2014) The microRNA-21/PTEN pathway regulates the sensitivity of HER2-positive gastric cancer cells to trastuzumab. *Ann Surg Oncol* **21**: 343–350.
48. K Eto, M Iwatsuki, M Watanabe, T Ishimoto, S Ida, Y Imamura, S Iwagami, Y Baba, Y Sakamoto, Y Miyamoto, N Yoshida, H Baba (2014) The sensitivity of gastric cancer to trastuzumab is regulated by the miR-223/FBXW7 pathway. *Int J Cancer*.
49. W Bao, HJ Fu, QS Xie, L Wang, R Zhang, ZY Guo, J Zhao, YL Meng, XL Ren, T Wang, Q Li, BQ Jin, LB Yao, RA Wang, DM Fan, SY Chen, LT Jia, AG Yang (2011) HER2 interacts with CD44 to up-regulate CXCR4 via epigenetic silencing of microRNA-139 in gastric cancer cells. *Gastroenterology* **141**: 2076–2087.
50. Y Esaki, R Hirayama, K Hirokawa (1990) A comparison of patterns of metastasis in gastric cancer by histologic type and age. *Cancer* **65**: 2086–2090.
51. D Marrelli, F Roviello, G de Manzoni, P Morgagni, A Di Leo, L Saragoni, A De Stefano, S Folli, C Cordiano, E Pinto, Italian Research Group for Gastric Cancer (2002) Different patterns of recurrence in gastric cancer depending on Lauren's histological type: Longitudinal study. *World J Surg* **26**: 1160–1165.
52. HJ Wang, HJ Ruan, XJ He, YY Ma, XT Jiang, YJ Xia, ZY Ye, HQ Tao (2010) MicroRNA-101 is down-regulated in gastric cancer and involved in cell migration and invasion. *Eur J Cancer* **46**: 2295–2303.
53. S Varambally, Q Cao, RS Mani, S Shankar, X Wang, B Ateeq, B Laxman, X Cao, X Jing, K Ramnarayanan, JC Brenner, J Yu, JH Kim, B Han, P Tan, C Kumar-Sinha, RJ Lonigro, N Palanisamy, CA Maher, AM Chinnaiyan (2008) Genomic loss of microRNA-101 leads to overexpression of histone methyltransferase EZH2 in cancer. *Science* **322**: 1695–1699.
54. J Carvalho, NC van Grieken, PM Pereira, S Sousa, M Tijssen, TE Buffart, B Diosdado, H Grabsch, MA Santos, G Meijer, R Seruca, B Carvalho, C Oliveira (2012) Lack of microRNA-101 causes E-cadherin functional deregulation through EZH2 up-regulation in intestinal gastric cancer. *J Pathol* **228**: 31–44.
55. Z Li, Y Cao, Z Jie, Y Liu, Y Li, J Li, G Zhu, Z Liu, Y Tu, G Peng, DW Lee, SS Park (2012) MiR-495 and miR-551a inhibit the migration and invasion of human gastric cancer cells by directly interacting with PRL-3. *Cancer Lett* **323**: 41–47.
56. J Wang, J Zhang, J Wu, D Luo, K Su, W Shi, J Liu, Y Tian, L Wei (2012) MicroRNA-610 inhibits the migration and invasion of gastric cancer cells by suppressing the expression of vasodilator-stimulated phosphoprotein. *Eur J Cancer* **48**: 1904–1913.

57. Q Yao, Z Cao, C Tu, Y Zhao, H Liu, S Zhang (2013) MicroRNA-146a acts as a metastasis suppressor in gastric cancer by targeting WASF2. *Cancer Lett* **335**: 219–224.
58. N Sakamoto, Y Naito, N Oue, K Sentani, N Uraoka, H Zarni Oo, K Yanagihara, K Aoyagi, H Sasaki, W Yasui (2014) MicroRNA-148a is down-regulated in gastric cancer, targets MMP7, and indicates tumor invasiveness and poor prognosis. *Cancer Sci* **105**: 236–243.
59. L Chen, MH Lu, D Zhang, NB Hao, YH Fan, YY Wu, SM Wang, R Xie, DC Fang, H Zhang, CJ Hu, SM Yang (2014) miR-1207-5p and miR-1266 suppress gastric cancer growth and invasion by targeting telomerase reverse transcriptase. *Cell Death Dis* **5**: e1034.
60. L Xu, Y Li, D Yan, J He, D Liu (2014) MicroRNA-183 inhibits gastric cancer proliferation and invasion via directly targeting Bmi-1. *Oncol Lett* **8**: 2345–2351.
61. B Jiang, Z Li, W Zhang, H Wang, X Zhi, J Feng, Z Chen, Y Zhu, L Yang, H Xu, Z Xu (2014) miR-874 Inhibits cell proliferation, migration and invasion through targeting aquaporin-3 in gastric cancer. *J Gastroenterol* **49**: 1011–1025.
62. J Gong, J Li, Y Wang, C Liu, H Jia, C Jiang, Y Wang, M Luo, H Zhao, L Dong, W Song, F Wang, W Wang, J Zhang, J Yu (2014) Characterization of microRNA-29 family expression and investigation of their mechanistic roles in gastric cancer. *Carcinogenesis* **35**: 497–506.
63. Z Jin, FM Selaru, Y Cheng, T Kan, R Agarwal, Y Mori, AV Olaru, J Yang, S David, JP Hamilton, JM Abraham, J Harmon, M Duncan, EA Montgomery, SJ Meltzer (2011) MicroRNA-192 and -215 are upregulated in human gastric cancer in vivo and suppress ALCAM expression in vitro. *Oncogene* **30**: 1577–1585.
64. J Liu, X Wang, X Yang, Y Liu, Y Shi, J Ren, B Guleng (2014) miRNA423-5p regulates cell proliferation and invasion by targeting trefoil factor 1 in gastric cancer cells. *Cancer Lett* **347**: 98–104.
65. M Iwatsuki, K Mimori, T Yokobori, H Ishi, T Beppu, S Nakamori, H Baba, M Mori (2010) Epithelial-mesenchymal transition in cancer development and its clinical significance. *Cancer Sci* **101**: 293–299.
66. B De Craene, G Berx (2013) Regulatory networks defining EMT during cancer initiation and progression. *Nat Rev Cancer* **13**: 97–110.
67. KW Hsu, AM Wang, YH Ping, KH Huang, TT Huang, HC Lee, SS Lo, CW Chi, TS Yeh (2014) Downregulation of tumor suppressor MBP-1 by microRNA-363 in gastric carcinogenesis. *Carcinogenesis* **35**: 208–217.
68. J Kurashige, H Kamohara, M Watanabe, Y Hiyoshi, M Iwatsuki, Y Tanaka, K Kinoshita, S Saito, Y Baba, H Baba (2012) MicroRNA-200b regulates cell

proliferation, invasion, and migration by directly targeting ZEB2 in gastric carcinoma. *Ann Surg Oncol* **19 Suppl 3**: S656–S664.
69. L Zhang, X Wang, P Chen (2013) MiR-204 down regulates SIRT1 and reverts SIRT1-induced epithelial-mesenchymal transition, anoikis resistance and invasion in gastric cancer cells. *BMC Cancer* **13**: 290.
70. SM Ahn, JY Cha, J Kim, D Kim, HT Trang, YM Kim, YH Cho, D Park, S Hong (2012) Smad3 regulates E-cadherin via miRNA-200 pathway. *Oncogene* **31**: 3051–3059.
71. SM Weis, DA Cheresh (2011) Tumor angiogenesis: Molecular pathways and therapeutic targets. *Nat Med* **17**: 1359–1370.
72. J Dai, J Wang, L Yang, Y Xiao, Q Ruan (2015) miR-125a regulates angiogenesis of gastric cancer by targeting vascular endothelial growth factor A. *Int J Oncol* **47**: 1801–1810.
73. H Chen, L Li, S Wang, Y Lei, Q Ge, N Lv, X Zhou, C Chen (2014) Reduced miR-126 expression facilitates angiogenesis of gastric cancer through its regulation on VEGF-A. *Oncotarget* **5**: 11873–11885.
74. X Zhang, J Tang, X Zhi, K Xie, W Wang, Z Li, Y Zhu, L Yang, H Xu, Z Xu (2015) miR-874 functions as a tumor suppressor by inhibiting angiogenesis through STAT3/VEGF-A pathway in gastric cancer. *Oncotarget* **6**(3): 1605–17.
75. SH Lee, YD Jung, YS Choi, YM Lee (2015) Targeting of RUNX3 by miR-130a and miR-495 cooperatively increases cell proliferation and tumor angiogenesis in gastric cancer cells. *Oncotarget* **6**: 33269–33278.
76. P Mehlen, A Puisieux (2006) Metastasis: a question of life or death. *Nat Rev Cancer* **6**: 449–458.
77. G Francia, W Cruz-Munoz, S Man, P Xu, RS Kerbel (2011) Mouse models of advanced spontaneous metastasis for experimental therapeutics. *Nat Rev Cancer* **11**: 135–141.
78. B Zheng, L Liang, C Wang, S Huang, X Cao, R Zha, L Liu, D Jia, Q Tian, J Wu, Y Ye, Q Wang, Z Long, Y Zhou, C Du, X He, Y Shi (2011) MicroRNA-148a suppresses tumor cell invasion and metastasis by downregulating ROCK1 in gastric cancer. *Clin Cancer Res* **17**: 7574–7583.
79. B Zheng, L Liang, S Huang, R Zha, L Liu, D Jia, Q Tian, Q Wang, C Wang, Z Long, Y Zhou, X Cao, C Du, Y Shi, X He (2012) MicroRNA-409 suppresses tumour cell invasion and metastasis by directly targeting radixin in gastric cancers. *Oncogene* **31**: 4509–4516.
80. M Wang, C Li, H Nie, X Lv, Y Qu, B Yu, L Su, J Li, X Chen, J Ju, Y Yu, M Yan, Q Gu, Z Zhu, B Liu (2012) Down-regulated miR-625 suppresses invasion and metastasis of gastric cancer by targeting ILK. *FEBS Lett* **586**: 2382–2388.

81. J Tie, Y Pan, L Zhao, K Wu, J Liu, S Sun, X Guo, B Wang, Y Gang, Y Zhang, Q Li, T Qiao, Q Zhao, Y Nie, D Fan (2010) MiR-218 inhibits invasion and metastasis of gastric cancer by targeting the Robo1 receptor. *PLoS Genet* **6** :e1000879.
82. R Feng, X Chen, Y Yu, L Su, B Yu, J Li, Q Cai, M Yan, B Liu, Z Zhu (2010) miR-126 functions as a tumour suppressor in human gastric cancer. *Cancer Lett* **298**: 50–63.
83. S Liang, L He, X Zhao, Y Miao, Y Gu, C Guo, Z Xue, W Dou, F Hu, K Wu, Y Nie, D Fan (2011) MicroRNA let-7f inhibits tumor invasion and metastasis by targeting MYH9 in human gastric cancer. *PLoS One* **6**: e18409.
84. Y Xu, F Zhao, Z Wang, Y Song, Y Luo, X Zhang, L Jiang, Z Sun, Z Miao, H Xu (2012) MicroRNA-335 acts as a metastasis suppressor in gastric cancer by targeting Bcl-w and specificity protein 1. *Oncogene* **31**: 1398–1407.
85. X Zhao, W Dou, L He, S Liang, J Tie, C Liu, T Li, Y Lu, P Mo, Y Shi, K Wu, Y Nie, D Fan (2013) MicroRNA-7 functions as an anti-metastatic microRNA in gastric cancer by targeting insulin-like growth factor-1 receptor. *Oncogene* **32**: 1363–1372.
86. J Kurashige, K Mima, G Sawada, Y Takahashi, H Eguchi, K Sugimachi, M Mori, K Yanagihara, M Yashiro, K Hirakawa, H Baba, K Mimori (2015) Epigenetic modulation and repression of miR-200b by cancer-associated fibroblasts contribute to cancer invasion and peritoneal dissemination in gastric cancer. *Carcinogenesis* **36**: 133–141.
87. P Gao, AY Xing, GY Zhou, TG Zhang, JP Zhang, C Gao, H Li, DB Shi (2013) The molecular mechanism of microRNA-145 to suppress invasion-metastasis cascade in gastric cancer. *Oncogene* **32**: 491–501.
88. Y Takei, M Takigahira, K Mihara, Y Tarumi, K Yanagihara (2011) The metastasis-associated microRNA miR-516a-3p is a novel therapeutic target for inhibiting peritoneal dissemination of human scirrhous gastric cancer. *Cancer Res* **71**: 1442–1453.
89. X Li, Y Zhang, H Zhang, X Liu, T Gong, M Li, L Sun, G Ji, Y Shi, Z Han, S Han, Y Nie, X Chen, Q Zhao, J Ding, K Wu, F Daiming (2011) miRNA-223 promotes gastric cancer invasion and metastasis by targeting tumor suppressor EPB41L3. *Mol Cancer Res* **9**: 824–833.
90. SS Lo, PS Hung, JH Chen, HF Tu, WL Fang, CY Chen, WT Chen, NR Gong, CW Wu (2012) Overexpression of miR-370 and downregulation of its novel target TGFbeta-RII contribute to the progression of gastric carcinoma. *Oncogene* **31**: 226–237.
91. Q Wu, Z Yang, Y An, H Hu, J Yin, P Zhang, Y Nie, K Wu, Y Shi, D Fan (2014) MiR-19a/b modulate the metastasis of gastric cancer cells by targeting the tumour suppressor MXD1. *Cell Death Dis* **5**: e1144.

Chapter 17

microRNA-based Novel Therapeutic Development in Gastrointestinal Cancer

Andrew Fesler and Jingfang Ju

Abstract

Non-coding RNAs, and microRNAs (miRNAs) in particular, have emerged as important molecules in the cell that help to regulate proper cellular function. Since their discovery, miRNAs have been found to play important roles in cancer development and progression. miRNAs can target essential genes in the cell to regulate their expression. They have been identified as both oncogenes and tumor suppressors in many different types of cancers. Many miRNAs have been found to have altered expression in cancer tissues compared to normal tissue. Based on the important cancer-related functions that have been identified for miRNA, there is great interest in their therapeutic potential. Some miRNAs have shown promise in preclinical studies and miR-34 has advanced to clinical trials. miRNAs also have potential as cancer biomarkers which may further help in the management of cancer. In this chapter, we review the potential clinical applications of miRNAs in gastrointestinal cancers both as therapeutics and biomarkers.

Introduction

Non-coding RNAs are important molecules that comprise the majority of RNAs in the cell and are essential for proper cellular functions. One type of non-coding RNA that has received great interest and shown great promise for potential therapeutic applications is microRNA (miRNA). miRNAs are short (19–21 nucleotide) non-coding RNAs. Some miRNAs are derived from non-coding regions of the genome, while others are derived from the introns of coding genes.[1] The biogenesis and functions of miRNAs associated with cancer therapeutics are illustrated in Figure 1. The first miRNA to be identified was lin-4, identified in 1993 in *C. elegands*.[2] It would be 7 years before it was appreciated that miRNAs are conserved and found in other organisms, including humans.[3] In the time since the discovery of miRNAs, we have learned a great deal about their functions and the important biological roles they play. The primary function of miRNA is the regulation of target mRNA. This regulation is the result of complementarity between the 3′-UTR of the target mRNA and the miRNA. In particular, the 2–7 nucleotides of the miRNA are important for this interaction and are considered the seed sequence of the miRNA.[4] This interaction between the miRNA and the mRNA, in conjunction with the RISC complex, leads to mRNA degradation. Additionally, an miRNA can disrupt the translation of an mRNA, inhibiting the expression of the target.[5] An individual miRNA can have multiple different targets, and thus can regulate a network of genes. As we have developed a deeper understanding of miRNA functions, our appreciation for the critical roles they play in the cell has grown.

It was not long after miRNAs were identified in human cells, before it was discovered that they play a role in human diseases, and cancer in particular. In 2002, Calin *et al.* discovered that genomic deletions in the region encoding two miRNAs, miR-15 and miR-16, were associated with chronic lymphocytic leukemia.[6] This discovery would be the first of many showing the important roles of miRNAs in cancer. In the last 14 years, the miRNA-cancer field has exploded; a search on PubMed for miRNA and cancer reveals over 21,000 papers on this topic. In this time, miRNAs have been found to regulate many different genes that are important in cancer development. The expression of some miRNAs is also regulated by important genes associated with cancer. miRNAs have a diverse array of effects on the cell; while some have been identified as tumor suppressors, others seem to

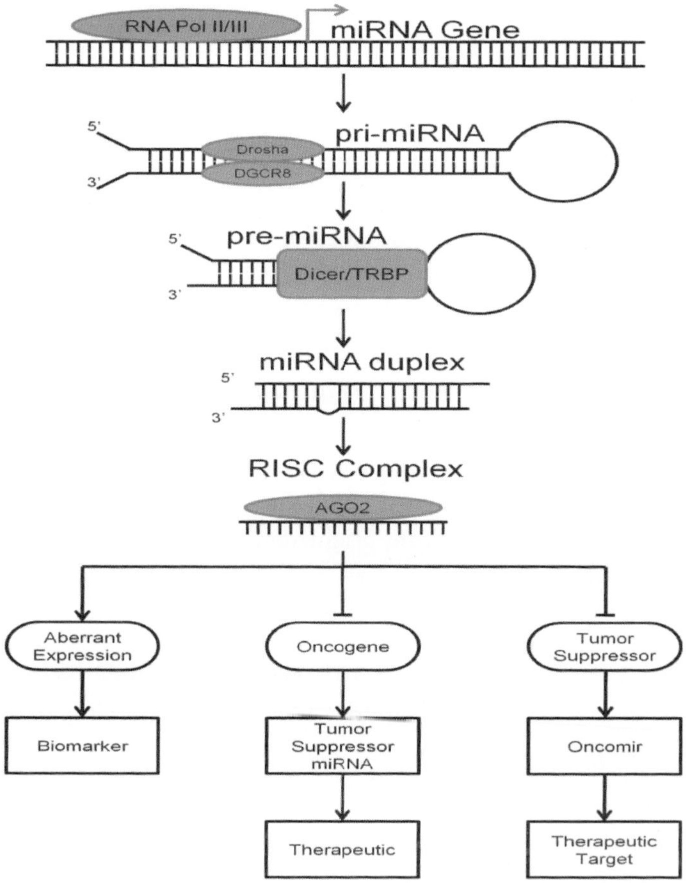

Figure 1. miRNA biogenesis and functions associated with therapeutics. miRNAs are transcribed by RNA Pol II or III. The miRNA precursor is processed first by Drosha and DGCR8 and then by Dicer/TRBP. miRNA associate with the RISC complex including AGO2 to target mRNA. Aberrant miRNA expression contributes to their roll in cancer and their potential as biomarkers. miRNAs that regulate tumor suppressors act as oncomiRs and are potential therapeutic targets. miRNAs that target oncogenes act as tumor suppressors and have potential as therapeutics.

be more oncogenic. These roles can be cell-type and tissue specific, due to different targets having more importance in different cellular contexts. In addition to what has been discovered thus far, the field continues to grow with new connections between miRNAs and different targets and pathways being discovered.

With the great appreciation that has developed in the last decade for the important functions of miRNAs and the significance they have in cancer treatment, attention has turned to their therapeutic potential. Indeed, some miRNAs show promise as therapeutics to be used in conjunction with traditional chemotherapy to improve treatment efficacy and patient outcomes. OncomiRs are being investigated as important therapeutic targets, the disruption of which may improve patient survival. In addition to this therapeutic angle, expression profiling has found that differences in the miRNA expression can be associated with cancer development as well as progression. Thus, there is also promise for miRNA-based biomarkers that may help with patient diagnosis or prognosis. This is further supported by the presence of miRNAs in circulation, which could make for very efficient non-invasive cancer screening. There are still challenges left to face in the development of miRNA-based therapeutics. However, this is an exciting frontier in cancer therapeutics, and the prospects are bright that miRNAs will have important roles in cancer treatment in the future.

Significant Functions of miRNA in Gastrointestinal (GI) Cancers

The important functional roles that miRNAs have in cancer are the result of miRNA targeting important oncogenic and tumor suppressor genes. Disruptions of miRNA expression can lead to changes in the expression of these important genes, promoting cancer development. In GI cancers as well as other cancers, miRNAs have been shown to regulate cell cycle progression and cell proliferation. There are also examples of miRNA regulating cancer metastasis, epithelial–mesenchymal transition (EMT), and chemoresistance. It is not only in cancer cells that aberrant miRNA expression can promote cancer development, but disruptions of miRNA expression in the tumor stromal cells and infiltrating immune cells can also contribute to cancer development and progression. Although the roles of some miRNAs remain difficult to classify, other miRNAs have clearly emerged as tumor suppressors or oncomiRs .

OncomiRs

As one might expect, when you consider the diverse genes, that miRNAs can regulate, some miRNAs seem to promote cancer formation and are considered oncomiRs. These miRNAs generally show increased expression in cancerous tissue when compared to normal tissue, and largely target tumor suppressor genes. miR-21 has been identified as an oncomiR in several different types of cancers. In esophageal cancer, miR-21 targets tumor suppressor, PTEN, and inhibition of miR-21 in cancer cells leads to a decrease in cell invasion.[7] In colorectal cancer, PDCD4 is another tumor suppressor targeted by miR-21.[8] These two targets have also been confirmed in gastric, liver, and pancreatic cancers.[9–11] In gastric cancer, this regulation has been linked to resistance to cisplatin. In pancreatic cancer, miR-21 regulation of these targets is associated with resistance to 5-fluorouracil (5-FU).[11] miR-21 expression is also elevated in fibroblast-like cells in colorectal cancer stroma. This overexpression inhibits the expression of RECK contributing to increased invasion of the colorectal cancer cells.[12] Clearly, miR-21 can have important influences on the development and progression of all of these GI-related cancers. It represents a strong example of an oncogenic miRNA in GI cancers. miR-155 is another miRNA that has been characterized as an oncomiR in GI cancers. In these cancers, miR-155 generally has been found to be overexpressed. In colon cancer, MLH1, MSH2, and MSH6, all of which are important genes in the mismatch repair pathway, have been identified as targets. The disruption of the expression of these genes by overexpression of miR-155 is associated with microsatellite instability and errors in DNA replication.[13] miR-155 also promotes cell proliferation, invasion, and is increased in colon cancer stem cells (CSCs). MLH1 has also been identified as a target of miR-155 in pancreatic cancer.[14] In liver cancer, miR-155 has been linked to cancer stemness, through targeting TP53INP.[15] Another miRNA that has been found to have oncogenic functions in GI cancers is miR-106b. In the case of miR-106b, in colon cancer and esophageal cancer, p21 has been identified as an important target.[16,17] In esophageal cancer, the inhibition of miR-106b reduced tumorigenesis *in vivo*.[16] In colon cancer, the inhibition of p21 as well as PTEN by miR-106b is associated with resistance to radiation therapy.[17] PTEN has also been verified as a target of miR-106b in gastric cancer-associated fibroblasts, and its inhibition by increased expression of miR-106b seems to promote migration and invasion.[18] In liver cancer, miR-106b targets APC and its overexpression promotes cell cycle progression, and is associated with poor prognosis.[19] miR-221/222 are also widely recognized as oncomiRs in GI cancers. In pancreatic cancer, the expression of these miRNAs promotes cell proliferation, enhances cell cycle progression, invasion, and inhibits apoptosis. miR-221/222 target TIMP-2, which in turn leads to the up-regulation of MMP-2 and MMP-9.[20] In liver, miR-221/222 have been found to target p27 and DDIT4. These miRNAs promote cell growth as well as tumorigenesis.[21] In the colon, evidence shows that the expression of these oncomiRs is regulated by oncogenic KRAS, and they are overexpressed in colon cancer tissue compared to normal colon tissue.[22] In both colon and gastric cancers, these miRNAs have been shown to target PTEN, and regulate proliferation and resistance to radiation therapy.[22,23] These are just a few examples of miRNAs that demonstrate oncogenic functions in GI cancers. These miRNAs may be valuable targets for therapeutic interventions going forward.

Tumor suppressor miRNAs

In addition to these miRNAs that have been identified as oncomiRs, there are also many miRNAs that have tumor suppressor functions. These miRNAs are generally downregulated in cancer compared to normal, and primarily target oncogenes. miR-34 is one of the best characterized tumor suppressor miRNAs. miR-34 is a direct transcriptional target of p53. The decreased expression of miR-34 in several cancers has been linked to methylation of the miR-34 promoter region.[24] In gastric cancer, miR-34 shows decreased expression compared to normal, and restoration of miR-34 inhibits cell growth and promotes apoptosis. Important for CSCs, miR-34 inhibits tumor sphere formation. Antiapoptotic BCL2 has been identified as a target of miR-34 in gastric cancer.[25] miR-34 also targets Ying Yang 1 (YY1), a transcription factor which effects the expression of Sox-2 and Oct-4. Overexpression of YY1 contributes to carcinogenesis, and miR-34 is able to ablate some of these effects.[26] miR-34 also regulates Wnt signaling by targeting several genes in this pathway. The loss of miR-34 repression of this pathway contributes to the development of colon cancer.[27] miR-34 in pancreatic cancer cells seems to inhibit self-renewal of CSCs, and is reduced in cells with more stem-like properties.[28] In liver cancer, miR-34 deregulation contributes to increased recruitment of regulatory T cells, which may contribute to tumor escape from immune surveillance.[29] Although let-7 was one of the first miRNAs discovered, in *C. elegands*, it was later determined to be found in many different species, including humans. Let-7 has been identified as a tumor suppressor gene in human GI cancers. In colon cancer cells, let-7 seems to reduce proliferation.[30] In gastric cancer, let-7 reduces colony formation, proliferation, invasion, and targets PKM2.[31] In esophageal cancer, HMGA2 plays an important role in metastasis when its regulation is disrupted by loss of let-7.[32] In pancreatic cancer, there is evidence that a long non-coding RNA, H19, inhibits let-7 allowing for increased expression of HMGA2 promoting cancer progression.[33] Another miRNA shown to be an important tumor suppressor is miR-101. In colon cancer, COX-2 and EZH2 are important targets, and miR-101 can inhibit Wnt signaling.[34] miR-101 shows lower expression in gastric cancer and also targets EZH2 and COX-2. The loss of miR-101 promotes invasion and migration.[35] An interesting recent finding in esophageal cancer shows that miR-101 can target the long non-coding RNA MALAT1. Through the targeting of MALAT1, miR-101 can inhibit proliferation, cell cycle progression, invasion, and migration.[36] In liver cancer, ZEB1, a key regulator of EMT, is targeted by miR-101 and can inhibit its ability to promote EMT.[37] There are many more examples of miRNA that exert tumor-suppressor-like functions in GI cancers. The loss of expression of these miRNAs contributes to cancer development, progression, or ability to resist chemotherapeutic intervention. Just as the oncomiRs represent important potential targets for drug intervention, these miRNAs have potential to be used as therapeutics themselves. If we can re-express the miRNAs that are lost in GI cancers, it may help to improve patient outcomes.

Therapeutic potential of miRNA: Therapeutics

With the preponderance of evidence that has been gathered in the last 14 years, showing that miRNAs have important regulatory functions and play significant roles in cancer, there is a great hope for the potential of miRNA-based therapeutics as well as targeting miRNA for therapy. 5-FU, which targets thymidylate synthase (TS) and disrupts DNA replication, targeting proliferating cells, is one of the key components of chemotherapeutic treatment of GI cancers. While treatments have improved patient outcomes, there remain challenges associated with the development of chemoresistance as well as recurrence. These challenges may be associated with the presence of CSCs, which may be resistant to traditional therapeutics and responsible for recurrence. miRNA-based treatments may help to alleviate some of these issues by working in conjunction with chemotherapeutic agents to improve efficacy. The ability of miRNA to regulate multiple different targets also makes them promising for overcoming resistance as they can effect multiple gene networks. For miRNAs that seem to be tumor suppressors, mimics or modified version of the miRNA can be reintroduced into the tumor to restore regulation of target oncogenes. For miRNAs that are overexpressed and seem to be oncogenic, they can be targeted with miRNA inhibitors. This will alleviate the excess repression of tumor suppressor genes regulated by these miRNAs. The potential therapeutic miRNA candidates in various stages of development including those in the preclinical pipeline and those that have shown potential in mouse studies are listed in Table 1. Perhaps unsurprisingly, one of the most well-studied and characterized miRNA, miR-34, is leading the charge in miRNA therapeutics. A treatment based on a miR-34 mimic encapsulated in a liposomal nanoparticle, branded MRX34 is currently in phase I clinical trials, with the hopes of determining the safe dosing level for treatment of liver cancer and other solid tumors. As described previously, miR-34 has been found to act as a tumor suppressor in a wide array of cancers, and targets many important oncogenes. miR-34 has also shown potential in mouse models of cancer. In gastric cancer xenograft models, tumors which express miR-34 through adenoviral vector, exhibited smaller tumors compared to control xenografts. In investigations of metastasis, through a tail vein injection model, the inhibition of miR-34 led to increased tumor formation in the lungs.[26] Xenografts with pancreatic cancer cells transfected with miR-34 mimic also inhibited tumor formation and growth.[28] There is great hope that MRX34 will break through and become the first miRNA-based cancer therapeutic. Beyond miR-34, there are additional miRNA-based therapeutics in the pipeline for clinical application such as miR-101, miR-215, and let-7. miR-101 has shown promise in mouse experimental models. In colon cancer xenografts, miR-101 reduced tumor growth compared to control and also improved response to paclitaxel.[38] MiR-215 in colon cancer cells has been shown to improve sensitivity to 5-FU and target several important genes.[39,40] The development of these miRNAs for therapeutic use is all in the preclinical stage. All of these miRNAs target important oncogenes. There is also interest in developing therapeutics based on targeting oncomiRs. The hope is to inhibit the expression of these

Table 1. miRNAs with potential as therapeutics or therapeutic targets in GI cancers.

microRNA	OncomiR/tumor suppressor	Important targets	Tumor type	References
miR-34	Tumor suppressor	BCL2, Notch, HMGA2, YY1, WNT1, WNT3, LRP6, β-catenin, LEF1	Gastric, colon, liver, pancreatic	(25–28)
Let-7	Tumor suppressor	PKM2, HMGA2	Esophageal, gastric, colon, pancreatic	(30–32)
miR-101	Tumor suppressor	EZH2, COX-2, Mcl-1, Fos, MALAT1, ZEB1	Esophageal, gastric, colon, liver	(34–37)
miR-215	Tumor suppressor	TYMS, DTL, DHFR	Colon	(39, 40)
miR-140	Tumor suppressor	SMAD2, HDAC4	Colon	(41)
miR-129	Tumor suppressor	BCL2, TS, E2F3	Colon	(42)
miR-181b	Tumor suppressor	BCL2	Pancreatic	(43)
miR-21	OncomiR	PTEN, PDCD4,	Esophageal, gastric, colon, liver pancreatic	(7–11)
miR-155	OncomiR	MLH1, MLH2, MSH6, TP53INP	Colon, liver, pancreatic	(13–15)
miR-106b	OncomiR	p21, PTEN, APC	Esophageal, gastric, colon, liver	(16–19)
miR-221/222	OncomiR	TIMP-2, p27, DDIT4, PTEN	Gastric, colon, liver, pancreatic	(20–23)

miRNAs in cancer patients. Targeting of miR-21 and miR-221 is being investigated in liver cancer. As explained above, these miRNAs promote tumorigenesis and target important tumor suppressors.

Given that we are only in the early stages of the development of miRNA therapeutics, we must rely on the experimental data we have from *in vivo* mouse models to consider which additional miRNAs have potential to follow miR-34 through the therapeutics pipeline. In colon cancer, miR-140 may have some potential, as it has been shown to inhibit the tumor formation of colon CSCs in xenograft models. miR-140 also reduced metastasis of these colon CSCs in tail vein injection models. miR-140 inhibits proliferation and invasion of colon cancer cells.[41] miR-129 is another potential candidate that has shown preclinical potential. This miRNA suppresses a number of key targets such as TS, E2F3, and BCL2 in colorectal cancer. In mouse xenograft models, miR-129 reduces tumor growth as well as enhances chemotherapeutic effects of 5-FU.[42] miR-181b has shown potential in pancreatic cancer mouse xenografts, where miR-181 expressing tumor cells showed more sensitivity to gemcitabine and had smaller tumor size.[43] These are just a few of the miRNAs that have shown potential in preclinical studies and may be candidates to advance in the pipeline for clinical development. There are many miRNAs that have potential, and without a doubt more will be identified.

While the prospect of miRNA therapeutics continues to inch closer to reality, the application of miRNA-based therapeutics is not without its challenges. Some of these challenges are inherent to the nature of miRNAs, while others are technical challenges in implementing their clinical use. The ultimate goal of cancer therapeutics is to be able to kill the cancer cells while doing as little harm as possible to healthy cells in order to limit the toxic effects on patients. Part of reducing toxicity is involved with limiting off-target effects. miRNAs represent a double-edged sword when it comes to this; because miRNAs can regulate multiple targets, this makes them a powerful tool to regulate cellular networks. At the same time, this raises additional concerns for off-target effects. A particular miRNA may target some oncogenes but may also target some tumor suppressor genes, complicating the interpretation of its overall function. It is not yet clear in the field if the targeting of one or a few major targets or a wide network of targets is more important for the major functions of miRNAs.[44] This is something that needs to be carefully considered in developing any therapeutic that utilizes miRNA or targets an miRNA. There needs to be thorough investigation to be sure that there are no additional targets that may have effects that undermine the treatment or affect the patient adversely. Another similar challenge is that miRNA can have diverse functions in different tissues. This is also the result of miRNA affecting multiple different targets. In a particular cellular context, one target may be key and dictate the overall functional output of the miRNA. However, in a different context another target may dominate and lead to different functional effects. miR-125b is an important example of an miRNA that seems to have different functions in different cancers. In hepatocellular carcinoma (HCC), miR-125b targets Mcl-1 and acts as a tumor suppressor.[45] Meanwhile, in pancreatic cancer, miR-125b seems to be overexpressed.[46] In addition, miR-125b has been found to target pro-apoptotic genes such as p53 and Bak1 as well as antiapoptotic genes such as BCL2 in different cancers.[47] The challenges associated with miRNA targeting tie into some of the technical challenges associated with miRNA therapeutics. The potential for off-target effects highlights the importance of being able to deliver miRNA therapeutics to the target organ with limited delivery to other organs in order to limit negative side effects and toxicity.

In order for miRNA to be efficient therapeutics, the ability to deliver the miRNA or miRNA inhibitor to the target tissue is essential. Several potential approaches have come forward as delivery options and each have different pros and cons to their implementations. One such technology is nanoparticles. Nanoparticles can be composed of several different types of materials, and various different nanoparticle types have been shown to effectively deliver miRNA *in vivo*. There has been work showing that gold nanoparticles can deliver miR-122 intracellularly to liver cancer cells.[48] Cationic lipid nanoparticles have also been shown to be effective for delivering miR-122 to HCC cells in mouse liver cancer xenograft models.[49] Since miRNAs have great potential to supplement more traditional chemotherapy to increase efficacy and combat resistance, the prospect of delivery of miRNA in conjunction with other therapy is of great interest. Using nanoparticles composed of poly(ethylene glycol) and poly(ε-caprolactone) linked by a gelatinase cleavable peptide, the simultaneous delivery of Docetaxel and miR-200c to gastric cancer cells was possible and in xenograft studies reduced tumor growth.[50] There are various other examples of nanoparticles composed of different materials being used for miRNA delivery. They can be modified with different compounds to help target the release of the miRNA they are carrying to the tumor, or help to hide them from an immune response.[51] Some of these modifications help to address some of the shortcomings of nanoparticles such as limited circulation time and effects on healthy cells.

Liposomal delivery of miRNA is another possible option that has been investigated and shown promise in various types of cancers. Systemic delivery of a miR-34 mimic with a liposome has been shown to be effective in orthotopic liver cancer mouse xenograft studies. This treatment decreased tumor growth with xenografts from multiple different cell lines. In immune competent mice, this treatment was also found to not illicit an immune response.[52] A different liposomal-based delivery system has been shown to be effective in delivering miR-499 to mouse colon cancer xenografts when administered systemically. Importantly, these miRNA–liposome complexes showed accumulation in the tumor with little accumulation in the liver.[53] There are many different liposomal formulations that have shown they are effective for miRNA delivery. Modifications to the surface of liposomes can help with targeting to tumor cells.[54]

Exosomes have also emerged as a potential miRNA delivery system. Exosomes are vesicles that are produced by cells, and are found in circulation, that contain miRNA. These vesicles seem to be a natural mechanism by which cells can transfer miRNAs.[55] Being that exosomes are naturally produced by the body, they should offer minimal challenge when it comes to eliciting an immune response. Some work has showed efficient delivery of exosomes produced by marrow stromal cells containing miRNA to tumor cells, and the reduction of tumor growth in xenograft models.[56]

Viral-based delivery is also an option for miRNA therapeutics. There are several different viral vector-based options for delivery, which include lentivirus, adenovirus, and adeno-associated virus (AAV). Each has its own plusses and minuses; generally, they exhibit efficient transduction, but have potential to elicit some immune response which may pose a problem. For lentivirus, the integration of the viral genome into the host genome leads to the stable expression of the miRNA of interest. This, however, also presents a problem as there is potential for this integration to further disrupt the host genome, particularly if a healthy cell is infected. Lentiviral delivery of miR-101, via tail vein injection is effective for reducing HCC tumor growth with no acute liver toxicity observed.[57] Adenoviral vectors have less genotoxic concerns than lentivirus as they do not integrate into the genome. However, as a result, their effects can be transient. They also have the potential to elicit an immune response which may hamper their effectiveness.[58] In HCC mouse xenografts, adenoviral vectors expressing both miR-34 and IL-24, delivered via intratumoral injection, resulted in complete tumor regression with no recurrence.[59] AAV vectors are capable of stable expression, and in addition, due to different serotypes, there is a potential for targeting different cell types.[60] However, as with the other viral vectors, there is some potential for immune responses.

One interesting application of therapeutics associated with miRNA is using the aberrant expression of miRNA to regulate oncolytic viral therapy. An example of this is that miR-148a and miR-216a are highly expressed in normal pancreatic cells, but their expression is greatly reduced in pancreatic cancer cells. By engineering target sites for these miRNAs into an adenoviral genome to regulate the replication of the virus by the expression of these miRNA, the effects of the virus can be limited to only those cells that do not express these miRNAs. This approach not only produces the virus that retains antitumor effects but also limits excessive pancreatic damage.[61]

Although we are in the early stages of research in miRNA therapeutics for cancer, there is a great potential for miRNA to have significant impacts on cancer treatments. Hopefully, as the field develops, miRNA therapy will improve patient outcomes. There are many candidate miRNAs that have shown preclinical promise, and hopefully these miRNAs will follow miR-34 into the clinical pipeline and delivery technology will continue to mature.

Therapeutic potential of miRNA: Biomarkers

One of the most promising potential clinical applications for miRNA is as cancer biomarkers. As we have clearly seen in looking at oncogenic and tumor suppressor miRNAs, many miRNAs show differential expression between cancer and normal tissue. Evidence has suggested that miRNA may have potential as both diagnostic and prognostic biomarkers. From a prognostic prospective, differences in miRNA expression have been associated with differences in patient survival; there are also correlations between miRNA expression and responsiveness to chemotherapy. Thus, by assessing the miRNA expression profile of a cancer patient sample, some insight can be provided to suggest what types of treatment as well as how aggressive the patients' cancer might be. Potential miRNA-based biomarkers in GI cancer are listed in Table 2. One advantage of miRNA is the fact that miRNAs are stable in FFPE tissue, and thus their expression can be accessed from patient samples processed in this manner.[62] In gastric cancer, low expression of both miR-21 and miR-181b are associated with response to S-1.[63] In pancreatic cancer, overexpression of miR-21, miR-100, and miR-99a associate with poor response to chemotherapy. Elevated expression of these miRNAs also correlates with worse patient survival.[64] There are many similar examples of miRNA whose expression in patient samples associates with patient survival and response to chemotherapy. miRNAs from patient samples can also be useful for the diagnosis of cancers of unknown origin. Using a binary decision tree along with k-nearest-neighbor algorithms, and a microarray of 64 miRNAs, cancer tissue origin could be identified accurately with high specificity and sensitivity.[65] If we can standardize some of these correlations, perhaps with a panel of miRNAs for a particular cancer, it may greatly improve our ability to treat patients, and will at least provide clinicians more information on which to base patient treatment decisions.

These studies looking at miRNA expression from patient samples can provide a significant amount of prognostic insight; however, they do not help with early diagnosis. miRNAs also have potential as diagnostic biomarkers. In particular, miRNA expression levels in circulation may provide insight and suggest further investigation for patient diagnosis. Already, there are various miRNAs that have shown potential as circulating biomarkers for different GI cancers. In the liver, multiple groups have found that circulating miR-21 may be associated with HCC. The expression is higher in the plasma of patients with HCC than healthy subjects. In one study, the increased expression of miR-21 in plasma exhibited a sensitivity of 87.3 and 92% specificity.[66] In pancreatic cancer, plasma expression of miR-483-3p, miR-221, and miR-182 have been found to be elevated.[67–69] The combination of serum expression of three miRNAs, namely miR-193a-3p, miR-23a, and miR-338-5p, associates with colorectal cancer, with 80.0% sensitivity, 84.4% specificity, and 83.3% accuracy.[70] Perhaps not surprising, elevated miR-21

Table 2. Potential miRNA biomarkers in GI cancers.

microRNA	Tissue/circulation	Expression	Cancer type	References
Let-7	Tissue	Decreased	Esophageal, gastric, colon	(30–32)
miR-181b	Tissue	Increased	Gastric	(63)
miR-21	Tissue/circulating	Increased	Esophageal, gastric, colon, liver, pancreatic	(7, 10, 63, 64, 66, 67, 71)
miR-100	Tissue	Increased	Pancreatic	(64)
miR-99a	Tissue	Increased	Pancreatic	(64)
miR-483-3p	Circulating	Increased	Pancreatic	(67)
miR-221	Tissue/circulating	Increased	Pancreatic	(68)
miR-182	Circulating	Increased	Pancreatic	(69)
miR-193a-3p	Circulating	Increased	Colon	(70)
miR-23a	Circulating	Increased	Colon	(70)
miR-338-5p	Circulating	Increased	Colon	(70)

was also found in the serum of colorectal cancer patients.[71] These are just a few examples of miRNAs that have been found in the circulation and may be useful for diagnosis. The enthusiasm for the prospect of miRNA-based biomarkers is reflected in clinical trials. There are about15 different clinical trials in GI cancers that are aimed at looking at expression profiles of miRNAs. Clearly, this is an important push to leverage our understanding of miRNAs and their regulation and dysregulation in cancer. There are some challenges that need to be addressed to enable miRNA diagnostics to be utilized for patients. As we can see from these examples, the serum expression of some miRNAs, such as miR-21, has been associated with multiple different cancers. In order for such an expression to be utilized effectively, we need to focus on those miRNAs which can indicate a particular type of cancer rather than those that may be associated with an assortment of different cancers. In deploying these types of markers in the clinical setting, isolation techniques need to be optimized and standardized so that repeatable standards can be established. If we can standardize some circulating miRNA profiles that can be associated with particular cancers, it will be a great advantage, as this would allow for non-invasive cancer screening. Based on miRNA profiles, a patient can be recommended for further screening. This has the potential to greatly improve early diagnosis. Given that early diagnosis is important to patient outcomes, this has great potential to have a significant impact and may improve our ability to treat cancers.

Conclusion

Based on the extensive research efforts in the last decade, we have revealed the profound impact of miRNAs on cancer. The research has also recently been expanded to other types of non-coding RNAs such as lncRNAs and circular RNAs. A number of promising miRNA-based therapeutics have been validated in preclinical models and are ready for clinical trials. The superior stability of miRNAs in tissues and body fluids makes miRNA-based biomarker discovery and validation an attractive cancer diagnostic and prognostic tool. We are witnessing the emergence of miRNA-based GI cancer diagnostics and prognostics in future clinical management. Many technical hurdles for miRNA-based therapeutics have been overcome by recent advancements in drug delivery technologies. Along with a better understanding of the functional impact of miRNAs on GI cancer in terms of targets and gene regulatory networks, we can better design rationalized combinations of miRNAs for future therapeutics development. In the near future, miRNA-based cancer therapeutics will impact and improve patient survival from GI cancers and other cancer types.

Acknowledgments

This study was supported by National Institute of Health/National Cancer Institute under grant numbers R01CA155019 (J. Ju) and R33CA147966 (J. Ju).

References

1. A Rodriguez, S Griffiths-Jones, JL Ashurst, A Bradley (2004) Identification of mammalian microRNA host genes and transcription units. *Genome Res* **14**: 1902–1910.
2. RC Lee, RL Feinbaum, V Ambros (1993) The C. elegans heterochronic gene lin-4 encodes small RNAs with antisense complementarity to lin-14. *Cell* **75**: 843–854.

3. M Lagos-Quintana, R Rauhut, W Lendeckel, T Tuschl (2001) Identification of novel genes coding for small expressed RNAs. *Science* **294**: 853–858.
4. BP Lewis, IH Shih, MW Jones-Rhoades, DP Bartel, CB Burge (2003) Prediction of mammalian microRNA targets. *Cell* **115**: 787–798.
5. Y Zeng, R Yi, BR Cullen (2003) MicroRNAs and small interfering RNAs can inhibit mRNA expression by similar mechanisms. *Proc Natl Acad Sci USA* **100**: 9779–9784.
6. GA Calin, CD Dumitru, M Shimizu, R Bichi, S Zupo, E Noch, H Aldler, S Rattan, M Keating, K Rai, L Rassenti, T Kipps, M Negrini, F Bullrich, CM Croce (2002) Frequent deletions and down-regulation of micro- RNA genes miR15 and miR16 at 13q14 in chronic lymphocytic leukemia. *Proc Natl Acad Sci USA* **99**: 15524–15529.
7. P Li, WM Mao, ZG Zheng, ZM Dong, ZQ Ling (2013) Down-regulation of PTEN expression modulated by dysregulated miR-21 contributes to the progression of esophageal cancer. *Dig Dis Sci* **58**: 3483–3493.
8. IA Asangani, SA Rasheed, DA Nikolova, JH Leupold, NH Colburn, S Post, H Allgayer (2008) MicroRNA-21 (miR-21) post-transcriptionally downregulates tumor suppressor Pdcd4 and stimulates invasion, intravasation and metastasis in colorectal cancer. *Oncogene* **27**: 2128–2136.
9. SM Yang, C Huang, XF Li, MZ Yu, Y He, J Li (2013) miR-21 confers cisplatin resistance in gastric cancer cells by regulating PTEN. *Toxicology* **306**:162–168.
10. F Meng, R Henson, H Wehbe-Janek, K Ghoshal, ST Jacob, T Patel (2007) MicroRNA-21 regulates expression of the PTEN tumor suppressor gene in human hepatocellular cancer. *Gastroenterology* **133**: 647–658.
11. X Wei, W Wang, L Wang, Y Zhang, X Zhang, M Chen, F Wang, J Yu, Y Ma, G Sun (2016) MicroRNA-21 induces 5-fluorouracil resistance in human pancreatic cancer cells by regulating PTEN and PDCD4. *Cancer Med.*
12. MD Bullock, KM Pickard, BS Nielsen, AE Sayan, V Jenei, M Mellone, R Mitter, JN Primrose, GJ Thomas, GK Packham, AH Mirnezami (2013) Pleiotropic actions of miR-21 highlight the critical role of deregulated stromal microRNAs during colorectal cancer progression. *Cell Death Dis* **4**: e684.
13. N Valeri, P Gasparini, M Fabbri, C Braconi, A Veronese, F Lovat, B Adair, I Vannini, F Fanini, A Bottoni, S Costinean, SK Sandhu, GJ Nuovo, H Alder, R Gafa, F Calore, M Ferracin, G Lanza, S Volinia, M Negrini, MA McIlhatton, D Amadori, R Fishel, CM Croce (2010) Modulation of mismatch repair and genomic stability by miR-155. *Proc Natl Acad Sci USA* **107**: 6982–6987.
14. WJ Liu, YP Zhao, TP Zhang, L Zhou, QC Cui, WX Zhou, L You, G Chen, H Shu (2013) MLH1 as a direct target of MiR-155 and a potential predictor of favorable prognosis in pancreatic cancer. *J Gastrointest Surg* **17**: 1399–1405.

15. F Liu, X Kong, L Lv, J Gao (2015) TGF-beta1 acts through miR-155 to down-regulate TP53INP1 in promoting epithelial-mesenchymal transition and cancer stem cell phenotypes. *Cancer Lett* **359**: 288–298.
16. T Kan, F Sato, T Ito, N Matsumura, S David, Y Cheng, R Agarwal, BC Paun, Z Jin, AV Olaru, FM Selaru, JP Hamilton, J Yang, JM Abraham, Y Mori, SJ Meltzer (2009) The miR-106b-25 polycistron, activated by genomic amplification, functions as an oncogene by suppressing p21 and Bim. *Gastroenterology* **136**: 1689–1700.
17. L Zheng, Y Zhang, Y Liu, M Zhou, Y Lu, L Yuan, C Zhang, M Hong, S Wang, X Li (2015) MiR-106b induces cell radioresistance via the PTEN/PI3K/AKT pathways and p21 in colorectal cancer. *J Transl Med* **13**: 252.
18. TS Yang, XH Yang, X Chen, XD Wang, J Hua, DL Zhou, B Zhou, ZS Song (2014) MicroRNA-106b in cancer-associated fibroblasts from gastric cancer promotes cell migration and invasion by targeting PTEN. *FEBS Lett* **588**: 2162–2169.
19. G Shen, H Jia, Q Tai, Y Li, D Chen (2013) miR-106b downregulates adenomatous polyposis coli and promotes cell proliferation in human hepatocellular carcinoma. *Carcinogenesis* **34**: 211–219.
20. Q Xu, P Li, X Chen, L Zong, Z Jiang, L Nan, J Lei, W Duan, D Zhang, X Li, H Sha, Z Wu, Q Ma, Z Wang (2015) miR-221/222 induces pancreatic cancer progression through the regulation of matrix metalloproteinases. *Oncotarget* **6**: 14153–14164.
21. P Pineau, S Volinia, K McJunkin, A Marchio, C Battiston, B Terris, V Mazzaferro, SW Lowe, CM Croce, A Dejean (2010) miR-221 overexpression contributes to liver tumorigenesis. *Proc Natl Acad Sci USA* **107**: 264–269.
22. T Tsunoda, Y Takashima, Y Yoshida, K Doi, Y Tanaka, T Fujimoto, T Machida, T Ota, M Koyanagi, M Kuroki, T Sasazuki, S Shirasawa (2011) Oncogenic KRAS regulates miR-200c and miR-221/222 in a 3D-specific manner in colorectal cancer cells. *Anticancer Res* **31**: 2453–2459.
23. Z Chun-Zhi, H Lei, Z An-Ling, F Yan-Chao, Y Xiao, W Guang-Xiu, J Zhi-Fan, P Pei-Yu, Z Qing-Yu, K Chun-Sheng (2010) MicroRNA-221 and microRNA-222 regulate gastric carcinoma cell proliferation and radioresistance by targeting PTEN. *BMC Cancer* **10**: 367.
24. M Vogt, J Munding, M Gruner, ST Liffers, B Verdoodt, J Hauk, L Steinstraesser, A Tannapfel, H Hermeking (2011) Frequent concomitant inactivation of miR-34a and miR-34b/c by CpG methylation in colorectal, pancreatic, mammary, ovarian, urothelial, and renal cell carcinomas and soft tissue sarcomas. *Virchows Arch* **458**: 313–322.
25. Q Ji, X Hao, Y Meng, M Zhang, J Desano, D Fan, L Xu (2008) Restoration of tumor suppressor miR-34 inhibits human p53-mutant gastric cancer tumorspheres. *BMC Cancer* **8**: 266.

26. AM Wang, TT Huang, KW Hsu, KH Huang, WL Fang, MH Yang, SS Lo, CW Chi, JJ Lin, TS Yeh (2014) Yin Yang 1 is a target of microRNA-34 family and contributes to gastric carcinogenesis. *Oncotarget* **5**: 5002–5016.
27. NH Kim, HS Kim, NG Kim, I Lee, HS Choi, XY Li, SE Kang, SY Cha, JK Ryu, JM Na, C Park, K Kim, S Lee, BM Gumbiner, JI Yook, SJ Weiss (2011) p53 and microRNA-34 are suppressors of canonical Wnt signaling. *Sci Signal* **4**: ra71.
28. Q Ji, X Hao, M Zhang, W Tang, M Yang, L Li, D Xiang, JT Desano, GT Bommer, D Fan, ER Fearon, TS Lawrence, L Xu (2009) MicroRNA miR-34 inhibits human pancreatic cancer tumor-initiating cells. *PLoS One* **4**: e6816.
29. P Yang, QJ Li, Y Feng, Y Zhang, GJ Markowitz, S Ning, Y Deng, J Zhao, S Jiang, Y Yuan, HY Wang, SQ Cheng, D Xie, XF Wang (2012) TGF-beta-miR-34a-CCL22 signaling-induced Treg cell recruitment promotes venous metastases of HBV-positive hepatocellular carcinoma. *Cancer Cell* **22**: 291–303.
30. Y Akao, Y Nakagawa, T Naoe (2006) let-7 microRNA functions as a potential growth suppressor in human colon cancer cells. *Biol Pharm Bull* **29**: 903–906.
31. R Tang, C Yang, X Ma, Y Wang, D Luo, C Huang, Z Xu, P Liu, L Yang (2016) MiR-let-7a inhibits cell proliferation, migration, and invasion by down-regulating PKM2 in gastric cancer. *Oncotarget.*
32. Q Liu, T Liu, S Zheng, X Gao, M Lu, I Sheyhidin, X Lu (2014) HMGA2 is down-regulated by microRNA let-7 and associated with epithelial-mesenchymal transition in oesophageal squamous cell carcinomas of Kazakhs. *Histopathology* **65**: 408–417.
33. C Ma, K Nong, H Zhu, W Wang, X Huang, Z Yuan, K Ai (2014) H19 promotes pancreatic cancer metastasis by derepressing let-7's suppression on its target HMGA2-mediated EMT. *Tumour Biol* **35**: 9163–9169.
34. A Strillacci, MC Valerii, P Sansone, C Caggiano, A Sgromo, L Vittori, M Fiorentino, G Poggioli, F Rizzello, M Campieri, E Spisni (2013) Loss of miR-101 expression promotes Wnt/beta-catenin signalling pathway activation and malignancy in colon cancer cells. *J Pathol* **229**: 379–389.
35. HJ Wang, HJ Ruan, XJ He, YY Ma, XT Jiang, YJ Xia, ZY Ye, HQ Tao (2010) MicroRNA-101 is down-regulated in gastric cancer and involved in cell migration and invasion. *Eur J Cancer* **46**: 2295–2303.
36. X Wang, M Li, Z Wang, S Han, X Tang, Y Ge, L Zhou, C Zhou, Q Yuan, M Yang (2015) Silencing of long noncoding RNA MALAT1 by miR-101 and miR-217 inhibits proliferation, migration, and invasion of esophageal squamous cell carcinoma cells. *J Biol Chem* **290**: 3925–3935.
37. S Zhao, Y Zhang, X Zheng, X Tu, H Li, J Chen, Y Zang, J Zhang (2015) Loss of MicroRNA-101 Promotes epithelial to mesenchymal transition in hepatocytes. *J Cell Physiol* **230**: 2706–2717.

38. MB Chen, L Yang, PH Lu, XL Fu, Y Zhang, YQ Zhu, Y Tian (2015) MicroRNA-101 down-regulates sphingosine kinase 1 in colorectal cancer cells. *Biochem Biophys Res Commun* **463**: 954–960.
39. V Boni, N Bitarte, I Cristobal, R Zarate, J Rodriguez, E Maiello, J Garcia-Foncillas, E Bandres (2010) miR-192/miR-215 influence 5-fluorouracil resistance through cell cycle-mediated mechanisms complementary to its post-transcriptional thymidilate synthase regulation. *Mol Cancer Ther* **9**: 2265–2275.
40. B Song, Y Wang, MA Titmus, G Botchkina, A Formentini, M Kornmann, J Ju (2010) Molecular mechanism of chemoresistance by miR-215 in osteosarcoma and colon cancer cells. *Mol Cancer* **9**: 96.
41. H Zhai, A Fesler, Y Ba, S Wu, J Ju (2015) Inhibition of colorectal cancer stem cell survival and invasive potential by hsa-miR-140-5p mediated suppression of Smad2 and autophagy. *Oncotarget* **6**: 19735–19746.
42. M Karaayvaz, H Zhai, J Ju (2013) miR-129 promotes apoptosis and enhances chemosensitivity to 5-fluorouracil in colorectal cancer. *Cell Death Dis* **4**: e659.
43. B Cai, Y An, N Lv, J Chen, M Tu, J Sun, P Wu, J Wei, K Jiang, Y Miao (2013) miRNA-181b increases the sensitivity of pancreatic ductal adenocarcinoma cells to gemcitabine in vitro and in nude mice by targeting BCL-2. *Oncol Rep* **29**: 1769–1776.
44. EC Lai (2015) Two decades of miRNA biology: Lessons and challenges. *RNA* **21**: 675–677.
45. HY Jia, YX Wang, WT Yan, HY Li, YZ Tian, SM Wang, HL Zhao (2012) MicroRNA-125b functions as a tumor suppressor in hepatocellular carcinoma cells. *Int J Mol Sci* **13**: 8762–8774.
46. M Bloomston, WL Frankel, F Petrocca, S Volinia, H Alder, JP Hagan, CG Liu, D Bhatt, C Taccioli, CM Croce (2007) MicroRNA expression patterns to differentiate pancreatic adenocarcinoma from normal pancreas and chronic pancreatitis. *JAMA* **297**: 1901–1908.
47. YM Sun, KY Lin, YQ Chen (2013) Diverse functions of miR-125 family in different cell contexts. *J Hematol Oncol* **6**: 6.
48. Y Yuan, X Zhang, X Zeng, B Liu, F Hu, G Zhang (2014) Glutathione-mediated release of functional miR-122 from gold nanoparticles for targeted induction of apoptosis in cancer treatment. *J Nanosci Nanotechnol* **14**: 5620–5627.
49. SH Hsu, B Yu, X Wang, Y Lu, CR Schmidt, RJ Lee, LJ Lee, ST Jacob, K Ghoshal (2013) Cationic lipid nanoparticles for therapeutic delivery of siRNA and miRNA to murine liver tumor. *Nanomedicine* **9**: 1169–1180.
50. Q Liu, RT Li, HQ Qian, J Wei, L Xie, J Shen, M Yang, XP Qian, LX Yu, XQ Jiang, BR Liu (2013) Targeted delivery of miR-200c/DOC to inhibit cancer stem cells and cancer cells by the gelatinases-stimuli nanoparticles. *Biomaterials* **34**: 7191–7203.

51. X Deng, Y Wang, F Zhang, Z Yin, Q Hu, X Xiao, Z Zhou, Y Wu, W Sheng, Y Zeng (2016) Acidic pH-induced charge-reversal nanoparticles for accelerated endosomal escape and enhanced microRNA modulation in cancer cells. *Chem Commun* **52**: 3243–3246.
52. CL Daige, JF Wiggins, L Priddy, T Nelligan-Davis, J Zhao, D Brown (2014) Systemic delivery of a miR34a mimic as a potential therapeutic for liver cancer. *Mol Cancer Ther* **13**: 2352–2360.
53. H Ando, T Asai, H Koide, A Okamoto, N Maeda, K Tomita, T Dewa, T Minamino, N Oku (2014) Advanced cancer therapy by integrative antitumor actions via systemic administration of miR-499. *J Control Release* **181**: 32–39.
54. HY Lee, KA Mohammed, F Kaye, P Sharma, BM Moudgil, WL Clapp, N Nasreen (2013) Targeted delivery of let-7a microRNA encapsulated ephrin-A1 conjugated liposomal nanoparticles inhibit tumor growth in lung cancer. *Int J Nanomed* **8**: 4481–4494.
55. H Valadi, K Ekstrom, A Bossios, M Sjostrand, JJ Lee, JO Lotvall (2007) Exosome-mediated transfer of mRNAs and microRNAs is a novel mechanism of genetic exchange between cells. *Nat Cell Biol* **9**: 654–659.
56. M Katakowski, B Buller, X Zheng, Y Lu, T Rogers, O Osobamiro, W Shu, F Jiang, M Chopp (2013) Exosomes from marrow stromal cells expressing miR-146b inhibit glioma growth. *Cancer Lett* **335**: 201–204.
57. F Zheng, YJ Liao, MY Cai, TH Liu, SP Chen, PH Wu, L Wu, XW Bian, XY Guan, YX Zeng, YF Yuan, HF Kung, D Xie (2015) Systemic delivery of microRNA-101 potently inhibits hepatocellular carcinoma in vivo by repressing multiple targets. *PLoS Genet* **11**: e1004873.
58. BD Brown, G Sitia, A Annoni, E Hauben, LS Sergi, A Zingale, MG Roncarolo, LG Guidotti, L Naldini (2007) *In vivo* administration of lentiviral vectors triggers a type I interferon response that restricts hepatocyte gene transfer and promotes vector clearance. *Blood* **109**: 2797–2805.
59. W Lou, Q Chen, L Ma, J Liu, Z Yang, J Shen, Y Cui, XW Bian, C Qian (2013) Oncolytic adenovirus co-expressing miRNA-34a and IL-24 induces superior antitumor activity in experimental tumor model. *J Mol Med* (*Berl*) **91**: 715–725.
60. M Della Peruta, A Badar, C Rosales, S Chokshi, A Kia, D Nathwani, E Galante, R Yan, E Arstad, AM Davidoff, R Williams, MF Lythgoe, AC Nathwani (2015) Preferential targeting of disseminated liver tumors using a recombinant adeno-associated viral vector. *Hum Gene Ther* **26**: 94–103.
61. X Bofill-De Ros, M Gironella, C Fillat (2014) miR-148a- and miR-216a-regulated oncolytic adenoviruses targeting pancreatic tumors attenuate tissue damage without perturbation of miRNA activity. *Mol Ther* **22**: 1665–1677.

62. Y Xi, G Nakajima, E Gavin, CG Morris, K Kudo, K Hayashi, J Ju (2007) Systematic analysis of microRNA expression of RNA extracted from fresh frozen and formalin-fixed paraffin-embedded samples. *RNA* **13**: 1668–1674.
63. J Jiang, X Zheng, X Xu, Q Zhou, H Yan, X Zhang, B Lu, C Wu, J Ju (2011) Prognostic significance of miR-181b and miR-21 in gastric cancer patients treated with S-1/Oxaliplatin or Doxifluridine/Oxaliplatin. *PLoS One* **6**: e23271.
64. SA Dhayat, B Abdeen, G Kohler, N Senninger, J Haier, WA Mardin (2015) MicroRNA-100 and microRNA-21 as markers of survival and chemotherapy response in pancreatic ductal adenocarcinoma UICC stage II. *Clin Epigenetics* **7**: 132.
65. E Meiri, WC Mueller, S Rosenwald, M Zepeniuk, E Klinke, TB Edmonston, M Werner, U Lass, I Barshack, M Feinmesser, M Huszar, F Fogt, K Ashkenazi, M Sanden, E Goren, N Dromi, O Zion, I Burnstein, A Chajut, Y Spector, R Aharonov (2012) A second-generation microRNA-based assay for diagnosing tumor tissue origin. *Oncologist* **17**: 801–812.
66. Y Tomimaru, H Eguchi, H Nagano, H Wada, S Kobayashi, S Marubashi, M Tanemura, A Tomokuni, I Takemasa, K Umeshita, T Kanto, Y Doki, M Mori (2012) Circulating microRNA-21 as a novel biomarker for hepatocellular carcinoma. *J Hepatol* **56**: 167–175.
67. M Abue, M Yokoyama, R Shibuya, K Tamai, K Yamaguchi, I Sato, N Tanaka, S Hamada, T Shimosegawa, K Sugamura, K Satoh (2015) Circulating miR-483-3p and miR-21 is highly expressed in plasma of pancreatic cancer. *Int J Oncol* **46**: 539–547.
68. T Kawaguchi, S Komatsu, D Ichikawa, R Morimura, M Tsujiura, H Konishi, H Takeshita, H Nagata, T Arita, S Hirajima, A Shiozaki, H Ikoma, K Okamoto, T Ochiai, H Taniguchi, E Otsuji (2013) Clinical impact of circulating miR-221 in plasma of patients with pancreatic cancer. *Br J Cancer* **108**: 361–369.
69. Q Chen, L Yang, Y Xiao, J Zhu, Z Li (2014) Circulating microRNA-182 in plasma and its potential diagnostic and prognostic value for pancreatic cancer. *Med Oncol* **31**: 225.
70. FL Yong, CW Law, CW Wang (2013) Potentiality of a triple microRNA classifier: miR-193a-3p, miR-23a and miR-338-5p for early detection of colorectal cancer. *BMC Cancer* **13**: 280.
71. G Basati, A Emami Razavi, S Abdi, A Mirzaei (2014) Elevated level of microRNA-21 in the serum of patients with colorectal cancer. *Med Oncol* **31**: 205.

Chapter 18

Unraveling the Relationship between Autophagy and microRNA in Gastrointestinal Cancer

Yuanyuan Yin, Peiqi Wang, Yaxin Zheng, Yi Chen, and Jinhui Wang

Abstract

microRNAs (miRNAs), small and non-coding RNAs of 22–24 nucleotides in length, have been found to participate in a wide range of cellular processes including proliferation and cell death. The dysregulated expression of miRNAs plays a vital role in the initiation and progression of human cancers, including gastrointestinal cancer. Autophagy, an intracellular self-digestive process, is involved in the lysosomal degradation of dysfunctional proteins and damaged organelles in cytoplasm. Autophagy could be either a cytoprotective mechanism or a means of cell death for cancer cells. Accumulating evidence has shown that miRNAs can modulate autophagy via different targets in gastrointestinal cancer. In this chapter, we focus on the interaction of miRNAs with autophagy, thereby unraveling the relationship between miRNAs and autophagy in gastrointestinal cancer, which may shed light on miRNA-based therapeutics for cancer treatment.

Introduction

The term autophagy is from Greek "auto" (self) and "phagy" (to eat), which represents a series of evolutionarily conserved cellular processes. According to the difference of the delivery mode to the lysosome, autophagy can be classified into at least three types, including macroautophagy, microautophagy, and chaperone-mediated autophagy.[1] The term "autophagy" usually refers to macrophagy, through which cells can digest long-lived proteins and damaged organelles by lysosomal degradation as well as recycling the ingredients to promote cell survival. In normal circumstances, autophagy maintains at a relatively low level to keep cellular homeostasis. Autophagy can be induced under stressful conditions such as starvation and endoplasmic reticulum (ER) stress, exhibiting cytoprotective effects.[2] However, if the cellular stress leads to hyperactivation of autophagy, autophagic cell death would ensue.[3] In cancer cells, autophagy could be either a biological mechanism for temporary survival or a means of cell death by modulating autophagy-related genes (ATGs) and their regulators.[4]

microRNAs (miRNAs) are a class of highly conserved, small, and non-coding RNAs of 22–24 nucleotides in length, which have been estimated to regulate approximately 30% human coding genes.[5] During the synthetic process, miRNAs are firstly transcribed as primary miRNAs (pri-miRNAs) by polymerase II within the nucleus. These pri-miRNAs are cleaved into hairpin-shaped precursor miRNAs (pre-miRNAs) by the ribonuclease Drosha. Subsequently, pre-miRNAs are transported into cytoplasm by a RANGTP-dependent transporter named Exportin. In the cytoplasm, these pre-miRNAs are cleaved and processed into mature miRNAs by RNase III enzyme Dicer and TRBP (the human immunodeficiency virus transactivating response RNA-binding protein), which produces a duplex molecule consisting of a single-stranded mature miRNA and RNA fragments. In addition, the mature miRNA molecules are integrated into the RNA-induced silencing complex and function by binding to the 3′UTR (3′ untranslated region) of target message RNAs (mRNAs).[6] The regulation of miRNAs on targeted genes depends on the degree of miRNA–mRNA complementarity. Sufficient complementarity results in Ago-catalyzed cleavage of targeted miRNA, whereas incomplete complementarity excludes this kind of cleavage but suppresses mRNA translation.

Lin-4 was the first miRNA discovered in 1993 by Lee *et al.*[7] The small RNA encoded by lin-4 could regulate protein lin-14, resulting in an impact on the developmental timing of the nematode. However, only when let-7 was identified and determined to be reserved in model organisms, the significance of miRNAs in the physiological and pathological processes began to emerge.[8] Ever since then, miRNAs have been found to participate in a wide range of cellular processes including cell proliferation and cell death.[9]

Accumulating evidence has shown that the dysregulated expression of miRNAs in human cancers plays a vital role in cancer, including initiation, progression, metastasis, as well as therapeutic sensitivity. miR-15 and miR-16, two miRNAs located in a region of chromosome 13 with tumor suppressive functions in chronic lymphocytic leukemia, are the first miRNAs that were discovered to highlight the links between miRNAs and cancer.[10] miR-155, the first identified oncogenic miRNA, was found to be overexpressed in hematopoietic system cancers. Since then, miRNAs have shown tight connections with tumor occurrence and development, serving as either oncogenes or tumor suppressive genes.[11]

Because of the differential expression patterns of miRNAs between normal and cancer cells, miRNAs are being exploited for the diagnosis and classification of tumors, as well as for prognosis prediction. In addition, a single miRNA can simultaneously modulate multiple targets and biological signaling networks, which provides a significant advantage from a clinical perspective. Furthermore, increasing data have confirmed that miRNAs are involved in the development of chemoresistance or radioresistance in many cancers, such as gastrointestinal cancer including gastric cancer (GC), colorectal cancer, pancreatic cancer, and hepatocellular carcinoma (HCC), making miRNA-based cancer therapies attractive to researchers. However, the interplay of miRNAs and autophagy in other gastrointestinal cancers such as gallbladder cancer, gastric stromal tumor, and small intestine carcinoma still remains to be clarified.

In this chapter, we mainly focus on the regulatory role of miRNAs in autophagy and the molecular mechanisms of the interaction between autophagy and miRNAs in gastrointestinal cancer, including GC, colorectal cancer, pancreatic cancer, and hepatocellular cancer, which are common and lethal diseases that pose a serious threat to human health. Unraveling the relationship between miRNAs and autophagy may spark off better understanding of miRNA-based therapeutic strategies for gastrointestinal cancer treatment.

miRNAs Regulate Autophagy

In general, the whole autophagic process can be divided into five different stages: induction, vesicle nucleation, vesicle elongation and completion, docking and fusion, and degradation and recycling.[12] miRNA-30a is the first miRNA that was found to attenuate autophagy activity by targeting Beclin-1 in TG98 cells treated with rapamycin.[13] Ever since then, an increasing number of miRNAs have been confirmed to play a role in modulating some members of ATGs and their regulators at different stages.

First, the induction of autophagy is initiated by activation of the ULK (unc-51 like kinase) complex composed of ULK1/2, ATG13, FIP200 (the focal adhesion kinase family interacting protein of 200 KD) and ATG101. Among them, ULK1 is the key initiator and can be inhibited by the mammalian target of rapamycin (mTOR). miR-290-295 cluster may suppress autophagic cell death enhanced by glucose starvation via targeting ULK1 and ATG7 in melanoma cells.[14] miR-20a and miR-106b expression can be downregulated by leucine deprivation, which suppresses their transcription factor c-myc, and their mimics could attenuate the autophagy activity induced by leucine deprivation in C2C12 myoblasts. The mechanistic study revealed that ULK1 is the direct target of miR-20a and miR-106b.[15] Isoliquiritigenin, a kind of chalconetype flavonoid and liquorice derivative, can downregulate the miR-25 expression in multidrug resistant MCF7 cells, and miR-25 inhibition could increase ULK1 expression, leading to autophagic cell death.[16] A recent study has shown that miR-885-3p could contribute to autophagy regulation by targeting ULK2, which is another autophagy initiator.[17]

Second, vesicle nucleation is characterized by the recruitment of proteins and lipids to construct the autophagosomal membrane, which depends on the activation of the class III PI3K/Beclin-1 complex. Bax-interacting factor-1 (BIF-1), ATG14L, UV irradiation resistance-associated gene (UVRAG), and Rubicon are important binding partners of this complex.[18] miRNA-30a/b, miRNA-376b, miR-216a, miR-17-5p, and miR-519a can suppress vesicle nucleation by inhibiting Beclin-1 expression. miR-630 and miR-374a can downregulate UVRAG expression. ATG14, a part of the class III PI3K/Beclin-1 complex, which plays a critical role in autophagosomal membrane nucleation, was discovered to be the target of miR-195. In addition, miRNA-101 has been identified as an autophagy inhibitor by targeting RAB5A, a small GTPase which can enhance autophagosome formation by interacting with hVPS34 and Beclin-1.

Third, vesicle elongation and completion require two ubiquitin-like conjugation systems including the ATG12–ATG5–ATG16L system and the ATG8/LC3 (microtubule-associated protein 1A/1B-light chain 3) system. Once the vesicle expansion is accomplished, ATG8/LC3 separates from phosphatidylethanolamine (PE) with the aid of ATG4.[12] miR-101 and miR-376b may inhibit the expression of ATG4C and ATG4D. miR-376a and 376b have the same seed sequence and targets such as ATG4C and Beclin-1. miR-375 can target ATG7 to suppress the conversion of LC3-I to LC3-II. miR-17 negatively regulates ATG7 expression in glioblastoma cell lines. Moreover, RAB5A is associated with ATG5–ATG12 conjugation as well; hence, miR-101 may function at both the vesicle nucleation stage and the elongation stage via RAB5A. Furthermore, miR-204 has been confirmed to regulate the autophagy process by targeting LC3B in renal clear cell carcinoma. miR-106B, miR-93, and miR142-3p may regulate autophagy through the modulation of ATG16L.

Fourth, docking and fusion is a process in which autophagosome matures and the autophagosomal contents break down, which requires proteins such as Rab7, LAMP1/2 (lysosome-associated membrane protein1/2), SKD1 (suppressor of K^+ transport growth defect1), and so on. ATG9A has been found to be the direct target of miR-34a and miRNA-130a may inhibit autophagy by targeting ATG2B.[19]

In the final step of degradation and recycling, cargoes inside the vesicle are digested, contributing to the nutrient and energy cycle. SQSTM1, (sequestosome 1) encoding the poly-ubiquitin binding protein p62 and binding to LC3, is regulated by the miR-17/20/93/106 family of miRNAs, which share the common seed sequence.[20]

Ever since miR-30a was discovered, the first autophagy-related miRNA was identified in 2009, an increasing number of studies have been conducted to elucidate the molecular mechanisms underlying miRNA-mediated autophagy regulation. Researchers have found that a multitude of miRNAs with various functions and their downstream genes form a complicated signaling network. miRNAs can inhibit different autophagic stages as well as enhance autophagy activity. In addition, miRNAs also play a role in the interconnection between apoptosis and autophagy.

The Relationship Between Autophagy and miRNAs in GC

GC ranks fourth in the most common cancers around the world and it is the second leading cause of death associated with cancer.[21] There are approximately 760,000 cases of GC across the world, with poor prognosis. The overall 5-year survival rate of GC is less than 35% and the death is primarily caused by terminal illness at the date of initial diagnosis, low response to the neoadjuvant or adjuvant therapy or tumor recurrence after surgical removal.[22] For the early stage of GC, surgery is the most preferred treatment option. However, with no effective techniques for early diagnosis, more than 60% of the patients are diagnosed with advanced stage disease. The first-line treatment for these patients is perioperative chemotherapy and a number of novel chemotherapeutic drugs have been employed in clinical practice. Nevertheless, this perioperative treatment fails when applied to some patients due to intrinsic or acquired drug resistance, especially the multidrug resistance (MDR).[23] The inner mechanisms of MDR have been extensively studied, which includes intracellular drug accumulation, drug targets alternation, DNA repair activity promotion, and cell death inactivation. Autophagy induction contributes to the occurrence of chemoresistance and radioresistance as well. miRNAs have been found to be involved in chemoresistance by regulating autophagy in GC, making them potential targets for the treatment of chemoresistant GC (Figure 1 and Table 1).

miRNAs downregulate autophagy in GC cancer

miR-23b-3p: ATG12 and HMGB2

To our knowledge, ATG12, one of the two ubiquitin-like proteins in the vesicle elongation and completion process, is of vital importance in the formation of autophagic vacuole. ATG12 conjugates with ATG5 and interacts with ATG16L, a small coiled-coil protein to form an

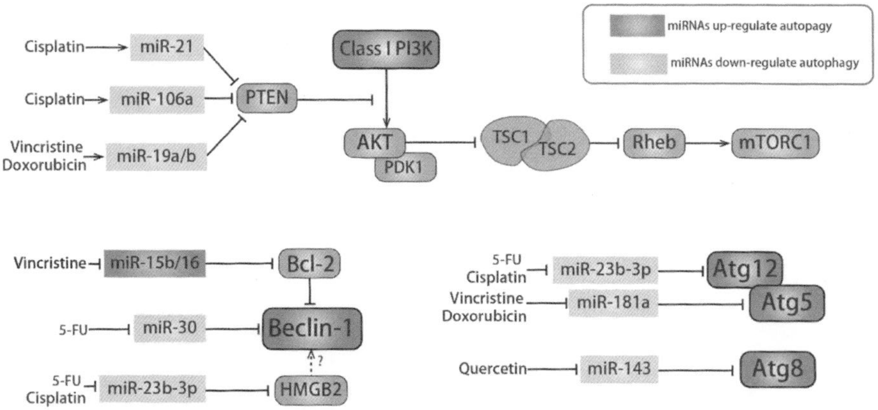

Figure 1. miRNAs regulate autophagy in GC.
Note: miRNAs including miR-23-3p, miR-143, miR-181a, miR-19a/b, miR-21, miR-106a, and miR-30 downregulate autophagy and other miRNAs including miR-15b and miR-16 upregulates autophagy.

ATG12–ATG5–ATG16L complex, in which ATG16L can lead the complex to the autophagic isolation membrane. In addition, the ATG8-PE conjugation reaction and the lipidation of ATG8 can be promoted by the ATG12–ATG5 conjugate, which has been identified as a ubiquitin-protein ligase (E3)-like enzyme. HMGB2 (high-mobility group box 2) is a kind of non-histone nuclear protein from the HMGB family, whose members include HMGB1, HMGB2, HMGB3, and HMGB4. Of note, HMGB1 enhances autophagy in multiple cancer types by interacting with Beclin1 displacing Bcl-2, resulting in a stabilized HMGB1–Beclin1 complex. And because of the high homology of HMGB2 with HMGB1, HMGB2 might play a similar role in autophagy regulation, but this speculation needs to be studied further.

Recently, An *et al.* found that miR-23b-3p could enhance the chemoresistance of GC cells through targeting ATG12 and HMGB2.[24] The overexpression of miR-23b-3p can not only reverse the sensitivity of cancer cells to a series of chemotherapy drugs *in vitro*, but also sensitize those tumors to chemotherapy *in vivo*. miR-23b-3p functions by directly targeting ATG12 and HMGB2, which are closely related to autophagy occurrence. Moreover,

Table 1. miRNAs regulate autophagy and their targets in gastrointestinal cancer.

Stimulus	miRNA	Expression in patients or tissues	Confirmed targets	Function of miRNA	Cell line(s); animals	References
Gastric cancer						
Vincristine	miR-23b-3p	Decreased	TG12, HMGB2	Inhibit autophagy, increase chemosensitivity (*in vitro*); sensitize tumors to chemotherapy (*in vivo*)	SGC7901, SGC7901/VCR; nude mice	(24)
Quercetin	miR-143	Decreased	ATG8	Inhibit autophagy, increase chemosensitivity (*in vitro*)	AGS/MNK28	(25)
Cisplatin	miR-181a	—	ATG5	Inhibit autophagy, increase chemosensitivity (*in vitro*); reduce the volumes of xenograft tumor in cisplatin-resistant nude mice (*in vivo*)	SGC7901/CDDP; nude mice	(26)
Vincristine, Doxorubicin	miR-19a/b	Increased	PTEN/PI3K/Akt	Inhibit autophagy and apoptosis, increase chemoresistance (*in vitro*)	SGC7901, SGC7901/VCR, SGC7901/ADR	(28)
Cisplatin	miR-21	Increased	PTEN/PI3K/Akt	Inhibit autophagy and apoptosis, increase chemoresistance (*in vitro*)	SGC7901, SGC7901/DDP	(29)

Cisplatin	miR-106a	Increased	PTEN/PI3K/Akt	Inhibit autophagy and apoptosis, increase chemoresistance (*in vitro*)	SGC7901, SGC7901/DDP	(30)
Vincristine	miR-15b, MiR-16	Increased	Bcl-2	Enhance autophagy and apoptosis (*in vitro*)	SGC7901, SGC7901/VCR	(31)
5-FU	miR-30	—	BECN1	Inhibit autophagy; 5-FU suppresses miR-30 to up-regulate Beclin-1 to induce autophagic cell death and cell proliferation arrest (*in vitro*)	SNU-5	(32)
Colorectal cancer						
Hypoxia/HIF-1α	miR-210	—	BCL-2	Enhance autophagy, decrease radiosensitivity (*in vitro*)	SW480, SW620	(35)
Radiation	miR-18	Increased	ATM3, mTORC1	Enhance autophagy and ionize radiation-induced autophagy (*in vitro*)	HCT116	(36)
—	miR-18	Increased	hnRNP A1 E2	Induce apoptosis via the autophagolysosomal degradation of hnRNP A1 E2 (*in vitro*); inhibited colon cancer progression (*in vivo*)	SW620; nude mice	(37)

(*Continued*)

Table 1. (*Continued*)

Stimulus	miRNA	Expression in patients or tissues	Confirmed targets	Function of miRNA	Cell line(s); animals	References
—	miR-502	Decreased	Rab1B, p53	Inhibit autophagy, colon cancer cell growth and cell-cycle progression (*in vitro*); inhibit cancer growth in a mouse tumor xenografts model (*in vivo*)	HCT116; mouse	(38)
Paclitaxel	miR-22	—	PTEN/PI3K/Akt	Inhibit autophagy, decrease cell proliferation and survival, induce cell apoptosis in the p53-mutated colon cancer cells (*in vitro*)	p53-mutated HT-29 and HCT-15	(39)
5-FU	miR-22	Decreased	BTG1	Inhibit autophagy, promote apoptosis, increase 5-FU sensitivity (*in vitro*)	SW620, RKO	(40)
Starvation	miR-106b	—	ATG16L1, BECN1, ATG12	Inhibit autophagy (*in vitro*)	HCT116	(41)
Pancreatic cancer						
Radiation	miR-23b	Decreased	ATG12	Inhibit autophagy, increase radiosensitivity (*in vitro*)	BxPC3, PANC-1	(44)
Radiation	miR-216a	Decreased	BECN1	Inhibit autophagy, increase radiosensitivity (*in vitro*)	PANC-1	(45)

Hepatocellular cancer						
—	miR-100	Decreased	IGF-1R, mTOR	Enhance autophagy, induce mitochondrial apoptotic cell death (*in vitro*); inhibit tumor growth (*in vivo*)	SK-Hep1, MHCC97-L, SMMC-7721, HCCLM3, Huh7, Hep3B, HepG2	(47)
Sorafenib	miR-423-5p	Increased	ATG7	Enhance autophagy (*in vitro*)	HUH7, HepG2	(48)
Hypoxia	miR-375	Decreased	ATG7	Inhibit autophagy, induce mitochondrial apoptotic cell death (*in vitro*); xenograft tumors with larger areas of necrosis and slower growth speed (*in vivo*)	HCC; mice	(49)
Cisplatin	miR-199a-5p	Decreased	ATG7	Inhibit autophagy and cell proliferation, increase chemosensitivity (*in vitro*)	Huh7, HepG2, HEK 293	(50)
Cisplatin	miR-101	Decreased	RAB5A, STMN1, ATG4D, mTOR	Inhibit autophagy, promote apoptotic cell death, increase chemosensitivity (*in vitro*)	HepG2	(53)
5-FU, Doxorubicin	miR-101	Decreased	EZH2	Inhibit autophagy, promote apoptotic cell death, increase chemosensitivity (*in vitro*)	HepG2, Hep3B, SNU-18	(54)
Baculovirus	miR-17, miR-20a	Decreased	ULK1, ATG7, p62	Inhibit autophagy (*in vitro*)	Mahlavu	(55)
HBV-infection	miR-30a	Decreased	BECN1	Inhibit autophagy (*in vitro*)	HBV infected HCC	(58)

the response of GC cells to chemotherapy could be enhanced when autophagy or the gene expressions of ATG12 and HMGB2 were downregulated. This is the first report that identifies miR-23b-3p as a key chemosensitivity regulator. Previous studies have reported that miR-23b-3p was dysregulated in many types of cancer with inconsistent or even conflicting roles. Besides, chemoresistant patients exhibit inhibited levels of miR-23b-3p, and their overall survival is correlated with miR-23b-3p expression.

miR-143: ATG8

GABARAPL1 is also known as ATG8, another ubiquitin-like protein required in the process of vesicle elongation and completion. ATG8 plays a fundamental role in the autophagosome membrane formation. The process of soluble ATG8 converting to membrane bound ATG8 is called lipidation and ATG8 is widely used as an autophagy biomarker. Researchers have found that miR-143 could promote the chemosensitivity of Quercetin by targeting GABARAPL1 and inhibiting autophagy in GC.[25] miR-143, a tumor suppressor identified in several types of cancers, has been found to be significantly downregulated in both GC tissues and cell lines when compared with the normal samples. Moreover, when combined with miR-143, the chemosensitivity of Quercetin in AGS/MNK28 cells could also be enhanced.

miR-181a: ATG5

ATG5, a component of the ATG12–ATG5–ATG16L complex, is associated with the process of elongation. According to the recent study conducted by Zhao *et al.*, miR-181a could suppress autophagy by targeting ATG5, resulting in enhanced chemosensitivity of SGC7901/CDDP cells to cisplatin.[26] The volumes of xenograft tumor in cisplatin-resistant nude mice were reduced by the artificially enforced expression of miR-181a as well. Therefore, miR-181a was identified to inhibit autophagy activity, thus increasing the toxicity of the cisplatin, and increasing chemosensitivity in GC cells. This is consistent with a previous study conducted by Tekirdag *et al.*, who showed that autophagy induced by starvation and rapamycin could be attenuated in MCF-7, Huh-7, and K562 cells.[27] By targeting ATG5, miR-181a inhibits autophagy primarily through affecting the formation of autophagosome membrane formation.

miR-19a/b, miR-21, miR-106a: PTEN/PI3K/Akt

The aforementioned miRNAs including miR-23b-3p, 143, and 181a directly target ATGs, resulting in enhanced chemosensitivity. Additionally, studies have shown that miRNAs can promote chemoresistance mainly by inhibiting apoptotic cell death with downregulated autophagy involved in the signal pathway. Wang *et al.* demonstrated that miR-19a/b was upregulated in both the Vincristine-resistant gastric cell line and the Doxorubicin-resistant gastric cell line, which suppressed drug-induced apoptosis and promoted drug resistance via targeting phosphatase and tensin homolog (PTEN).[28] Besides, it has also been shown that the level of miR-21 was increased in cisplatin-resistant GC cells and miR-21 enhanced chemoresistance by regulating PTEN.[29] In addition, upregulated miR-106a was also demonstrated to mediate the resistance of GC cells to cisplatin by targeting PTEN.[30] miR-19a/b, miR-21, miR-106a, can all attenuate autophagy and apoptosis through PTEN/PI3K/Akt pathway, which is frequently activated in several cancers and plays a vital role in cell survival, tumor metastasis, as well as chemoresistance. PTEN can negatively regulate PI3K/Akt pathway, while upregulated miRNAs can activate PI3K/Akt by targeting PTEN, resulting in inhibited autophagy, reduced apoptosis, and enhanced chemoresistance.

miR-15b and miR-16: Bcl-2

Bcl-2, the primary member in the Bcl-2 family has been identified to suppress apoptosis. Additionally, Bcl-2 can interact with Beclin-1 by binding to the BH3 domain of Beclin-1, thus decreasing the activity of PI3KIII, which significantly prevents autophagy induction, leading to downregulated autophagy. Xia *et al.* found that downregulated miR-15b and miR-16 in a Vincristine-resistant gastric cell line resulted in decreased autophagy and apoptosis, which increased the chemoresistance of SGC7901 cells.[31] The enforced expression of miR-15b or miR-16 could enhance autophagy and apoptosis by targeting Bcl-2.

miR-30: BECN1

Interestingly, enhanced autophagy could not only result in chemoresistance, which favors cancer cell survival, but also induce autophagic cell death. Fluorouracil (5-FU), an adjuvant drug applied in chemotherapy, improves the survival of GC patients by triggering autophagic cell death. Bioinformatics analysis revealed that miR-30 inhibited autophagy by binding to the 3′UTR of BECN-1, a key autophagy gene. Researchers have found that miR-30 could be downregulated by Fluorouracil, resulting in autophagic cell death in SNU-5 cell line.[32] This is another example of miRNAs downregulating autophagy in GC. miR-30 is a family formed by four clusters which locate in different genomic regions including miR-30a, miR-30c-2, miR-30b, and miR-30d, miR-30e, and miR-30c-1. Previous research has identified miR-30a as a negative regulator of autophagy by targeting BECN1 in human breast cancer, lung cancer, and glioma. Besides, downregulated miR-30d has been found in anaplastic thyroid carcinoma (ATC), which leads to enhanced autophagy and decreased chemosensitivity of cells to cisplatin.[33] The function of miR-30 in ATC is consistent with the current study conducted in GC cells.

The Relationship Between Autophagy and miRNAs in Colorectal Cancer

Colorectal cancer (CRC), one of the most common cancer types, is the third leading cause of cancer-related death all over the world.[34] The occurrence and development of CRC is closely related to genetic and epigenetic abnormalities. Conversely, accumulating evidence has shown that the aberrant expression of non-coding RNAs is involved in tumorigenesis by regulating autophagy in CRC as well (Figure 2, Table 1).

miRNAs upregulate autophagy in CRC

miR-210: Bcl-2

Recently, Sun *et al.* has demonstrated that autophagy induced by hypoxia is associated with the HIF-1α/miR-210/Bcl-2 pathway in colon cancer cell

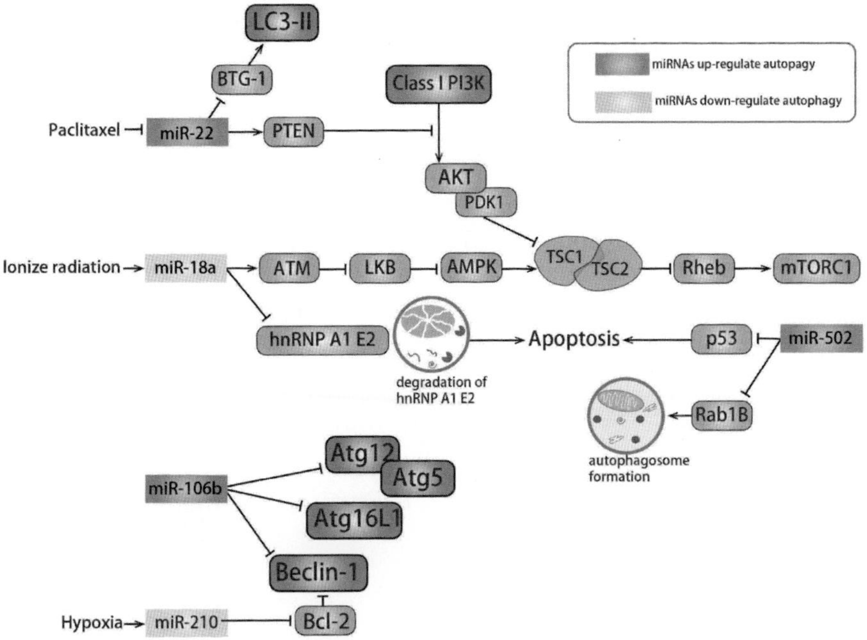

Figure 2. miRNAs regulate autophagy in CRC.
Note: miRNAs including miR-210 and miR-18a upregulate autophagy and other miRNAs including miR-502, miR-22, and miR-106b downregulate autophagy.

lines SW480 and SW620.[35] HIF-1α, a member of hypoxia-inducible factors (HIFs), can cause the overexpression of miR-210 during hypoxia, and miR-210 enhances autophagy by suppressing the expression of Bcl-2. miR-210 has been found to be particularly sensitive to oxygen deprivation and overexpressed in many cancers, such as lung cancer. As we have mentioned before, Bcl-2 can modulate Beclin1-PI3KIII/Vps34 and attenuate autophagy activity by binding to Beclin-1. Therefore, we can conclude that miR-210 can enhance autophagy by targeting Bcl-2.

miR-18a: ATM

Ataxia telangiectasia mutated (ATM) belongs to the phosphoinositide 3-kinase (PI3K)-related protein kinase (PIKK) family. When cells are exposed to agents that can induce DNA damage, especially ionizing radiation, ATM can phosphorylate its downstream substrates that involve in cell cycle arrest, apoptosis, and DNA repair to maintain genomic stability. In addition, ATM has been found to enhance the autophagy of cell response to genotoxic and oxidative stimuli by the LKB/AMPK/TSC2 pathway. AMPK can phosphorylate TSC2 and increase the GTPase activity of TSC2, which leads to the stabilization of TSC2/TSC1 complex and the inactivation of mTORC1. And mTORC1 plays a vital role in autophagy suppression.

miR-18a is a family member of the miR-17-92 cluster, which processes a common precursor transcript into six miRNAs and involves in tumorigenesis including small cell lung cancer and diffuse large B cell lymphoma. miR-18a has been reported to promote autophagy by targeting ATM in HCT116 cells.[36] The overexpression of miR-18a could increase the expression of ATM and inhibit mTORC1 activity, resulting in enhanced autophagy.

miR-18a: hnRNP A1 E2

In addition to regulating ATM expression by modifying the translation of ATM mRNA, miR-18a can also bind to heterogeneous nuclear ribonucleoprotein A1 (hnRNP A1) E2 directly and induce subsequent apoptosis via the autophagolysosomal degradation in colon cancer cells.[37] HnRNP A1 has been identified to negatively regulate apoptosis by stabilize the miRNAs of cyclin D1 and CTGF and increase their expression, which are closely related to the evasion of apoptosis. Transfected miR-18a was found to form a complex with hnRNP A1 in the cytoplasma and then enhance the autophagic process to degrade hnRNP A1, which conversely promoted cancer cell apoptosis. This is a novel function of miR-18a demonstrated by the study of Fujiya *et al.*[37] Therefore, miR-18a, which modulates gene expression as well as protein degradation, is a multifunctional molecule in cancer progression. Besides, this is also the first report that shows a miRNA suppresses cancer progression by directly binding to a RNA-binding protein, inducing autophagolysosomal degradation of this complex, and eventually apoptosis of cancer cells, which may shed light on new therapeutic strategies.

miRNAs downregulate autophagy in CRC

miR-502: Rab1B

Rab1, a monomeric GTPase and a member of Ras super family, plays a vital role in controlling the traffic from ER to Golgi and is necessary for the formation of autophagosome under both starvation and rapamycin treatment. The colocalization of Ran1b-labeled vesicles occurs upon the induction of autophagy. The enforced expression of miR-502 has been found to suppress autophagy by inhibiting Rab1B, a significant mediator of autophagy, in both HCT116 (p53 +/+) and HCT116 (p53 –/–) cells *in vitro*.[38] Moreover, the tumor growth in a mouse tumor xenograft model was also inhibited. Except for being known as an important tumor suppressive gene, p53 is a key regulator of autophagy as well. miR-502 has a potential p-53 binding site in the promoter region; thus, p53 suppresses the expression of miR-502 at a transcriptional level. Furthermore, researchers found that forced expression of miR-502 could downregulate the expression of p53 protein at post-transcriptional level. Therefore, there is a functional reciprocal inhibition between miR-502 and p53. Thus, miR-502 serves as a promising tumor suppressor by downregulating autophagy through both Rab1 and p53.

miR-22: PTEN

As we know, the activation of PTEN/PI3K/Akt pathway can inactivate mTORC1 and enhance autophagy by inhibiting the expression of TSC1/TSC2 complex. Li *et al.* reported that miR-22, a tumor suppressive miRNA, could activate PTEN signaling and reverse the chemoresistance induced by Paclitaxel in p53-mutated colon cancer cells.[39] PTEN expression subsequently inhibited Akt Ser473 phosphorylation and MTDH (metadherin) expression, and increased the levels of Bax and active caspase-3. This is the first time to identify a suppressive role of miR-22 in autophagy through the PTEN/PI3K/Akt pathway.

miR-22: BTG1

Recently, researchers have reported that miR-22 could promote 5-FU sensitivity via suppressing autophagy and enhancing apoptosis in CRC cell lines

SW620 and RKO.[40] B-cell translocation gene 1 (BTG1) was identified as a novel target of miR-22. In this study, the overexpression of miR-22 was found to repress LC3-II formation, and BTG1 could reverse this impact in SW620 cells in which miR-22 was overexpressed. Therefore, by targeting BTG1, miR-22 could inhibit autophagy via suppressing LC3-II formation in CRC cells.

Previously, miR-22 was first identified to play a tumor suppressive role in HeLa cells, and then miR-22 was found in different kinds of tissues with several targets, including PTEN, Max as well as oncogene c-myc. The downregulation of miR-22 has been observed in colon tumor tissues. The overexpression of miR-22 could inhibit angiogenesis in colon cancer by targeting HIF1-α and suppress the migration and invasion of CRC cell by decreasing the expression of TIAM1 (T-cell lymphoma invasion and metastasis-inducing protein 1), MMP2 (matrix metalloproteinase-2), and MMP9 (matrix metalloproteinase-2). Taken together, miR-22 plays an important role in CRC, and miR-22 based therapeutic strategies may be potential candidates for gastrointestinal cancer treatment.

miR-106b: *ATG16L1*

The protein conjugation system which consists of ATG12, ATG5, and ATG16L1 is of vital importance for the formation of autophagosome. miR-106b was demonstrated to regulate autophagy in CRC cells, and part of the mechanism was to directly interact with the ATG16L1 3′UTR.[41] miR-106b is a member of the miR-17 family, which includes miR-17, -20a, -20b, -93, and -106b. miR-106b and miR-106a could regulate other genes such as BECN1 and ATG12, but the autophagy regulation function of miR-106a may not be associated with ATG16L1. Besides, the miR-17 family could all regulate autophagy by targeting multiple genes, and the underlying mechanisms require further investigation.

miRNA profiling in CRC during 5-FU-induced autophagy

Hou *et al.* have investigated the expression profile of miRNAs in human colon cancer cells in response to 5-FU treatment or nutrient starvation by miRNA microarray analysis.[42] They identified and selected 27 upregulated miRNAs and downregulated miRNAs as potential regulators of autophagy in human cancer cells. They proposed that these miRNAs could be potentially used to regulate autophagy induced by 5-FU in CRC. Among these upregulated miRNAs, one of the predicted targets for hsa-miR-99b-5p was mTOR, and the expression of hsa-miR-99b-5p was significantly increased under both 5-FU treatment and starvation induced autophagy induction. Besides, the Bcl-2 family was shown to be the target of hsa-let-7c-5p, hsa-miR-195-5p, hsa-miR-23a-3p, hsa-miR-15a-5p, hsa-miR-98-5p, and hsa-miR-181a-5p. Among these downregulated miRNAs, the mTOR signaling pathway was proved to be of regulatory importance. In addition to the Bcl-2 family and mTOR, autophagy core genes were predicted target genes as well. Further studies to identify the precise targets of upregulated or downregulated miRNAs are warranted.

The Relationship Between Autophagy and miRNAs in Pancreatic Cancer

Pancreatic cancer is one of the most common causes of cancer-related death with a 5-year survival rate <5%, lacking effective therapeutic methods.[34] Surgical resection is the most effective and curative treatment, but only 10 to 20% of patients are eligible for resection at the time of diagnosis.[43] About 40% of patients with locally advanced pancreatic cancer receive chemo or radiation therapy. However, the radioresistance of pancreatic cancer significantly affects the therapeutic effect of radiotherapy in clinical practice. Therefore, understanding the molecular mechanisms of radioresistance may improve the outcomes of radiotherapy (Figure 3, Table 1).

miRNAs downregulate autophagy in pancreatic cancer

miR-23b: ATG12

miR-23b has been identified to regulate the expression of a series of genes in different cell types and be involved with the development of cancer in different organs. Compared with other miRNAs that exhibited dysregulated expression, miR-23b decreased most in radioresistant cells. Wang *et al.* have identified that miRNA-23b could inhibit autophagy by targeting ATG12 and improve the radiosensitivity of pancreatic cancer cells.[44] ATG12, as we mentioned before, is a ubiquitin-like protein and plays a vital role in the formation of autophagic vacuole. They found that the level of miR-23b was reduced and autophagy was increased to enhance radioresistance in pancreatic cancer cells. The forced expression of miR-23b sensitized pancreatic cancer cells to irradiation by inhibiting autophagy. This is the first report that confirms the regulatory role of mi-23b in autophagy in pancreatic cancer.

miR-216a: BECN1

Recently, another miRNA, miR-216a, has been reported to regulate autophagy-induced radioresistance of pancreatic cancer cells as well.[45] Researchers found downregulated miR-216a and enhanced autophagy in pancreatic cancer cells. The forced expression of miR-216a could inhibit autophagy by directly targeting BECN1 and sensitize pancreatic cancer cells to radiation treatment, which is consistent with the role of miR-23b in pancreatic cancer.

The Relationship Between Autophagy and miRNAs in HCC

HCC is the fifth most common malignancies and one of the leading causes of cancer death worldwide, with more than 500,000 new cases diagnosed every year.[46] It is the most frequently reported type of primary liver cancers as well. A number of risk factors are closely related to the occurrence of HCC, which include the infection of chronic hepatitis B virus (HBV) or chronic hepatitis C virus, the misuse of alcohol, and so on. Most patients of HCC are diagnosed at an advanced tumor stage with limited therapeutic options and extremely poor prognosis. Therefore, further studies are needed to uncover the molecular mechanisms underlying HCC and develop an effective therapy for HCC patients (Figure 3, Table 1).

miRNAs upregulate autophagy in HCC

miR-100: IGF-1R, mTOR

IGF-1R (type I insulin-like growth factor receptor) can activate the PI3K/AKT/mTOR and Ras/Raf/MAPK signaling pathways. There are two types

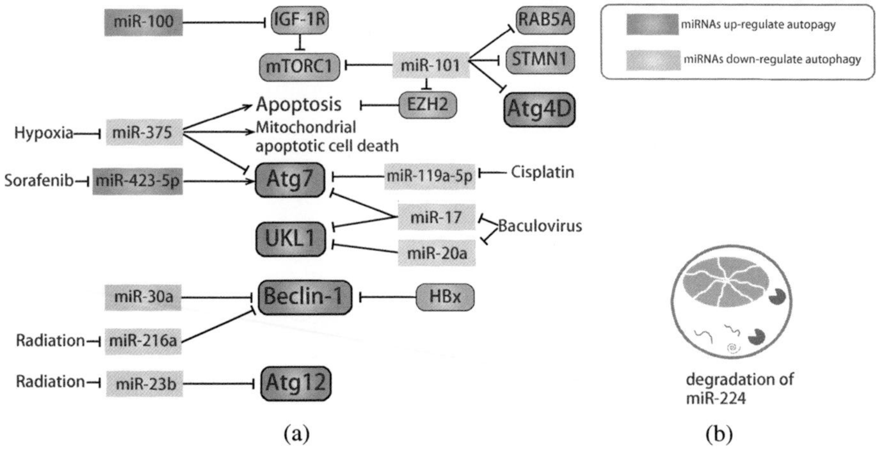

Figure 3. miRNAs regulate autophagy in pancreatic cancer and hepatocellular carcinoma. (a) In pancreatic cancer, miR-23b and miR-216a downregulate autophagy. In HCC, miR-100 and miR-423-5p upregulate autophagy; other miRNAs including miR-375, 199a-5p, miR-101, miR-17, miR-20a and miR-30a down-regulate autophagy. (b) Autophagy downregulates miR-224 by autophagic degradation.

of mTOR in mammals, but only mTORC1 plays a vital role in suppressing autophagy activation. AKT (protein kinase B), AMPK (mitogen-activated protein kinase), and its downstream regulators can destabilize TSC2, leading to the activation of mTORC1.

The expression of miR-100 is context-dependent in different cancer types, which is upregulated in GC and pediatric acute myeloid leukemia, while downregulated in several malignancies including HCC. Hitherto, the majority of studies about miR-100 have been focused on the regulatory role in cell proliferation in various cancer types. Researchers have identified that miR-100 could suppress the cell growth of HCC, but little is known about the impact of miR-100 on autophagy. Ge *et al.* found a close link between the downregulation of miR-100 and decreased autophagy in human HCC tissues.[47] Restoration of miR-100 could enhance autophagy, induce subsequent apoptotic cell death, and suppress the *in vivo* growth of HCC cells; the expression of IGF-1R and mTOR was suppressed by miR-100 binding to their 3'UTR. This report identifies a novel biological function of miR-100 on autophagy. In addition, the up-regulation of autophagy by miR-100 may trigger mitochondrial apoptotic cell death as well. Therefore, mi-100 was shown to suppress HCC development through multiple mechanisms, which makes it a potential target for HCC therapy.

miR-423-5p: ATG7

ATG7, an E1-like activating enzyme, can regulate two ubiquitin-like conjugation systems that are required for autophagosome expansion: ATG7/ATG10 mediates the conjugation of ATG12 onto ATG5; ATG7/ATG3 mediates the conjugation of ATG8 (LC3) onto PE. Recently, miR-423-5p was reported to promote autophagy by increasing the expression of ATG7 in HCC cells and Sorafenib treatment could upregulate the serum level of miR-423-5p in HCC patients.[48] Studies have shown that miR-423-5p played a role in cell cycle inhibition and autophagy enhancement in HCC cells. The serum level of miR-423-5p in HCC patients was increased after the treatment with Sorafenib, the only approved drug for patients at the late stage of HCC. Researchers suggest that miR-423-5p may serve as a predictive biomarker of the response of HCC patients to Sorafenib.

miRNAs downregulate autophagy in HCC

miR-375: ATG7

Chang *et al.* investigated the relationship between downregulated miR-375 and enhanced autophagy under hypoxia in HCC.[49] They found that overexpressed miR-375 inhibited autophagy by directly targeting ATG7, which plays a vital role in autophagosome formation and elongation as we have mentioned before. In addition, the downregulation of ATG7 could also inhibit mitochondrial autophagy (mitophagy), and the accumulation of damaged mitochondria lead to increased release of apoptotic proteins, which severely impairs viability of HCC cells. The forced expression of miR-375 in mice xenograft tumors resulted in fewer autophagic cells, increased necrosis rate, and growth speed. Besides, previous studies have shown that miR-375 can modulate glucose metabolism by regulating myotrophin and PDK1 (pyruvate dehydrogenase kinase1), as well as promote apoptosis by targeting genes related to the apoptosis. Therefore, miR-375 has been identified to be involved in the dysregulation of glucose metabolism, apoptosis, and autophagy, which are key factors in the occurrence, metastasis, and prognosis of HCC. Taken together, miR-375 has shown multiple effects in tumor suppression. The restoration of miR-375 expression may be a promising adjuvant treatment when combined with some chemotherapy drugs which lose efficacy because of autophagy induction, such as Sorafenib.

miR-199a-5p: *ATG7*

Deregulated miR-199a-5p has been identified in several cancer types, including HCC, breast cancer, and testicular cancer, which suggest the biological functions of miR-199a-5p. Recent studies have shown that miR-199a-5p may play a suppressive role in liver cancer and testicular cancer. Both reduced miR-199a-5p and activated autophagy were found in cisplatin-treated HCC patients and human HCC cell lines.[50] Xu *et al.* identified that the forced expression of miR-199a-5p could inhibit autophagy by targeting ATG7 and promote the inhibition of cell proliferation mediated by cisplatin. Besides, autophagy inhibition reversed cell proliferation induced by the downregulation of miR-199a-5p. This study suggests that miR-199a-5p may sensitize HCC cells to cisplatin by inhibiting cytoprotective autophagy.[50]

miR-101: *RAB5A, STMN1, ATG4D, and mTOR*

Stathmin, a cytosolic phosphoprotein, can destabilize microtubules as well as regulate cell cycle. Stathmin has been identified as an autophagy regulator in a siRNA-based screen, but the precise mechanism of its role in autophagy regulation remains unknown and requires further study.[51] RAB5A, a small GTPase and an important regulator of early endocytosis, is associated with the formation of LC3-positive autophagic vesicles and the conjugation of ATG5–ATG12. In addition, it can interact with Beclin-1 when PI3-kinase Vps34 is present.[52] These findings suggest a vital role for RAB5A in the early stage of autophagosome formation. Finally, ATG4D is a kind of cysteine protease from the ATG4 family, which plays a crucial role in autophagosome biogenesis. The ATG4 family processes LC3 and subsequently conjugates to PE, which facilitates the fusion of autophagosome and lysosome, as well as LC3 recycling.

miR-101 has been observed to be downregulated in several cancer types. In GC, miR-101 could induce apoptosis and inhibit the occurrence, metastasis, and invasion of tumor cells. *In vivo* studies have shown that miR-101 could increase the sensitivity of HCC cells to apoptosis by targeting myeloid cell leukemia sequence1 (Mcl-1). Moreover, the expression of miR-101 could be enhanced though the activation ERK signaling pathway induced by TPA (12-O-tetradecanoylphorbol 13-acetate) in HepG2 cells. According to a study conducted by Xu *et al.*, miR-101 was identified to suppress autophagy by targeting RAB5A, STMN1, and ATG4D, as well as promote cisplatin-induced apoptotic death in the HepG2 cell line.[53] In addition to RAB5A, STMN1 (stathmin1), and ATG4D, mTOR was found to be another target of miR-101. The inhibition of mTOR leads to autophagy activation, which seems to be contradictory to the fact that miR-101 suppressed autophagy. Xu *et al.* suggest that this may be that, although there were four targets for miR-101, the comprehensive effect of miR-101 on autophagy was primarily mediated by targeting RAB5A, STMN1, and ATG4D. This study indicates that the overexpression of miR-101 can improve the chemosensitivity of HCC cells to cisplatin by inhibiting autophagy.

miR-101: *EZH2*

Apart from AB5A, STMN1, ATG4D, and mTOR, miR-101 has also been reported to directly target oncogene EZH2 and down regulate its expression, leading to suppressed autophagy and increased drug sensitivity in HCC cells.[54] Enhancer of zeste homolog 2 (EZH2), an epigenetic enzyme, serves as a transcriptional suppressor that silencing genes by chromatin modification. The overexpression of EZH2 is frequently observed in tumors, including HCC. miR-101 has been identified to repress the proliferation, colony formation, and invasion of tumor cells, and these effects may be ascribed to miR-101 mediated EZH2 silencing. In this study, Xu *et al.* uncovered that miR-101-induced EZH2 silencing lead to the accumulation of autophagosomes and suppressed the fusion of autophagosome and lysosome, which resulted in cell death and promoted cytostatic drug sensitivity in HCC. However, the molecular mechanisms of how EZH2 inhibition affects the autophagy need further investigation.

miR-17: ULK1, ATG7, and p62

miR-20a: ULK1 and p62

Chen *et al.* have confirmed that Baculovirus could upregulate PTENP1 and PTEN, which inhibited the oncogenic PI3K/AKT pathway, leading to suppressed cell proliferation and migration, as well as enhanced autophagy and apoptosis in HCC cells.[55] PTENP1, a long non-coding RNA (lncRNA), is a pseudogene of PTEN and shares high homology with PTEN in 3′UTR. PTENP1 decoyed miRNAs, including miR-17, miR-19b, and miR-20a that would otherwise target PTEN, thus elevated the levels of PTEN. They found that miR-17 significantly suppressed the expression of ULK1, ATG7, and p62, while miR-20a effectively downregulated ULK1 and p62 in HCC cells. They are all core autophagy genes which are of vital importance in the initiation and completion of autophagy. Therefore, their study suggests that miR-17 and miR-20a negatively regulate autophagy via targeting ULK1, ATG7, and p62 in HCC cells.

miR-30a: BECN1

HCC is one of the liver complications that chronically infected HBV patients may get. Chronic HBV infection is associated with the development of HCC. HBV X protein (HBx), an HBV-encoding protein, has been reported to be involved in regulating several host genes to enhance cell proliferation, suppress apoptosis, and activate some signaling pathways to promote the progression of HCC.[56] One of the mechanisms HBV employs for its survival has been identified to be autophagy. Autophagy was confirmed to be activated during HBV infection, which facilitated the replication of HBV with little effect on RNA transcription in hepatoma cells and mice.[57] HBV may enhance an autophagy response without increasing the degradation of autophagic proteins, which requires HBx to promote the activity of PI3KC3 by binding to it.

Recently, Kumar *et al.* have demonstrated that HBx could induce autophagosome formation by increasing the expression of Beclin-1, while the overexpression of miR-30a could significantly suppress Beclin-1 expression which was promoted by HBx in hepatic cells.[58] HBx can transactivate the

Beclin-1 promoter, which has binding sites for transcription factors that are responsive to HBx, thus increasing the expression of Beclin-1, whereas, miR-30a can directly target Beclin-1 by binding to its 3′UTR and attenuate autophagy activity. Besides, previous study has confirmed a positive role of miR-30a in regulating apoptosis. Therefore, Kumar *et al.* proposed that miR-30a could significantly suppress the procarcinogenic effects of HBx and protect hepatic cells from HBV infection by its role in proapoptosis and antiautophagy.

Autophagy downregulates miR-224

The autophagic process involves both non-selective and selective degradation pathways. Metabolic stresses, such as starvation can activate the non-selective degradation pathway to degrade dysfunctional organelles or proteins. Meanwhile, the selective degradation pathway can selectively degrade proteins, infective pathogens, and unnecessary organelles. Increasing data have confirmed that the selective autophagic degradation can modulate several signaling pathways associated with the occurrence and progression of cancer, including apoptosis and WTN signaling.

There have been a number of studies showing that miRNAs can regulate autophagy by various targets in cancer cells, while little is known about how autophagy can modulate miRNAs. Lan *et al.* for the first time identified the regulatory role of autophagy on miR-224.[59] They uncovered that autophagy could downregulate the expression of miR-224 through the selective autophagic degradation pathway. Previously, both upregulated the expression of miR-224 and impaired autophagy have been observed in HCC. In this study, researchers confirmed that in HBV-induced HCC, reduced autophagy resulted in the accumulation of miR-224, downregulated the expression of Smad4, and eventually increased cell migration as well as tumor formation. Besides, miR-224 was preferentially recruited into the autophagosome and then degraded by lysosome. RNA-binding proteins can bind to miRNA and then regulate miRNA maturation. Therefore, they speculated that miR-224 could be recognized by certain RNA-binding protein and subsequently recruited into the autophagosome for degradation with the assistance of autophagy adapter proteins. Further studies are required to clarify the molecular mechanisms underlying it.

miRNAs Regulate the Crosstalk Between Autophagy and Apoptosis in Gastrointestinal Cancer

Both autophagy and apoptosis are evolutionarily conserved and genetically modulated processes, which play vital roles in cell proliferation and cell death. There are some common upstream signaling pathways that are involved in both autophagy and apoptosis. Autophagy and apoptosis can be attenuated by the overexpression of miR-19a/b, miR-21, and miR-106a in GC cells through PTEN/PI3K/Aktpathway.[28–30] miR-15b or miR-16 has been identified to enhance autophagy and apoptosis by targeting Bcl-2.[31] miR-18a has been reported to induce autophagy by upregulating ATM and suppressing mTORC1 in colon cancer cells.[36] Besides, miR-18a directly binds to hnRNP A1 E2 and induces subsequent apoptosis through autophagolysosomal degradation in the same type of cancer cells as well.[37] miR-22 suppresses autophagy by activating the PTEN/PI3K/Akt pathway in CRC cells.[39] Inhibited autophagy and enhanced apoptosis can also be induced by miR-22 via its novel target, BTG1.[40] Mitochondrial apoptotic cell death can be triggered by miR-100 in HCC cells.[47] miR-375 has been demonstrated to inhibit autophagy by targeting ATG7, leading to the accumulation of dysfunctional mitochondria and increased release of apoptotic proteins in HCC.[49]

Conclusion

miRNAs are potential candidates as diagnostic, therapeutic, and prognostic molecular biomarkers in clinical practice, because the expression patterns of miRNAs can be easily assessed in different samples and miRNAs present high stability and tissue specificity. Studies have confirmed that the expression of miRNAs is altered in different types of cancers, including gastrointestinal carcinoma. Therefore, extensive studies are focused on investigating miRNA-based therapies for cancer treatment lately.

Autophagy plays a double-edged sword role in the initiation and progression of malignant tumors via the clearance of damaged or dysfunctional proteins and organelles. The effects of autophagy depend on the histological type of cancer, the context as well as the location. In GC, CRC, and pancreatic cancer, autophagy is upregulated to exert its cytoprotective effects, which facilitates tumor progression. However, in HCC, autophagy has usually been found to be suppressed, and autophagic cell death induced by the overexpression of some miRNAs can block cancer development. In GC and pancreatic cancer, enhanced autophagy is closely related to chemoresistance, and the forced expression of miRNAs can increase the chemosensitivity of GC or pancreatic cells by suppressing autophagy. Upregulation of miR-204-5p, 106b, 502, and 124 were identified to inhibit autophagy and tumor growth in CRC cells. In addition, miR-18a has been reported to increase cancer cell death by either inducing apoptosis via autophagolosomal degradation of hnRNP A1 or upregulating autophagy via ATM. In HCC, the overexpression of miR-423-5p and miR-100 was demonstrated to inhibit cancer progression by inducing autophagic cell death. Moreover, mitophagy inhibition by miR-375 could lead to mitochondrial apoptotic cell death and tumor inhibition under hypoxia. Of note, Lan *et al.* has reported that autophagy could downregulate miRNA expression through the selective autophagic degradation pathway, revealing the regulatory role of autophagy in miRNA in HCC for the first time. The alteration of miRNAs in different cancers appears to be dependent on the histological type of cancer. Identifying the exact alteration of miRNAs in gastrointestinal cancer and their roles in autophagy regulation may provide reference for clinic treatment.

Intrinsic or acquired resistance to chemo and radiotherapy is a huge obstacle in clinical cancer treatment, which results in metastasis and recurrence in the majority of malignant tumors. Extensive studies about the mechanisms of chemoresistance and radioresistance, such as increased drug efflux, inactivation of detoxification enzymes, target gene mutation, dysfunction of proapoptotic proteins as well as enhancement of DNA repair activity, have been reported. However, the molecular mechanisms underlying it remain unclear. Upregulated or downregulated miRNA has been demonstrated to be involved in the development of chemoradioresistance in different cancer types, including gastrointestinal cancer. Moreover, in most of chemotherapy and radiotherapy, autophagy plays a cytoprotective role by degrading dysfunctional proteins and organelles to provide energy resources and promote cell survival. Autophagy partially determines how cancer cells respond to therapy and its induction can lead to chemoresistance and radioresistance. In GC, downregulated miR-181a, 143, 30, and 23b-3p were found to be associated with autophagy induction induced by drug treatment in either cancer cells or cancer tissues. The overexpression of these miRNAs could significantly reverse chemoresistance and sensitize GC cells to chemotherapy drugs, such as cisplatin, 5-FU, and Quercetin. In addition, miR-19a/b, miR-2, and miR-106a were found to be upregulated in drug-treated GC cells, which increase autophagy activity and contribute to chemoresistance. In CRC, miR-22 has been reported to increase 5-FU sensitivity and reverse Paclitaxel-induced chemoresistance by suppressing autophagy and inducing apoptosis in cancer cells. And, the radiosensitivity of colon cancer cells could be reduced by hypoxia-related autophagy, which was mediated by the HIF-1α/miR-210/Bcl-2 pathway. Moreover, in pancreatic cancer, radioresistance mediated by autophagy could be reversed by the upregulated expression of miR-23b and miR-216a. Furthermore, in HCC, both miR-101 and miR-199a-5p have demonstrated to play an inhibitive role in autophagy regulation and then increase the drug sensitivity of HCC cells.

Considering the regulatory role of miRNAs in autophagy as well as the oncogenic or tumor suppressive role of autophagy in cancer, miRNAs may be the targets of gene therapies to control the progression of gastrointestinal cancer and prevent the recurrence of tumor. Besides, they also have therapeutic potential for chemoresistant or radioresistant patients. Therefore, traditional therapies combined with miRNAs which inhibit autophagy may be promising strategies in gastrointestinal treatment.

References

1. Z Yang, DJ Klionsky (2010) Eaten alive: A history of macroautophagy. *Nat Cell Biol* **12**: 814–822.
2. N Mizushima, B Levine, AM Cuervo, DJ Klionsky (2008) Autophagy fights disease through cellular self-digestion. *Nature* **451**: 1069–1075.
3. AM Choi, SW Ryter, B Levine (2013) Autophagy in human health and disease. *N Engl J Med* **368**: 651–662.
4. B Liu, X Wen, Y Cheng (2013) Survival or death: Disequilibrating the oncogenic and tumor suppressive autophagy in cancer. *Cell Death Dis* **4**: e892.
5. DP Bartel (2004) MicroRNAs: Genomics, biogenesis, mechanism, and function. *Cell* **116**: 281–297.
6. J Winter, S Jung, S Keller, RI Gregory, S Diederichs (2009) Many roads to maturity: MicroRNA biogenesis pathways and their regulation. *Nat Cell Biol* **11**: 228–234.

7. RC Lee, RL Feinbaum, V Ambros (1993) The *C. elegans* heterochronic gene lin-4 encodes small RNAs with antisense complementarity to lin-14. *Cell* **75**: 843–854.
8. G Hutvagner, J McLachlan, AE Pasquinelli, E Balint, T Tuschl, PD Zamore (2001) A cellular function for the RNA-interference enzyme Dicer in the maturation of the let-7 small temporal RNA. *Science* **293**: 834–838.
9. DP Bartel (2009) MicroRNAs: Target recognition and regulatory functions. *Cell* **136**: 215–233.
10. GA Calin, CD Dumitru, M Shimizu, R Bichi, S Zupo, E Noch, *et al.* (2002) Frequent deletions and down-regulation of micro-RNA genes miR15 and miR16 at 13q14 in chronic lymphocytic leukemia. *Proc Natl Acad Sci USA* **99**: 15524–15529.
11. CH Lawrie (2007) MicroRNAs and haematology: Small molecules, big function. *Br J Haematol* **137**: 503–512.
12. X Wen, J Wu, F Wang, B Liu, C Huang, Y Wei (2013) Deconvoluting the role of reactive oxygen species and autophagy in human diseases. *Free Radic Biol Med* **65**: 402–410.
13. H Zhu, H Wu, X Liu, B Li, Y Chen, X Ren, *et al.* (2009) Regulation of autophagy by a beclin 1-targeted microRNA, miR-30a, in cancer cells. *Autophagy* **5**: 816–823.
14. Y Chen, R Liersch, M Detmar (2012) The miR-290-295 cluster suppresses autophagic cell death of melanoma cells. *Sci Rep* **2**: 808.
15. H Wu, F Wang, S Hu, C Yin, X Li, S Zhao, *et al.* (2012) MiR-20a and miR-106b negatively regulate autophagy induced by leucine deprivation via suppression of ULK1 expression in C2C12 myoblasts. *Cell Signal* **24**: 2179–2186.
16. Z Wang, N Wang, P Liu, Q Chen, H Situ, T Xie, *et al.* (2014) MicroRNA-25 regulates chemoresistance-associated autophagy in breast cancer cells, a process modulated by the natural autophagy inducer isoliquiritigenin. *Oncotarget* **5**: 7013–7026.
17. Y Huang, AY Chuang, EA Ratovitski (2011) Phospho-DeltaNp63alpha/miR-885-3p axis in tumor cell life and cell death upon cisplatin exposure. *Cell Cycle* **10**: 3938–3947.
18. C He, B Levine (2010) The Beclin 1 interactome. *Curr Opin Cell Biol* **22**: 140–149.
19. NR Christoffersen, R Shalgi, LB Frankel, E Leucci, M Lees, M Klausen, *et al.* (2010) p53-independent upregulation of miR-34a during oncogene-induced senescence represses MYC. *Cell Death Differ* **17**: 236–245.
20. A Meenhuis, PA van Veelen, H de Looper, N van Boxtel, IJ van den Berge, SM Sun, *et al.* (2011) MiR-17/20/93/106 promote hematopoietic cell expansion by targeting sequestosome 1-regulated pathways in mice. *Blood* **118**: 916–925.

21. A Jemal, F Bray, MM Center, J Ferlay, E Ward, D Forman (2011) Global cancer statistics. *CA Cancer J Clin* **61**: 69–90.
22. WB Robb, C Mariette (2012) Predicting the response to chemotherapy in gastric adenocarcinoma: Who benefits from neoadjuvant chemotherapy? *Recent Results Cancer Res* **196**: 241–268.
23. D Fan, X Zhang, X Chen, Z Mou, J Hu, S Zhou, *et al.* (2005) Bird's-eye view on gastric cancer research of the past 25 years. *J Gastroenterol Hepatol* **20**: 360–365.
24. Y An, Z Zhang, Y Shang, X Jiang, J Dong, P Yu, *et al.* (2015) miR-23b-3p regulates the chemoresistance of gastric cancer cells by targeting ATG12 and HMGB2. *Cell Death Dis* **6**: e1766.
25. F Du, Y Feng, J Fang, M Yang (2015) MicroRNA-143 enhances chemosensitivity of Quercetin through autophagy inhibition via target GABARAPL1 in gastric cancer cells. *Biomed Pharmacother* **74**: 169–177.
26. J Zhao, Y Nie, H Wang, Y Lin (2016) MiR-181a suppresses autophagy and sensitizes gastric cancer cells to cisplatin. *Gene* **576**: 828–833.
27. KA Tekirdag, G Korkmaz, DG Ozturk, R Agami, D Gozuacik (2013) MIR181A regulates starvation- and rapamycin-induced autophagy through targeting of ATG5. *Autophagy* **9**: 374–385.
28. F Wang, T Li, B Zhang, H Li, Q Wu, L Yang, *et al.* (2013) MicroRNA-19a/b regulates multidrug resistance in human gastric cancer cells by targeting PTEN. *Biochem Biophys Res Commun* **434**: 688–694.
29. SM Yang, C Huang, XF Li, MZ Yu, Y He, J Li (2013) miR-21 confers cisplatin resistance in gastric cancer cells by regulating PTEN. *Toxicology* **306**: 162–168.
30. Y Fang, H Shen, H Li, Y Cao, R Qin, L Long, *et al.* (2013) miR-106a confers cisplatin resistance by regulating PTEN/Akt pathway in gastric cancer cells. *Acta Biochim Biophys Sin (Shanghai)* **45**: 963–972.
31. L Xia, D Zhang, R Du, Y Pan, L Zhao, S Sun, *et al.* (2008) miR-15b and miR-16 modulate multidrug resistance by targeting BCL2 in human gastric cancer cells. *Int J Cancer* **123**: 372–379.
32. C Yang, Y Pan (2015) Fluorouracil induces autophagy-related gastric carcinoma cell death through Beclin-1 upregulation by miR-30 suppression. *Tumour Biol.*
33. Y Zhang, WQ Yang, H Zhu, YY Qian, L Zhou, YJ Ren, *et al.* (2014) Regulation of autophagy by miR-30d impacts sensitivity of anaplastic thyroid carcinoma to cisplatin. *Biochem Pharmacol* **87**: 562–570.
34. R Siegel, D Naishadham, A Jemal (2012) Cancer statistics, 2012. *CA Cancer J Clin* **62**: 10–29.
35. Y Sun, X Xing, Q Liu, Z Wang, Y Xin, P Zhang, *et al.* (2015) Hypoxia-induced autophagy reduces radiosensitivity by the HIF-1alpha/miR-210/Bcl-2 pathway in colon cancer cells. *Int J Oncol* **46**: 750–756.

36. AB Qased, H Yi, N Liang, S Ma, S Qiao, X Liu (2013) MicroRNA-18a upregulates autophagy and ataxia telangiectasia mutated gene expression in HCT116 colon cancer cells. *Mol Med Rep* **7**: 559–564.
37. M Fujiya, H Konishi, MK Mohamed Kamel, N Ueno, Y Inaba, K Moriichi, *et al.* (2014) microRNA-18a induces apoptosis in colon cancer cells via the autophagolysosomal degradation of oncogenic heterogeneous nuclear ribonucleoprotein A1. *Oncogene* **33**: 4847–4856.
38. H Zhai, B Song, X Xu, W Zhu, J Ju (2012) Inhibition of autophagy and tumor growth in colon cancer by miR-502. *Oncogene* **32**: 1570–1579.
39. J Li, Y Zhang, J Zhao, F Kong, Y Chen (2011) Overexpression of miR-22 reverses paclitaxel-induced chemoresistance through activation of PTEN signaling in p53-mutated colon cancer cells. *Mol Cell Biochem* **357**: 31–38.
40. H Zhang, J Tang, C Li, J Kong, J Wang, Y Wu, *et al.* (2015) MiR-22 regulates 5-FU sensitivity by inhibiting autophagy and promoting apoptosis in colorectal cancer cells. *Cancer Lett* **356**: 781–790.
41. Z Zhai, F Wu, AY Chuang, JH Kwon (2013) miR-106b fine tunes ATG16L1 expression and autophagic activity in intestinal epithelial HCT116 cells. *Inflamm Bowel Dis* **19**: 2295–2301.
42. N Hou, J Han, J Li, Y Liu, Y Qin, L Ni, *et al.* (2014) MicroRNA profiling in human colon cancer cells during 5-fluorouracil-induced autophagy. *PLoS One* **9**: e114779.
43. D Li, K Xie, R Wolff, JL Abbruzzese (2004) Pancreatic cancer. *Lancet* **363**: 1049–1057.
44. P Wang, J Zhang, L Zhang, Z Zhu, J Fan, L Chen, *et al.* (2013) MicroRNA 23b regulates autophagy associated with radioresistance of pancreatic cancer cells. *Gastroenterology* **145**: 1133–1143.
45. X Zhang, H Shi, S Lin, M Ba, S Cui (2015) MicroRNA-216a enhances the radiosensitivity of pancreatic cancer cells by inhibiting beclin-1-mediated autophagy. *Oncol Rep* **34**: 1557–1564.
46. M Schwartz, S Roayaie, M Konstadoulakis (2007) Strategies for the management of hepatocellular carcinoma. *Nat Clin Pract Oncol* **4**: 424–432.
47. YY Ge, Q Shi, ZY Zheng, J Gong, C Zeng, J Yang, *et al.* (2014) MicroRNA-100 promotes the autophagy of hepatocellular carcinoma cells by inhibiting the expression of mTOR and IGF-1R. *Oncotarget* **5**: 6218–6228.
48. P Stiuso, N Potenza, A Lombardi, I Ferrandino, A Monaco, S Zappavigna, *et al.* (2015) MicroRNA-423-5p promotes autophagy in cancer cells and is increased in serum from hepatocarcinoma patients treated with sorafenib. *Mol Ther Nucleic Acids* **4**: e233.

49. Y Chang, W Yan, X He, L Zhang, C Li, H Huang, *et al.* (2012) miR-375 inhibits autophagy and reduces viability of hepatocellular carcinoma cells under hypoxic conditions. *Gastroenterology* **143**: 177–187.
50. N Xu, J Zhang, C Shen, Y Luo, L Xia, F Xue, *et al.* (2012) Cisplatin-induced downregulation of miR-199a-5p increases drug resistance by activating autophagy in HCC cell. *Biochem Biophys Res Commun* **423**: 826–831.
51. LB Frankel, J Wen, M Lees, M Hoyer-Hansen, T Farkas, A Krogh, *et al.* (2011) microRNA-101 is a potent inhibitor of autophagy. *EMBO J* **30**: 4628–4641.
52. B Ravikumar, S Imarisio, S Sarkar, CJ O'Kane, DC Rubinsztein (2008) Rab5 modulates aggregation and toxicity of mutant huntingtin through macroautophagy in cell and fly models of Huntington disease. *J Cell Sci* **121**: 1649–1660.
53. Y Xu, Y An, Y Wang, C Zhang, H Zhang, C Huang, *et al.* (2013) miR-101 inhibits autophagy and enhances cisplatin-induced apoptosis in hepatocellular carcinoma cells. *Oncol Rep* **29**: 2019–2024.
54. L Xu, S Beckebaum, S Iacob, G Wu, GM Kaiser, A Radtke, *et al.* (2014) MicroRNA-101 inhibits human hepatocellular carcinoma progression through EZH2 downregulation and increased cytostatic drug sensitivity. *J Hepatol* **60**: 590–598.
55. CL Chen, YW Tseng, JC Wu, GY Chen, KC Lin, SM Hwang, *et al.* (2015) Suppression of hepatocellular carcinoma by baculovirus-mediated expression of long non-coding RNA PTENP1 and MicroRNA regulation. *Biomaterials* **44**: 71–81.
56. C Neuveut, Y Wei, MA Buendia (2010) Mechanisms of HBV-related hepatocarcinogenesis. *J Hepatol* **52**: 594–604.
57. J Li, Y Liu, Z Wang, K Liu, Y Wang, J Liu, *et al.* (2011) Subversion of cellular autophagy machinery by hepatitis B virus for viral envelopment. *J Virol* **85**: 6319–6333.
58. S Kumar, P Gupta, S Khanal, A Shahi, P Kumar, SK Sarin, *et al.* (2015) Overexpression of microRNA-30a inhibits hepatitis B virus X protein-induced autophagosome formation in hepatic cells. *FEBS J* **282**: 1152–1163.
59. SH Lan, SY Wu, R Zuchini, XZ Lin, IJ Su, TF Tsai, *et al.* (2014) Autophagy-preferential degradation of MIR224 participates in hepatocellular carcinoma tumorigenesis. *Autophagy* **10**: 1687–1689.

Index

C

D